CALCIFIED TISSUE

TOPICS IN MOLECULAR AND STRUCTURAL BIOLOGY

Series Editors

Stephen Neidle
Institute of Cancer Research
Sutton, Surrey, UK

Watson Fuller
Department of Physics
University of Keele, UK

Protein–Nucleic Acid Interaction
Edited by Wolfram Saenger and Udo Heinemann

Calcified Tissue
Edited by David Hukins

Oligodeoxynucleotides
Edited by Jack S. Cohen

Molecular Mechanisms in Muscular Contraction
Edited by John M. Squire

CALCIFIED TISSUE

Edited by

DAVID W. L. HUKINS

Department of Medical Biophysics
University of Manchester, UK

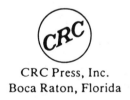

CRC Press, Inc.
Boca Raton, Florida

First published 1989

Published in the USA, its dependencies, and Canada by
CRC Press, Inc.
2000 Corporate Blvd., N.W.
Boca Raton, FL 33431, U.S.A.

Printed in Great Britain

Catalog #Z7115
ISBN 0–8493–7115–5
ISSN 0265–4377

Contents

Preface

The most obvious property of calcified tissues is their rigidity, which enables them to perform such mechanical functions as grinding food, in the case of teeth, and supporting the body, in the case of bones. However, they also contain macromolecules which are essential for their function and are implicated in the calcification process. Thus bone, for example, has a complex structure at both the histological and the macromolecular levels.

An understanding of the relationship between structure and function is essential for understanding the pathology of calcified tissues, and so is of practical as well as academic interest. For example, bone may be inappropriately formed, in rickets, or destroyed during ageing, in osteoporosis. These pathological processes involve cells, as well as the extracellular matrix, and emphasise that bone is a living tissue. Pathological calcification can also occur at sites which are not normally calcified. Deposition of minerals in joints is often associated with rheumatic diseases. Furthermore, hard 'stones' can be formed in many parts of the body – especially in the urinary tract. Minerals can also be deposited on foreign materials which are introduced into the body and so can interfere with the action of, for example, prosthetic heart valves. Therefore, the emphasis in this book is on aspects of calcification that are important in humans – although much of the research described here involves tissue from other mammals, and sometimes other vertebrates.

The aim of this book is not to present a comprehensive account of calcified tissues. In common with the rest of the series, it is intended to select some aspects of contemporary research – especially those in which attempts are being made to relate biological function to the structures and interactions of macromolecules. A consequence of this selection is that many of the chapters stress the importance of the extracellular matrix and the interactions of its macromolecules with mineral. Thus this book may be regarded as a sequel to Volume 5 of the series, *Connective Tissue Matrix*. Since much current research in calcified tissues is aimed at understanding events at the cellular level, the emphasis here on physical, rather than more obviously biological, techniques is unusual. I have attempted to redress the balance, to some extent, by the inclusion of Chapter 2, which provides a more conventionally biological introduction to the remaining chapters.

Nevertheless, there are important reasons for not neglecting the structure and physical properties of the calcified matrix. Interactions of macromolecules with minerals are an essential feature of the deposition and dissolution of calcified tissues. Furthermore, the most obvious functions of the tissues arise from their physical properties. I hope, therefore, that the selection of material presented here will provide an informative view of the more physical and physico-chemical aspects of contemporary calcified tissue research.

Manchester, 1989   D. W. L. H.

The contributors

P. Anderson
Department of Biochemistry
The London Hospital Medical College
Turner Street
London E1 2AD, UK

R. T. Bailey
Department of Chemistry
University of Strathclyde
Glasgow G1 1XL, UK

Adele L. Boskey
Department of Ultrastructural
    Biochemistry
The Hospital for Special Surgery
535 East 70th Street
New York
NY 10021, USA

R. Boakes
Department of Biochemistry
The London Hospital Medical College
Turner Street
London E1 2AD, UK

S. D. Dover
Department of Biophysics
King's College
26–29 Drury Lane
London WC2B 5RL, UK

J. C. Elliot
Department of Biochemistry
The London Hospital Medical College
Turner Street
London E1 2AD, UK

A. J. Freemont
Departments of Rheumatology and
    Pathology
University of Manchester
Stopford Building
Manchester M13 9PT, UK

J. E. Harries
SERC Daresbury Laboratory
Warrington WA4 4AD, UK

S. S. Hasnain
SERC Daresbury Laboratory
Warrington WA4 4AD, UK

C. Holt
Hannah Research Institute
Ayr KA6 5HL, UK

D. W. L. Hukins
Department of Medical Biophysics
University of Manchester
Stopford Building
Manchester M13 9PT, UK

M. J. J. M. van Kemenade
Van 't Hoff Laboratory
Transitorium 3, Padualaan 8
3548 CH Utrecht, The Netherlands

Sidney Lees
Bioengineering Department
Forsyth Dental Center
140 Fenway
Boston
MA 02115, USA

1
Mineral deposits in tissues

D. W. L. Hukins

INTRODUCTION

This chapter has two purposes. One is to provide background information on the minerals deposited in calcified tissues. The other is to summarise the techniques used to characterise them. An understanding of the range and scope of these techniques is essential for a critical evaluation of the material described in subsequent chapters. Furthermore, because of the complexity of many of the minerals, it is impossible to understand how their structures are defined without some appreciation of the techniques involved. Several techniques which are important subjects of current research are described in more detail in chapters devoted to them.

Characterisation of these mineral phases involves not only quantitative analysis of the ions present but also determination of their spatial relationships. There are several reasons why composition alone is inadequate to characterise biological minerals. Firstly, minerals are frequently deposited in association with other substances, and so the components would have to be separated before the composition of each could be determined (techniques which involve electron microscopy are an exception – see below). This separation would be very difficult in many cases; more importantly, the separation process could well affect the composition of the mineral phase. Physical techniques which rely on structure then provide a more reliable characterisation. Secondly, many biological minerals are non-stoichiometric. For example, mineral deposits described in the next section as hydroxyapatite (HAP; $Ca_5(PO_4)_3OH$) rarely have the expected molar Ca/P ratio of 1.67 and often incorporate other ions. Finally, minerals with the same chemical compositions may have different three-dimensional structures. For example, calcium pyrophosphate dihydrate ($Ca_2P_2O_7 . 2H_2O$), which is sometimes deposited in synovial joints (McCarty, 1976), can crystallise in either the monoclinic or the triclinic crystal forms (Okazaki et al., 1976). These two forms are expected to have different physical properties and may interact with their environment in different ways. Interactions of biological minerals, especially with macromolecules, will be a recurring theme in this book.

Calcium phosphates are the minerals most commonly deposited in tissues. Therefore, a brief summary of their chemistry follows the description of the techniques used to define mineral structures. Finally, the chapter concludes by summarising the problems which remain when the mineral phases have been characterised, and so serves as an introduction to the rest of the book. The next section summarises the importance of mineral deposition in tissues.

IMPORTANCE OF MINERAL DEPOSITS

The importance of mineral deposition for the biological function of certain tissues is most clearly demonstrated by the physical properties of bones and teeth; however, minerals are deposited during a variety of normal physiological and pathological processes. Like the rest of the book, this chapter emphasises those processes which are important in mammals – especially humans. Several less specialised reviews of mineral deposition in biological systems have been published (Lowenstam, 1981; Pautard and Williams, 1982; Mann, 1983; Weiner, 1986). Recent results on secretory granules formed by snails have emphasised the importance of amorphous calcium phosphate phases in certain biological processes, and demonstrate how they can incorporate other ions, such as manganese, into their structures (Taylor *et al.*, 1986, 1988). These investigations may provide useful model systems for mammalian mineralisation, as well as being of fundamental interest in their own right. For example, calcification of turkey leg tendons has been widely used as a simple system for investigating structural aspects of calcification of collagenous tissues (Eanes *et al.*, 1970; White *et al.*, 1977).

The mineral phase in bones and teeth resembles HAP (Boskey, 1980; Termine, 1972). However, the molar Ca/P ratio of bone mineral is less than 1.67 and it contains a variety of ions – especially carbonate. Furthermore, bone mineral can incorporate ions which may be present in the diet or (in the case of aluminium) can be inadvertently introduced during renal dialysis. As might be expected from its lack of stoichiometry, bone mineral is poorly crystalline (Wheeler and Lewis, 1977; Eanes *et al.*, 1981; Miller *et al.*, 1981). Since simple stoichiometry and regular crystallographic structure are not features of bone mineral, it can act as a reservoir of ions which can be exchanged with the environment (Raisz, 1982).

Minerals are deposited in the body in a range of pathological conditions (Gibson, 1974). Calcium phosphates, especially HAP and pyrophosphates, can be deposited in the cartilage and synovial fluid of joints; other minerals formed in joints include monosodium urate monohydrate (in gout), brushite ($CaHPO_4.2H_2O$) and calcium oxalate (Dieppe and Calvert, 1983). HAP is also deposited at pathological sites like atherosclerotic plaque (Schmid *et al.*, 1980); the related β-tricalcium phosphate (β-TCP; $Ca_3(PO_4)_2$) can also be deposited in the cardiovascular system (Bigi *et al.*, 1980, 1988). Furthermore, hard mineral 'stones' may be formed in some parts of the body. An example is provided by the 'corpora amylacea', which can form in the bovine mammary gland and may be expressed in the milk (Brooker, 1978). Renal calculi, which can contain HAP, brushite, calcium oxalate and struvite ($NH_4MgPO_4.6H_2O$), provide a more familiar example (Prien, 1963; Prien and Prien, 1968; Sutor, 1968; Sutor and Scheit, 1968; Smith, 1982). However, these stones do not consist solely of mineral and may contain proteins and carbohydrate (Boyce, 1968; Lian *et al.*, 1977; Smith, 1982). Mineralisation on the materials of artificial devices inserted into the body can interfere with their intended function. For example, poorly crystalline HAP can be deposited on prosthetic heart valves (Levy *et al.*, 1983), and urinary catheters frequently become blocked with a mixture of struvite and very poorly crystalline HAP as a result of colonisation of their surfaces by bacteria (Cox *et al.*, 1987, 1989).

CHARACTERISATION

Chemical composition

Clues to the identity of minerals deposited in tissues sometimes come from techniques which cannot provide detailed chemical compositions. Calcified deposits can often be seen in radiographs of affected joints, and the radiological appearance of calcium pyrophosphate deposits tends to be distinct from that of HAP deposits (Genant, 1976; Dieppe and Calvert, 1983; Watt, 1983). In histological sections of tissue, calcified deposits appear bright red when stained with the dye Alizarin Red (Gurr, 1971).

Colorimetry is simply a technique for measuring how much of a given ion is present from the intensity of coloration produced in reactions of this kind when they occur in solution. The formation of phosphomolybdic acid and its reduction to a blue compound (Allen, 1940) is still used to determine phosphorus concentrations.

However, the most common technique for quantitative analysis of the ions present in a material is atomic absorption spectroscopy, in which measurement of the absorbance of light, by a vaporised sample, at a selected wavelength, provides a measure of the concentration of the required element (Christian and Feldman, 1970; Slavin, 1978). A known mass of the material to be investigated is dissolved in a known volume of solvent, so that the concentration of the element can be calculated. The instrument is calibrated with solutions of known concentration and composition. However, two complications arise. 'Matrix interference' occurs if the physical nature of the sample solution (e.g. viscosity and volatility) is very different from that of the standard solution used as a calibrant; it can be controlled by matching the nature (solvent, temperature, concentration, etc.) of the standard solution as closely as possible to that of the sample solution. 'Chemical interference' occurs when atoms of the element being investigated combine with others in the flame used to vaporise the sample. For example, calcium combines with phosphate ions in a flame – unless excess lanthanum is added as a 'releasing agent'. Recently, ion chromatography has been used, as an alternative to atomic absorption spectroscopy, for the analysis of biological calcium phosphates (Holt *et al.*, 1987); its advantage is that the concentrations of most ions can be simply measured in a single experiment using about 1 mg of sample.

Analytical techniques which use the electron microscope enable the relative proportions of elements to be determined in a selected area of the image. Such techniques have the disadvantage that the electron beam cannot penetrate the depth of an intact sample, and so only its surface can be examined. Also, since only a small area is selected, the analysis is very sensitive to the features selected and so to contaminants. The technique most commonly used involves measurement of the intensity of X-rays emitted with a wavelength, which is characteristic of the element to be detected (Chandler, 1977). Concentrations of elements with an atomic number greater than that of carbon can be measured by this technique. However, characteristic X-rays from elements of lower atomic number are readily absorbed by the sample; this effect has to be allowed for if results are to be interpreted quantitatively (Roomans, 1981). Consequently, the technique has tended to be used qualitatively, to detect the presence of elements, or semi-quantitatively, to assess their relative proportions in investigations of biological minerals (e.g. Ali, 1985).

The remainder of this section on characterisation of minerals is concerned with defining structure, rather than simply determining elemental composition.

Crystal habit

Shapes of crystals depend on (1) the shapes of their unit cells and (2) the relative numbers of unit cells along the directions of the crystal axes. The second factor depends on the conditions under which the crystal grows. Thus crystals of the same structure (i.e. the same unit cell contents, and, hence, the same unit cell shapes) will tend to have the same habit (shape) when grown under reproducible conditions.

Individual crystals can often be examined in the light microscope.

Tissues in which crystals are embedded have either to be sectioned or else have their organic components digested before examination; the possibility exists that the crystals will be dissolved, or their compositions altered, by the preparative techniques involved. Consequently, light microscopy has proved most convenient for identifying the freely floating crystals in liquids, e.g. synovial fluid (Phelps *et al.*, 1968) and urine (Harrison, 1957).

If crystals are examined using polarised light, their optical anisotropies can be investigated to provide further information. In a 'positively birefringent' material, plane polarised light with its plane of polarisation parallel to the optic axis is propagated more slowly than when the plane of polarisation is perpendicular to the optic axis; the opposite is true for 'negatively birefringent' material. Further details are given in textbooks (e.g., Hartshorne and Stuart, 1969; Kerr, 1977); several brief accounts have also been published (e.g., Gatter, 1974; Fagan and Lidskey, 1974). In practice, the technique simply involves rotating the stage of the microscope and observing simple colour changes (Phelps *et al.*, 1968). The results can provide supplementary information to simple observation of crystal shape. Crystals of monosodium urate monohydrate, which are deposited in synovial fluid in gout (needle-like appearance), are strongly, negatively birefringent and so can be distinguished from both triclinic and monoclinic forms of calcium pyrophosphate dihydrate, deposited in chondrocalcinosis, or 'pseudo-gout' (as smaller needles or plates), which are both positively birefringent (Phelps *et al.*, 1968).

Scanning electron microscopy is an especially convenient method for examining crystal habit. Figure 1.1(a) shows a typical scanning electron micrograph of brushite, deposited in the presence of protein, which can be compared with the appearance, in figure 1.1(b), of HAP grown under similar conditions. (Whether brushite or HAP is precipitated is controlled by the pH of the solution.) However, figure 1.1(c) shows that in the absence of protein (but otherwise identical conditions), HAP is precipitated as granular aggregates (about 2 μm in diameter) rather than as a fluffy crust. Thus, crystals of the same substance might not appear the same if they were to grow under different conditions. The crystals shown in figure 1.1(b) were grown under conditions intended to mimic those occurring during encrustation of urinary catheters. Figure 1.1(d) shows the deposits on the surface of a naturally encrusted catheter; the fluffy deposits of HAP can then be distinguished from the relatively large, block-like crystals of struvite by their appearance (Cox and Hukins, 1989).

Transmission electron microscopy of thin sections of tissue has been used to investigate the interactions of mineral deposits with collagen (Weiner and Traub, 1986; Arsenault, 1988; Lees and Prostak, 1988). High-resolution transmission electron microscopy allows the lattice planes of crystals to be imaged; the technique therefore allows crystal domain sizes, crystal defects, etc., to be seen in calcified deposits (Mann, 1986).

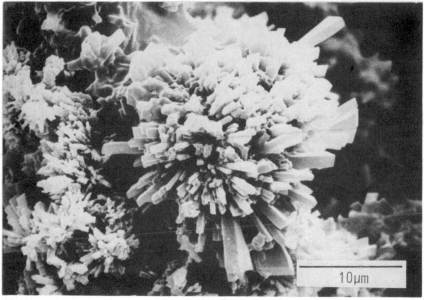

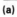
(a)

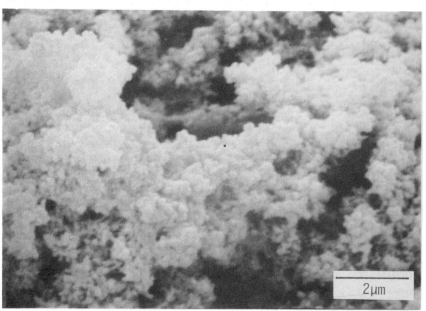
(b)

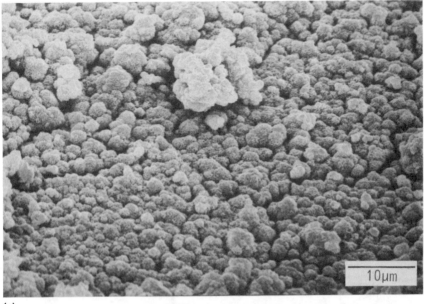

(c)

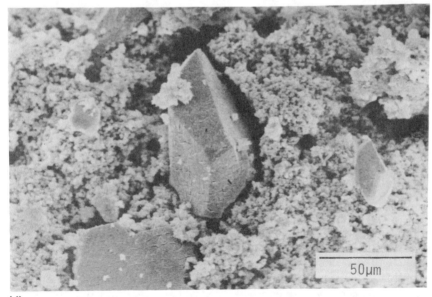

(d)

Figure 1.1   Scanning electron micrographs of: (a) brushite crystals grown in the presence of protein; (b) HAP crystals grown in the presence of protein; (c) HAP crystals grown in the absence of protein; (d) the surface of an encrusted urinary catheter, where block-like crystals of struvite are surrounded by fluffy deposits of HAP. (Micrographs courtesy of Dr A. J. Cox.)

Diffraction techniques

X-ray powder diffraction is the single most reliable technique for detecting and identifying crystalline phases is mineral deposits. Details of the experimental methods involved and of the principles of this technique are given in several books (Lipson and Steeple, 1970; Cullity, 1978; Hukins, 1981). A powder which consists of crystalline particles scatters X-rays along a series of coaxial conical paths, as shown in figure 1.2. Each cone is

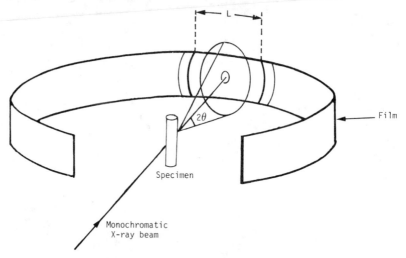

Figure 1.2   Schematic diagram showing the Debye–Scherrer method of recording an X-ray powder diffraction pattern. A strip of film is bent into a cylinder, of radius R, with the specimen on its axis. The polycrystalline powder scatters X-rays on the surfaces of cones of semi-vertical angle 2θ. One such cone is shown. Each cone intersects the film, to produce a pair of arcs. In the figure, a pair of arcs is separated by a distance L, when the film is flattened. The value of θ for this pair of arcs is then simply given, in radians, by $\theta = L/4R$.

characterised by its semi-vertical angle, $2\theta_{hkl}$, where h, k and l are integers which can be used to 'index' the cone. Allowed values of θ_{hkl} are given by

$$\theta_{hkl} = \sin^{-1}(\lambda/2d_{hkl}) \qquad (1.1)$$

where λ is the wavelength of the X-rays and is equal to 0.154 nm for the the (copper K_α) X-rays which are nearly always used to identify minerals. Values of d_{hkl} depend on the dimensions of the unit cell of the crystal. Consider a unit cell whose sides have lengths of a, b and c; the angles between pairs of these sides are denoted α (between b and c), β (between a and c), and γ (between a and b). The values of d_{hkl} for this unit cell are then given by the set of equations listed in table 1.1. Equation 1.1 is often referred to as 'Bragg's law'.

In practice, the values of d_{hkl} can be easily measured from the X-ray diffraction pattern of a crystalline powder. The scattered X-rays can be

Table 1.1 Equations required to calculate d_{hkl} values from the unit cell dimensions (a, b, c, α, β, γ) of a crystal

$$d_{hkl} = Q_{hkl}^{-1/2}$$
$$Q_{hkl} = h^2 a^{*2} + k^2 b^{*2} + l^2 c^{*2} + 2klb^*c^* \cos \alpha^* + 2lhc^*a^* \cos \beta^* + 2hka^*b^* \cos \gamma^*$$
$$a^* = V^{-1}bc \sin \alpha$$
$$b^* = V^{-1}ac \sin \beta$$
$$c^* = V^{-1}ab \sin \gamma$$
$$V = 2abc\{\sin s \sin (s - \alpha) \sin (s - \beta) \sin (s - \gamma)\}^{1/2}$$
$$s = (\alpha + \beta + \gamma)/2$$
$$\cos \alpha^* = (\cos \beta \cos \gamma - \cos \alpha)/(\sin \beta \sin \gamma)$$
$$\cos \beta^* = (\cos \gamma \cos \alpha - \cos \beta)/(\sin \gamma \sin \alpha)$$
$$\cos \gamma^* = (\cos \alpha \cos \beta - \cos \gamma)/(\sin \alpha \sin \beta)$$

recorded on a strip of photographic film bent into the arc of a circle centred on the specimen (the 'Debye–Scherrer' method), as shown in figure 1.2. Alternatively, the X-rays can be detected using a 'diffractometer', in which a counter measures their intensities directly, around the same arc. Figure 1.2 explains how θ_{hkl} can be measured; the corresponding value of d_{hkl} can then be calculated from equation 1.1.

The values of d_{hkl}, and the relative intensities of the X-rays scattered in

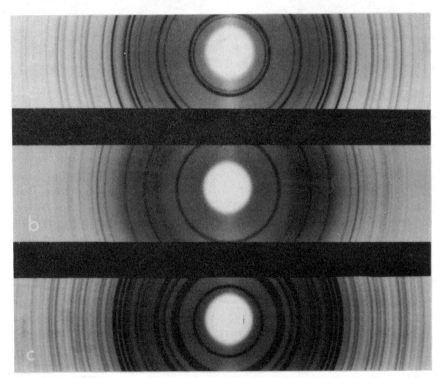

Figure 1.3   X-ray powder diffraction patterns of: (a) brushite; (b) calcium oxalate monohydrate; (c) struvite. The parts of the pattern which correspond to higher values of θ (see figure 1.2) are omitted.

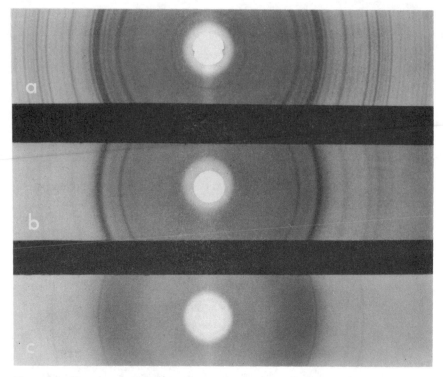

Figure 1.4   X-ray powder diffraction patterns of: (a) HAP; (b) poorly crystalline HAP; and (c) an amorphous calcium phosphate (ACP), which converts into poorly crystalline HAP unless it is carefully dried or chemically stabilised. The parts of the pattern that correspond to higher values of θ (see figure 1.2) are omitted.

the corresponding directions, can be used to identify the mineral. The relative intensities of the scattered X-rays depend on the arrangement of atoms in the unit cell. Figure 1.3 compares the Debye–Scherrer patterns of brushite, calcium oxalate and struvite. In each of these patterns, the positions of the lines depend on the dimensions of the unit cell, and their relative intensities depend on which elements are present in which positions within the unit cell. Thus the X-ray powder diffraction pattern acts as a 'fingerprint' of a crystal structure. Rather than compare diffraction patterns, it is often useful to tabulate d_{hkl} values and the corresponding relative intensities. An extensive set of tables, which is regularly updated, has been compiled by the American Society for Testing and Materials (Philadelphia, USA); more restricted tables, intended for specific applications, have also been published (e.g., Sutor and Scheit, 1968).

The appearance of an X-ray powder diffraction pattern can also be used to assess the extent of crystallinity of a sample. For example, the pattern of sharp lines in figure 1.4(a) is characteristic of crystalline HAP; in figure 1.4(b), the lines are more diffuse and tend to fade out at higher values of θ_{hkl} – indicating that the long-range order is not so highly developed in this sample; i.e., it could be described as 'poorly crystalline' (Woodhead–Galloway *et al.*, 1980). In figure 1.4(c), there are no obvious lines – indicating that the solid sample was 'amorphous'; i.e., that it resembled a glass with no long-range order. It is worth noting that X-ray diffraction is relatively insensitive to disordered phases and so may not detect them when they are mixed with crystalline material (see, e.g., Hukins *et al.*, 1986). Similarly, the technique is insensitive to minor components constituting less than about 10 per cent of a mixture of crystalline materials (Sutor, 1968).

X-ray diffraction may also be used to determine the positions of atoms in the unit cell. In this application of the technique, the sample is usually a single crystal of the synthetic compound or a geological mineral. Crystal structures of this kind have been reported for most of the minerals deposited in tissues (Young and Brown, 1982). In some of these examples, neutron, rather than X-ray, diffraction was used to solve the crystal structure; in either case, the principles and methods are closely similar (Bacon, 1962). More recently, a method (the 'Rietveld method') has been described for refining structural models for crystalline compounds from their powder diffraction patterns (Rietveld, 1969); this method has been applied to the structures of both fluorapatite and HAP which incorporates carbonate ions (Young *et al.*, 1977).

Electron diffraction has been used to investigate small crystals (dimensions measured in tens of nm) in the electron microscope (Mann, 1986).

Spectroscopic methods

Infrared (IR) spectroscopy has been widely used to characterise minerals deposited in biological systems and model compounds. A material will absorb only IR radiation whose frequency corresponds to the frequency of one of its interatomic vibrations. Thus the absorption frequencies depend on the chemical groups present within the material and on the way they are packed together. Thus, like an X-ray powder diffraction pattern, an IR spectrum can be used as a 'fingerprint' of a crystal structure. However, IR spectra of, for example, different calcium phosphates are much more similar than their X-ray diffraction patterns. The reason is that the vibrational frequencies of the phosphate groups are very similar in different crystal structures. Nevertheless, IR spectroscopy has been used to confirm the results of other techniques or to indicate the presence of chemical groups, such as carbonate (LeGeros *et al.*, 1964), within a sample (e.g., Bigi *et al.*, 1980). Furthermore, the appearance of the spectrum depends on the degree of crystallinity of a sample.

The sensitivity of IR spectroscopy has been greatly improved by Fourier transform techniques. As a result, it has the potential to provide more detailed information on the structures of calcified deposits from tissues and their model compounds, as described in Chapter 5. One very promising application of the technique is to detect the presence of HPO_4^{2-} ions in non-crystalline samples.

Nuclear magnetic resonance (NMR) spectroscopy has been used to investigate calcified deposits and their model compounds. ^{31}P NMR of solids is capable of distinguishing whether the phosphorus atoms are present in PO_4^{3-} or HPO_4^{2-} ions (Belton et al., 1988). An example is provided by the detection of mineral domains, which may resemble brushite in embryonic bone (Bonar et al., 1984).

X-ray absorption spectroscopy (XAS) is sensitive to the local environment of a selected-type atom or ion in a material. Thus it was considered to have considerable promise for investigating amorphous and poorly crystalline mineral deposits from biological systems, and their synthetic model compounds. Extended X-ray absorption fine-structure (EXAFS) spectra have been widely used to investigate calcium phosphates. While the technique can provide valuable information on the structures of bone mineral, micellar calcium phosphate from milk, and pathological deposits, it is not so sensitive to differences in the structures of amorphous calcium phosphates as had been anticipated. Further details are given in Chapter 4.

CALCIUM PHOSPHATES

Most of the calcium phosphates precipitated in the body can be considered as salts of orthophosphoric acid (H_3PO_4). Orthophosphoric acid dissociates in three stages:

$$H_3PO_4 \overset{1}{\rightleftharpoons} H^+ + H_2PO_4^- \overset{2}{\rightleftharpoons} 2H^+ + HPO_4^{2-} \overset{3}{\rightleftharpoons} 3H^+ + PO_4^{3-}$$

According to Le Chatelier's principle, the acid will be more highly dissociated when there are fewer H^+ ions in its environment; i.e., as the pH of its surroundings increases. The equilibrium position for each stage is given by the corresponding acid dissociation constant K_{a1}, K_{a2} and K_{a3}. For example K_{a2} is defined by

$$K_{a2} = [H^+][HPO_4^{2-}]/[H_2PO_4^-] \tag{1.2}$$

where brackets [] denote molar concentrations (i.e., concentrations measured in moles per litre). The dissociation constants are often quoted on a logarithmic scale, when they are denoted by pK_{a1}, pK_{a2} and pK_{a3}, defined, for example, by

$$pK_{a2} = -\log_{10} K_{a2} \tag{1.3}$$

This logarithmic scale can be useful because an acid is 50 per cent dissociated when the pH value of the surroundings equals its pK_a value. The pK_a values for orthophosphoric acid are: $pK_{a1} = 2.1$, $pK_{a2} = 7.2$, and $pK_{a3} = 12.7$. However, calculation of the precipitates which are likely to form in biological systems is not straightforward; calculations of ionic equilibria have been performed for milk (Holt *et al.*, 1981) and urine (Linder and Little, 1986). The forms of calcium phosphate precipitated under different conditions are more easily investigated experimentally. Examples include the effect of pH on the minerals deposited from urine (Elliot *et al.*, 1958), and the effects of gelatin and polyacrylamide gels on the crystallisation of calcium pyrophosphate (Harries *et al.*, 1983); further details are given by Nancollas (1982).

In many biological systems, PO_4^{3-} is precipitated with calcium as HAP; however, the mineral is frequently poorly crystalline, contains other ions (especially carbonate), and the positions of the lines in its X-ray powder diffraction may differ somewhat from those expected. Other apatites, in which fluoride and chloride ions (both present in the body) replace the OH^- ion of HAP, have very similar X-ray diffraction patterns. Carbonate ions may replace some of the phosphate in the HAP lattice, leading to a change in lattice dimensions and increased structural disorder (Harries *et al.*, 1987a). Furthermore, the X-ray powder diffraction pattern of HAP is closely similar to that of β-TCP, and, when the material is poorly crystalline, it is often difficult to distinguish between them with any certainty. β-TCP occurs naturally as the mineral whitlockite, when it invariably contains traces of magnesium (Frondel, 1941). Octacalcium phosphate (OCP; $Ca_8H_2(PO_4)_6 \cdot 5H_2O$) has been prepared which also has an X-ray powder diffraction pattern closely similar to that of HAP (Young and Brown, 1982). Crystal structures of many of these phases have been determined (Young and Brown, 1982). The conventional approach to this complexity seems to be to treat each of these structural variants as a unique chemical compound. Given the range of non-stoichiometry which exists in biological apatites, and their considerable structural disorder, this approach seems somewhat contrived. Although many deposits will resemble HAP more closely than β-TCP (and vice versa), some deposits may have structures which are intermediate between HAP and OCP or β-TCP, or which cannot be defined so precisely. Indeed, it would seem more profitable to consider the synthetic model compounds themselves as examples of the range of structures which can be adopted, rather than as discrete chemical compounds.

Several methods have been published for preparing amorphous calcium phosphate (ACP), which yields an X-ray powder diffraction pattern similar to that of figure 1.4(c) (Blumenthal *et al.*, 1972; Termine and Eanes, 1972; Nancollas, 1982; Harries *et al.*, 1987b). ACP gradually converts into a poorly crystalline form of HAP, unless it is carefully dried or chemically stabilised, e.g. with magnesium or citrate ions (Eanes and Posner, 1965; Walton *et al.*, 1967; Blumenthal *et al.*, 1972; Termine and Eanes, 1972; Nancollas, 1982; Harries *et al.*, 1987b). Although ACP can be prepared at a high pH value to ensure that it contains PO_4^{3-} ions (Harries *et al.*, 1987b), some preparations may include appreciable concentrations of HPO_4^{2-} ions (Termine and Eanes, 1972; Meyer and Eanes, 1978). Recently ACP samples have been prepared under neutral and slightly acidic conditions in which about half of the orthophosphate ions are present at HPO_4^{2-} (Holt *et al.*, 1988, 1989a). In milk there is an ACP, complexed to the phosphoprotein casein, whose solubility and chemical composition suggests that its structure is closely similar to these synthetic compounds (Holt *et al.*, 1989b).

Pyrophosphates contain the $P_2O_7^{4-}$ ion, which is produced during normal metabolic activity by the conversion of adenosine triphosphate (ATP) to adenosine monophosphate (McCarty, 1976; Dieppe and Calvert, 1983). It is usually converted into orthophosphates by enzymes called pyrophosphatases. However, calcium pyrophosphate dihydrate may crystallise in joints in either the triclinic or the monoclinic form (McCarty, 1976; Okazaki *et al.*, 1976; Dieppe and Calvert, 1983). There are no reports of amorphous pyrophosphates being synthesised or precipitated within the human body. However, amorphous pyrophosphates have been identified in secretory granules of snails (Taylor *et al.*, 1986, 1988).

REMAINING PROBLEMS

It is clear that there is no single technique which allows the structures of mineral deposits to be determined. Although diffraction techniques allow crystalline phases to be identified, and their structures to be determined, they are not so useful for characterising amorphous compounds and may not be able to provide much structural information for minerals which are associated with proteins. For example, complexes of phosphoproteins with calcium phosphates have yet to be crystallised, and the calcium phosphates within these complexes do not yield X-ray powder diffraction patterns consistent with their having an extended crystalline lattice. Further details are given in Chapter 8. Spectroscopic techniques may then be used in order to obtain at least some of the required structural information. X-ray absorption spectroscopy allows models to be developed for the environment of the calcium ions in poorly crystalline and amorphous mineral deposits. Unfortunately, for this approach to be successful, a crystalline model compound with a similar structure has to be identified – for the reasons described in Chapter 4. The chemical groups present in an amorphous phase can be determined by a variety of techniques, but it appears that Fourier transform infrared spectroscopy is likely to be especially useful, e.g. for determining the ratio of PO_4^{3-} and HPO_4^{2-} ions within a sample. The application of this technique to biological calcium phosphates and their synthetic model compounds is described in Chapter 5.

However, determination of the structure of the mineral phase alone is inadequate for defining the structure of a calcified tissue; it is also important to describe the interactions of the minerals with other tissue components, as well as to know how this system of interacting minerals and macromolecules is arranged in the tissue. The techniques used to investigate the interactions of calcium phosphates with phosphoproteins and phospholipids, as well as the conclusions which can be drawn from them, are described in Chapters 8 and 9, respectively.

Interactions of mineral with collagen are approached, in Chapter 6, with the emphasis on the velocity of propagation of ultrasound in mineralised tissues. Although the results from other techniques are discussed in the chapter, this approach is valuable because it links the structure of mineralised tissues to their mechanical properties. The mechanical properties of bones and teeth provide one of the clearest demonstrations of the biological functions of mineralisation. Thus the material of Chapter 6 provides a direct approach to relating an important aspect of the biological function of mineralised tissues to a simple description of structure. Although the simplicity of this approach is valuable for providing further understanding of the mechanical properties of cortical bone, a more sophisticated description of tissue structure is required to describe the normal physiological and pathological processes occurring in many tissues. Chapter 3 explains how high-resolution radiographic techniques can be used to provide much more detailed information on the structures of calcified tissues.

Although much of the emphasis in this book is structural, description of structure is useful only in so far as it provides an explanation of biological function – as well as a rational basis for describing pathology, and, hence, managing its consequences. Descriptions of specific structural aspects of calcified tissues in Chapters 6–9 are closely linked to biological function and pathological problems. However, the formation and destruction of calcified tissues are mediated by cells rather than being solely the consequence of structure. Chapter 2 provides a brief description of the histology of calcified tissues, with emphasis on the functions of its cells. Thus Chapters 1 and 2 together provide two alternative, but complementary, approaches to understanding calcified tissues. Chapter 1 emphasises the physical description of structure and function, while Chapter 2 adopts a more biological approach. Together, they provide an introduction to the material described in the remaining chapters.

ACKNOWLEDGEMENTS

I am most grateful to Drs A. J. Cox and C. Holt for discussions which have influenced the contents of this chapter, and to Miss K. E. Davies and Miss T. M. Westley for help with the illustrations.

REFERENCES

Ali, S. Y. (1985). Apatite-type crystal deposition in articular cartilage. *Scanning Electron Microsc.*, **IV**, 1555–66

Allen, R. J. L. (1940). The estimation of phosphorus. *Biochem. J.*, **34**, 858–65

Arsenault, A. L. (1988) Crystal–collagen relationships in calcified turkey leg tendons visualized by selected-area dark field electron microscopy. *Calcif. Tiss. Intl*, **43**, 202–12

Bacon, G. E. (1962). *Neutron Diffraction*, 2nd. edn, Clarendon Press, Oxford

Belton, P. S., Harris, R. K. and Wilkes, P. J. (1988). Solid-state phosphorus-31 NMR studies of synthetic inorganic calcium phosphates. *J. Phys. Chem. Solids*, **49**, 21–7

Bigi, A., Foresti, E., Incerti, A., Ripamonti, A. and Roveri, N. (1980). Structural and chemical characterization of the inorganic deposits in calcified human aortic wall. *Inorg. Chim. Acta*, **55**, 81–5

Bigi, A., Compostella, L., Fichera, A. M., Foresti, E., Gazzano, M., Ripamonti, A. and Roveri, N. (1988). Structural and chemical characterisation of inorganic deposits in calcified human mitral valve. *J. Inorg. Biochem.*, **37**, 75–82

Blumenthal, N. C., Posner, A. S. and Holmes, J. M. (1972). Effect of preparation conditions on the properties and transformation of amorphous calcium phosphate. *Mater. Res. Bull.*, **7**, 1181–90

Bonar, L. C., Grynpas, M. and Glimcher, M. J. (1984). Failure to detect crystalline brushite in embryonic chick and bovine bone by X-ray diffraction. *J. Ultrastruct. Res.*, **86**, 93–9

Boskey, A. L. (1980). Current concepts of the physiology and biochemistry of calcification. *Clin. Orthop.*, **157**, 225–57

Boyce, W. H. (1968). Organic matrix of human urinary concretions. *Am. J. Med.*, **45**, 673–83

Brooker, B. E. (1978). The origin, structure and occurrence of corpora amylacea in the bovine mammary gland and in milk. *Cell Tiss. Res.*, **191**, 525–538

Chandler, J. A. (1977). *X-Ray Microanalysis in the Electron Microscope*, North Holland, Amsterdam

Christian, G. D. and Feldman, F. J. (1970). *Atomic Absorption Spectroscopy – Applications in Agriculture, Biology and Medicine*, Wiley Interscience, New York

Cox, A. J. and Hukins, D. W. L. (1989). Morphology of mineral deposit on encrusted urinary catheters investigated by scanning electron microscopy. *J. Urol.*, submitted

Cox, A. J., Harries, J. E., Hukins, D. W. L., Kennedy, A. P. and Sutton, T. M. (1987). Calcium phosphate in catheter encrustation. *Brit. J. Urol.*, **59**, 159–163

Cox, A. J., Hukins, D. W. L. and Sutton, T. M. (1989). Infection of catheterised patients: bacterial colonisation of encrusted Foley catheters shown by scanning electron microscopy. *Urol. Res.*, submitted

Cullity, B. D. (1978). *Elements of X-Ray Diffraction*, 2nd edn, Addison-Wesley, London

Dieppe, P. and Calvert, P. (1983). *Crystals and Joint Disease*, Chapman & Hall, London

Eanes, E. D. and Posner, A. S. (1965). Kinetics and mechanism of conversion of noncrystalline calcium phosphate to hydroxyapatite. *Trans. NY Acad. Sci.*, **28**, 233–41

Eanes, E. D., Lundy, D. R. and Martin, G. N. (1970). X-Ray diffraction study of the mineralisation of turkey leg tendon. *Calcif. Tiss. Res.*, **6**, 239–48

Eanes, E. D., Powers, L. and Costa, J. L. (1981). Extended X-ray absorption fine structure (EXAFS) studies on calcium in crystalline and amorphous solids of biological interest. *Cell Calcium*, **2**, 251–61

Elliot, J. S., Quaide, W. L., Sharp, R. F. and Lewis, L. (1958). Mineralogical studies of urine: the relationship of apatite, brushite and struvite to urinary pH. *J. Urol.*, **80**, 269–71

Fagan, T. J. and Lidskey, M. D. (1974). Compensated polarized light microscopy using cellophane adhesive tape. *Arthr. Rheum.*, **17**, 256–62

Frondel, C. (1941). Whitlockite: a new calcium phosphate, $Ca_3(PO_4)_2$. *Amer. Mineral.*, **26**, 145–52

Gatter, R. A. (1974). The compensated polarized light microscope in clinical rheumatology. *Arthr. Rheum.*, **17**, 253–55

Genant, H. K. (1976). Roentgenographic aspects of calcium pyrophosphate dihydrate crystal deposition disease (pseudogout). *Arthr. Rheum.*, **19**, 307–28

Gibson, R. I. (1974). Descriptive human pathological mineralogy. *Amer. Mineral.*, **59**, 1177–82

Gurr, E. (1971). *Synthetic Dyes in Biology, Medicine and Chemistry*, Academic Press, London, pp. 234–5

Harries, J. E., Dieppe, P. A., Heap, P., Gilgead, J., Mather, M. and Shah, J. S. (1983). In vitro growth of calcium pyrophosphate crystals in polyacrylamide gels. *Ann. Rheum. Dis.*, **42** (Suppl. 1), 100–1

Harries, J. E., Hasnain, S. S. and Shah, J. S. (1987a). EXAFS study of structural disorder in carbonate-containing hydroxyapatite. *Calcif. Tiss. Intl*, **41**, 346–50

Harries, J. E., Hukins, D. W. L., Holt, C. and Hasnain, S. S. (1987b). Conversion of amorphous calcium phosphate into hydroxyapatite investigated by EXAFS spectroscopy. *J. Cryst. Growth*, **84**, 563–70

Harrison, G. A. (1957). *Chemical Methods in Clinical Medicine*, 4th edn, Churchill, London, pp. 107–16

Hartshorne, N. H. and Stuart, A. (1969). *Practical Optical Crystallography*, 2nd edn, Edward Arnold, London

Holt, C., Dalgleish, D. G. and Jenness, R. (1981). Calculation of the ion equilibria in milk diffusate and comparison with experiment. *Anal. Biochem.*, **113**, 154–63

Holt, C., Cox, A. J., Harries, J. E. and Hukins, D. W. L. (1987). In *Recent Developments in Ion Exchange* (eds P. A. Williams and M. J. Hudson), Elsevier Applied Science, Barking, 22–8

Holt, C., van Kemenade, M. J. J. M., Harries, J. E., Nelson, L. S., Bailey, R. T., Hukins, D. W. L., Hasnain, S. S. and de Bruyn, P. L. (1988). Preparation of amorphous calcium–magnesium phosphates at pH 7 and characterization by X-ray absorption and Fourier transform infrared spectroscopy. *J. Cryst. Growth*, **92**, 239–52

Holt, C., van Kemenade, M. J. J. M., Nelson, L. S., Hukins, D. W. L., Bailey, R. T., Harries, J. E., and Hasnain, S. S. and de Bruyn, P. L. (1989a). Amorphous calcium phosphates prepared at pH 6.5 and 6.0. *Mater. Res. Bull.*, **23**, 55–62

Holt, C., van Kemenade, M. J. J. M., Nelson, L. S., Sawyer, L., Harries, J. E., Bailey, R. T. and Hukins, D. W. L. (1989b). Composition and structure of micellar calcium phosphate. *J. Dairy Res.*, in press

Hukins, D. W. L. (1981). *X-Ray Diffraction by Disordered and Ordered Systems*, Pergamon, Oxford

Hukins, D. W. L., Cox, A. J. and Harries, J. E. (1986). EXAFS characterisation of poorly crystalline deposits from biological systems in the presence of highly crystalline material. *J. Physique.*, **47**, C8.1181–84

Kerr, P. F. (1977). *Optical Mineralogy*, 4th edn, McGraw-Hill, New York

Lees, S. and Prostak, K. (1988). The locus of mineral crystallites in bone. *Conn. Tiss. Res.*, **18**, 41–54

LeGeros, R. Z., LeGeros, J. P., Trautz, O. R. and Klein, E. (1964). Spectral properties of carbonate-containing apatites. *J. Dental Res.*, **43**, 752–60

Levy, R. J. Schoen, F. J., Levy, J. T., Nelson, A. C., Howard, S. L. and Oshry, L. J. (1983). Biologic determinants of dystrophic calcification and osteocalcin deposition in glutaraldehyde-preserved porcine aortic valve leaflets implanted subcutaneously in rats. *Am. J. Path.*, **113**, 143–55

Lian, J. B., Prien, E. L., Glimcher, M. J. and Gallup, P. M. (1977). The presence of protein-bound γ-carboxyglutamic acid in calcium containing renal stones. *J. Clin. Invest.*, **59**, 1151–7

Linder, P. W. and Little, J. C. (1986). Prediction by computer modelling of the precipitation of stone-forming solids from urine. *Inorg. Chim. Acta*, **123**, 137–45

Lipson, H. and Steeple, H. (1970). *Interpretation of X-Ray Powder Diffraction Patterns*, Macmillan, London

Lowenstam, H. A. (1981). Minerals formed by organisms. *Science*, **211**, 1126–31

McCarty, D. J. (1976). Calcium pyrophosphate deposition disease. *Arthr. Rheum.*, **19**, 275–85

Mann, S. (1983). Mineralization in biological systems. *Struct. Bond.*, **54**, 125–74

Mann, S. (1986). The study of biominerals by high resolution transmission electron microscopy. *Scanning Electron Microsc.*, **II**, 393–413

Meyer, J. L. and Eanes, E. D. (1978). A thermodynamic analysis of the amorphous to crystalline calcium phosphate transformation. *Calcif. Tiss. Res.*, **25**, 59–68

Miller, R. M., Hukins, D. W. L., Hasnain, S. S. and Lagarde, P. (1981). Extended X-ray absorption fine structure (EXAFS) studies of the calcium ion environment in bone mineral and related calcium phosphates. *Biochem. Biophys. Res. Commun.*, **99**, 102–6

Nancollas, G. H. (1982). Phase transformation during precipitation of calcium salts. In *Biological Mineralization and Demineralization* (ed. G. H. Nancollas), Springer, Berlin, 79–99

Okazaki, T., Saito, T., Mitomo, T. and Siota, Y. (1976). Pseudogout: clinical observations and chemical and analysis of deposits. *Arthr. Rheum.*, **19**, 293–305

Pautard, F. G. E. and Williams, R. J. P. (1982). Biological minerals. *Chemy. Brit.*, **18**, 188–93

Phelps, P., Steele, A. D. and McCarty, D. J. (1968). Compensated polarized light microscopy. Identification of crystals in synovial fluids from gout and pseudogout. *JAMA*, **203**, 508–12

Prien, E. L. (1963). Crystallographic analysis of urinary calculi: a 23-year survey study. *J. Urol.*, **89**, 917–24

Prien, E. L. and Prien, E. L. (1968). Composition and structure of urinary stone. *Am. J. Med.*, **45**, 654–72

Raisz, L. G. (1982). Mechanisms and regulation of normal and pathological demineralization. In *Biological Mineralization and Demineralization* (ed. G. H. Nancollas), Springer, Berlin, 287–301

Rietveld, H. M. (1969). A profile refinement method for nuclear and magnetic structures. *J. Appl. Crystallogr.*, **2**, 65–71

Roomans, G. M. (1981). Quantitative electron probe microanalysis of biological bulk specimens. *Scanning Electron Microsc.*, **II**, 345–56

Schmid, K., McSharry, W. O., Pameÿer, C. H. and Binette, J. P. (1980). Chemical and physicochemical studies on the mineral deposits of the human atherosclerotic aorta. *Artherosclerosis*, **37**, 199–210

Slavin, M. (1978). *Atomic Absorption Spectroscopy*, Wiley, New York

Smith, L. H. (1982). Abnormal calcification. In *Biological Mineralization and Demineralization* (ed. G. H. Nancollas), Springer, Berlin, 259–70

Sutor, D. J. (1968). Difficulties in the identification of components of mixed urinary calculi using the X-ray powder method. *Brit. J. Urol.*, **40**, 29–32

Sutor, D. J. and Scheidt, S. E. (1968). Identification standards for human urinary components using crystallographic methods. *Brit. J. Urol.*, **40**, 22–8

Taylor, M., Simkiss, K. and Greaves, G. N. (1986). Amorphous structure of intracellular mineral granules. *Biochem. Soc. Trans.*, **14**, 549–52

Taylor, M. G., Simkiss, K., Greaves, G. N. and Harries, J. (1988). Corrosion of intracellular granules and cell death. *Proc. R. Soc. Lond.*, **B234**, 463–76

Termine, J. D. (1972). Mineral chemistry and skeletal biology. *Clin. Orthop.*, **85**, 207–41

Termine, J. D. and Eanes, E. D. (1972). Comparative chemistry of amorphous and apatitic calcium phosphate preparations. *Calcif. Tiss. Res.*, **10**, 171–5

Walton, A. G., Bodin, W. J., Furedi, H. and Schwartz, A. (1967). Nucleation of calcium phosphate from solution. *Can. J. Chem.*, **45**, 2695–701

Watt, I. (1983). Radiology of the crystal-associated arthrides. *Ann. Rheum. Dis.*, **42** (Suppl. 1), 73–80

Weiner, S. and Traub, W. (1986). Organization of hydroxyapatite crystals within collagen fibrils. *FEBS Lett.*, **206**, 262–6

Wheeler, E. J. and Lewis, D. (1977). An X-ray study of the paracrystalline nature of bone apatite. *Calcif. Tiss. Res.*, **24**, 243–8

White, S. W., Hulmes, D. J. S., Miller, A. and Timmins, P. A. (1977). Collagen-mineral axial relationship in calcified turkey leg tendon by X-ray and neutron diffraction. *Nature, Lond.*, **266**, 421–5

Woodhead-Galloway, J., Young, W. H. and Hukins, D. W. L. (1980). Description of irregularity in biological structures. *Acta Crystallogr.*, **A36**, 198–205

Young, R. A. and Brown, W. E. (1982). Structures of biological minerals. In *Biological Mineralization and Demineralization* (ed. G. H. Nancollas), Springer, Berlin, 101–41

Young, R. A., Mackie, P. E. and von Dreele, R. B. (1977). Application of the pattern-fitting structure-refinement method to X-ray powder diffraction. *J. Appl. Crystallogr.*, **10**, 262–9

2

The histology of mineralised tissues

A. J. Freemont

INTRODUCTION

The reliance of so many organisms on mineralised tissues for support, protection, mineral stores, etc., is testimony to the importance of these tissues to normal body function. The diversity of mineralised tissue structure across the phylogenetic scale is too great for adequate discussion here, and so this description will be restricted to calcium-based minerals in representative organs of man (although many of the observations are pertinent to other organisms).

The most abundant of the calcified tissues in man is bone, which will form the basis of this review. Reference will also be made to calcified cartilage and to pathological tissue calcification.

BONE

After a long period of relative obscurity, there has been a recent upsurge of interest in bone structure and its regulation (Ellis, 1981). The standard against which these evolving concepts have to be judged is the observed morphology and histomorphometry of bone.

Bone (as opposed to *a* bone) has some striking histological characteristics. If one of the long bones of the appendicular skeleton is longitudinally or transversely sectioned, it will be seen (figure 2.1) to consist of two parts, an outer dense cylinder of bone (cortex) and an inner three-dimensional lattice of bone spicules (trabeculae).

Cortical bone itself has two zones. Most is made up of interlocking complete and incomplete spindle-shaped bone units. Each unit has a central longitudinally orientated canal, the Haversian canal, through which run blood vessels. Outside this Haversian bone lies periosteal bone formed of a series of thin concentric cylinders of bone covered by a fibrous tissue layer called periosteum from which they form (Pommer, 1925).

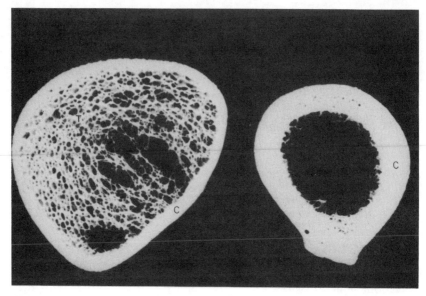

Figure 2.1   Microradiographs of bone showing dense cortical (C) and epicules of trabecular (T) bone.

In addition to the well-defined cortical and trabecular bone, there is also a zone known as subcortical bone, where trabecular bone merges with Haversian bone.

There are thus four zones or envelopes of bone: periosteal, Haversian, subcortical and trabecular (figure 2.2). These zones are conceptually and practically important because mineral turnover is different in each; these differences are important in considering age- and sex-related changes in bone mass. Periosteal bone is continuously deposited throughout life, whereas after middle age there is increased erosion in the subcortical envelope, resulting in a net loss of Haversian bone. The overall effect of these two changes is a slow but measurable increase in the external diameter of a long bone, while the overall thickness of the cortex is steadily reduced (Courpron *et al.*, 1977). Trabecular bone mass remains constant in women until the menopause and in men to late middle life, after which it gradually falls (figure 2.3). A similar age-related pattern of bone loss is seen within cortical bone, but, on average, it tends to occur somewhat later in life. Thus, from early adulthood to middle age, bone mass remains roughly constant, then a progressive reduction of cortical thickness commences with a loss of trabecular bone, followed by intra-cortical bone loss.

Much of the detailed understanding of bone structure and bone dynamics comes from the study of trabecular bone (Merz and Schenk, 1970; Melsen *et al.*, 1978), and surprisingly little is known of the other zones.

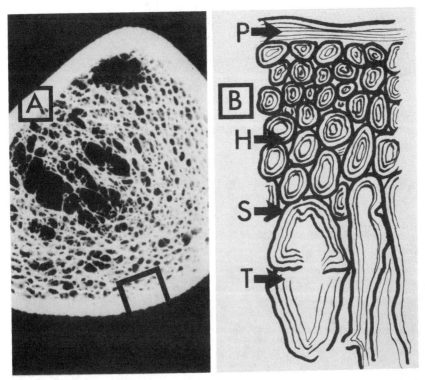

Figure 2.2   B is a diagnostic representation of the region of bone from the area within the box of A. P = periosteal, H = Haversian, S = subcortical and T = trabecular envelopes.

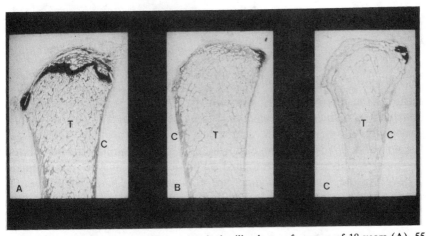

Figure 2.3   Representative sections through the iliac bone of women of 18 years (A), 55 years (B) and 85 years (C), showing progressive loss of trabecular (T) bone between B and A and cancellous and cortical bone (C) between A and C.

Histologically, bone can be considered to consist of four major components – collagen, non-collagenous organic matrix, mineral and cells.

Collagen

The collagen is predominantly type I. In 'normal' bone, it is arranged in layers of equal thickness (lamellae). Within a lamella, collagen fibres have a parallel orientation, which gives bone its characteristic striped appearance in polarised light (figure 2.4).

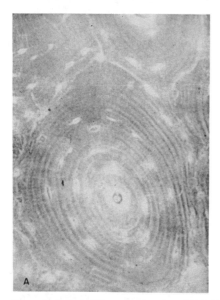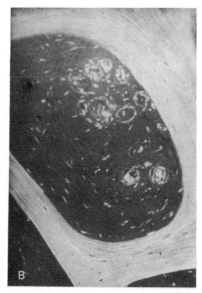

Figure 2.4   Polarising micrographs of (A) Haversian and (B) trabecular bone showing the lamellar arrangement of collagen fibres.

Non-collagenous organic matrix

Little of the composition of the non-collagenous organic component of bone can be defined histologically. It is known to contain various specific glycoproteins, one of which, osteocalcin (bone Gla protein) (Deftos and Catherwood, 1983), is believed to modulate matrix mineralisation. Even the most sophisticated histological techniques are, as yet, unhelpful in uncovering the diversity of macromolecules in these sites. (However, it must be admitted that this is a singularly neglected area of study.)

Mineral

The mineral phase is a complex inorganic crystalline salt, consisting mainly of calcium and phosphorus, which most closely resembles the mineral hydroxyapatite. Histological techniques are available for processing and studying 'undecalcified' bone (i.e., mineralised bone) (Anderson, 1982; Revell, 1983). Numerous histochemical techniques are available for identifying the components of the crystal lattice, which, particularly in disease, may include a variety of metals, including magnesium, strontium, aluminium (Denton *et al.*, 1984), etc. Despite the availability of these techniques, for reasons of ease of tissue handling, most bone is decalcified in acid or chelating agents, such as EDTA, prior to histological examination, but in so doing much of the information potentially available within the specimen is lost.

Bone cells

There are four types of bone cell – osteocytes, osteoblasts, osteoclasts and endosteal cells.

Osteocytes

Osteocytes are very abundant, but poorly understood. Their cell bodies lie within spaces deep inside bone known as lacunae. The lacunae are linked to one another and the bone surface by a series of narrow canals or canaliculi (figure 2.5). These contain osteocyte cytoplasmic processes, which communicate with the processes of other osteocytes. The role of the osteocyte is unclear. Studies of mineral clearance from bone of patients with renal failure indicate that mineral may be lost from deep within bone (Boyde, 1981), probably at the interface between the matrix and extracellular fluid within the osteocyte lacunae and canaliculi. Whether the osteocyte actively participates in this process, or whether passive ion exchange occurs between the mineral phase of bone and the extracellular fluid within the canaliculi, is not known. A second suggested role for the osteocyte relates to the known ability of bone to alter its structure in response to changing stress. According to this theory, the complex osteocyte network acts as a large differential pressure sensor, which can detect variations in bone loading and transmit information to the cells responsible for bone remodelling at bone surfaces (see below).

Osteoblasts

Bone is synthesised by osteoblasts. Production of bone occurs in two stages. Initially, osteoblasts deposit non-mineralised bone matrix (osteoid), which consists of collagen and non-collagenous organic matrix. This is later mineralised. Osteoid is deposited on the surface of a pre-existing calcified tissue, usually either mineralised bone or (particularly at epiphyseal growth plates) calcified cartilage. At any one time, approximately 12 per cent of the surface of the trabeculae is covered by osteoid.

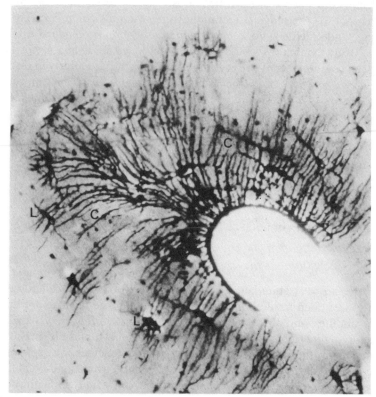

Figure 2.5   Bone stained to show osteocyte lacunae (L) and interconnecting canaliculi (C).

These thin layers of osteoid (osteoid seams) undergo mineralisation in a narrow zone at their interface with the calcified tissue (figure 2.6). Osteoblasts, including a few cells which become included within the osteoid, produce membrane-bound subcellular structures (matrix vesicles), which can be expelled into their immediate environment. Matrix vesicles are rich in calcium and phosphorus and are believed to migrate towards pre-existing calcified tissue where they act as a nidus about which passive mineralisation occurs (Revell, 1986). Passive mineralisation requires, among other things, an adequate concentration of calcium and phosphorus in the extracellular microenvironment. The control of extracellular free calcium is a complex interaction of various intercellular messengers, in particular 1,25-dihydroxy-vitamin D3 and the hormone parathormone produced by cells of the parathyroid gland. Inadequate concentrations of calcium result in a failure of osteoid mineralisation and a disease known in adults as osteomalacia and in children as rickets (Dent and Stamp, 1977). This disorder is characterised by thickening of the osteoid seams, which are

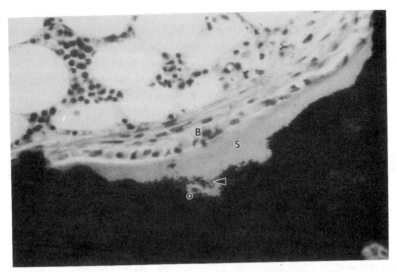

Figure 2.6 Undecalcified section of bone showing an osteoid seam (S) surmounted by osteoblasts (B). Stippled calcification (arrowed) is occurring about matrix vesicles secreted by an included osteoblast (O).

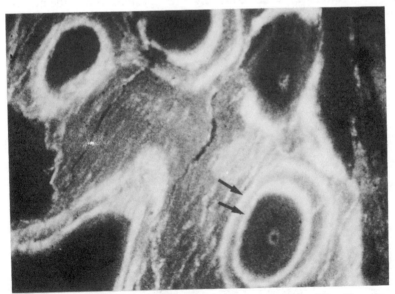

Figure 2.7 An unstained section of bone viewed in ultraviolet light. Two doses of tetracycline (arrowed) were given separated by an interval of ten days.

often formed normally but remain unmineralised, and, in severe cases, all bone surfaces can become covered in unmineralised osteoid. This bone is soft and under normal loads bends and twists.

In bone biopsies, mineralisation is assessed with the fluorochrome tetracycline, which, given orally or intravenously, is taken up *in vivo* into calcified tissues only at sites of active mineralisation. If unstained sections of a biopsy specimen taken shortly after a patient has been 'labelled' with tetracycline are examined in ultraviolet light, any mineralising fronts will be disclosed by tetracycline fluorescence (figure 2.7).

Osteoclasts

Osteoclasts are bone-resorbing, multinucleated giant cells. They are believed to form from the same marrow precursors as blood monocytes, under the influence of a variety of hormones including parathormone and vitamin D (Owen, 1980).

In crude terms, the osteoclast resembles a sucker. On a bone surface, it forms a 'seal' at its periphery, leaving an enclosed space between it and the bone (figure 2.8). The space is occupied by numerous osteoclast cytoplasmic processes (the ruffled border), and into this space the cell secretes high concentrations of hydrogen ions, lowering the pH to about 3. At this pH, demineralisation of the matrix occurs, effectively producing a layer of non-mineralised osteoid beneath the osteoclast. Osteoclasts synthesise a variety of proteinases, which could digest the proteins within the matrix. In addition, they produce neutral and acid phosphatases and a variety of other enzymes, including aryl sulphatase, β-galactosidase and β-glucosidase, which degrade the saccharide component of matrix glycopro-

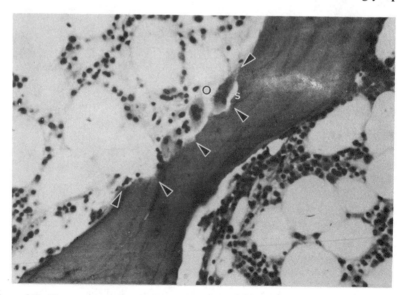

Figure 2.8 Transverse section through an osteoclast (O) showing peripheral areas of tight binding to bone and space so created into which hydrogen ions are pumped (S). The saucer-shaped depression eroded by the osteoclasts is marked by the arrows.

teins. All the enzymes can be demonstrated in tissue sections using histochemistry. Some, such as ATPase, succinic dehydrogenase and cytochrome oxidase, have been localised to the ruffled border area of the osteoclast using this technique (Chambers, 1985).

The number of osteoclasts is, under physiological conditions, inversely related to the concentration of free calcium in the serum. The osteoclasts do not respond directly to calcium, but are controlled by complex interactions between a variety of systemic and local hormones, of which the most important is parathormone. As the serum ionised calcium falls, the secretion of parathormone increases, as does the number of osteoclasts. It has been shown by *in vitro* studies that the osteoclast does not possess parathormone receptors, and that the effects of parathormone are mediated via an intermediate cell present either at bone surfaces or within the bone marrow immediately adjacent to bone. Possible candidates include osteoblasts and endosteal cells (Silve *et al.*, 1982).

Endosteal cells
Resting bone surfaces are covered by a layer of flattened, somewhat inconspicuous cells called endosteal cells, together with a thin layer of unmineralised collagen (figure 2.9). There is considerable controversy as to

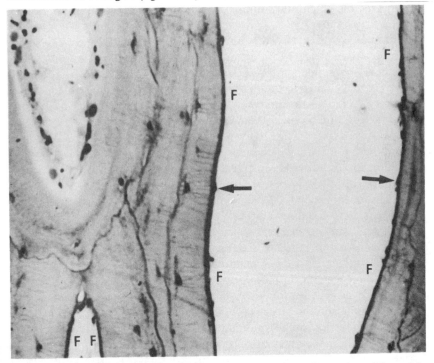

Figure 2.9   A section of bone stained to accentuate the layer of fibrous tissue (F) overlying resting bone surfaces. The nuclei of endosteal cells can just be discerned (arrowed).

whether this is osteoid or simply fibrous tissue (Vanderwiel, 1980), i.e. a form of collagen-based tissue in which the non-collagenous components do not promote local deposition of hydroxyapatite. The consensus view would seem to favour the latter concept. Except under extraordinary circumstances, osteoclasts are unable to excavate non-mineralised substances, and it has been suggested that this thin layer of collagen acts as a barrier to their gaining access to the mineralised bone matrix. It is proposed that, in response to appropriate stimuli (possibly parathormone), endosteal cells secrete collagenases which break down this collagen layer, exposing mineralised bone and thus facilitating osteoclastic resorption (Chambers, 1980). Although this concept is still speculative, there is no question that exposed mineralised material, wherever it may occur, is the single most potent stimulus to osteoclasis.

Modelling and remodelling

Often, one encounters bone trabeculae with osteoblasts on one side and osteoclasts on the other. This simultaneous bone removal from one side of a trabecula and deposition on the other leads to an overall change in shape of trabeculae. This is a continuous process throughout life, probably to accommodate altered stresses acting through the bone. It is most common during growth, when alterations of bone shape are essential for normal skeletal development.

Temporal coupling of osteoblasts and osteoclast activity in this way is known as modelling. More common in adults is the situation where osteoclasis at a single site precedes osteoblastic bone deposition, leading ultimately to a change in the matrix but not the shape of bone. This spatial coupling of osteoblastic and osteoclastic activity is known as remodelling.

The factors which link osteoblastic and osteoclastic activity in this way are unknown. However, one elegant explanation suggests that a substance present within bone, which acts as an inhibitor of osteoclasts and a stimulator of osteoblasts, is released from bone matrix and activated during osteoclastic bone resorption (Peck *et al.*, 1983).

As has been intimated, the complex interactions of osteoclasts and osteoblasts, both for the maintenance of skeletal integrity and for calcium homeostasis, are not just controlled at a local level. They are two of the effector cells of an intricate, interactive control system modulated by a group of systemic factors. The three most important of these are 1,25-dihydroxycholecalciferol, parathyroid hormone and calcitonin. Other factors include growth hormone, insulin, thyroid hormone, sex hormones, glucocorticoids and the vitamins A, C, K and E.

Bone cell activity can be modified by local and systemic factors released during pathological processes. The majority are cytokines released by a variety of inflammatory cells and include interleukin-1 (IL-1) and certain prostanoids.

A discussion of the complex effects of all the local and systemic factors that influence bone cell function is beyond the scope of this chapter, but these are well reviewed elsewhere (Parfitt, 1982; Raisy and Kream, 1983a, b; Runel *et al.*, 1983). Suffice it to say that bone cells exist in a complex chemical environment, and small changes in the balance of the composition of the environment can result in alterations of bone cell function.

CARTILAGE

Most cartilage is non-mineralised, but where it interfaces with bone, cartilage undergoes calcification.

Any cartilage can mineralise and then, by a process of modelling and remodelling, ossify (e.g., laryngeal cartilage). However, calcification of cartilage occurs predominantly in two areas: epiphyses and the interfaces between articular cartilage and adjacent subchondral bone.

Epiphyses

Epiphyses represent zones of growth of long bones. Although some animals such as rodents continue to grow throughout their lives, in man the epiphyseal growth plates cease to function and are replaced by bone during childhood and adolescence. The last close shortly after puberty. Epiphyses can be considered as areas of rapid synthesis of a suitable calcified matrix upon which new bone can be deposited. Chondrocytes in the epiphyseal plate divide in the superficial layers, enlarge in the mid-zone and line up to form vertical columns in the deeper zones (figure 2.10). Once these columns form, two simultaneous progressive processes begin. First, the chondrocytes produce matrix vesicles, which they export into the adjacent chondroid matrix, and, second, cell death occurs. Matrix vesicles are extruded into the matrix only at the lateral aspects of the cell columns, where they initiate matrix calcification. The end result is the production of alternating vertical bands of calcified and non-calcified cartilage, the latter containing spaces once occupied by chondrocytes. The non-calcified cartilage is then removed by blood vessel ingress from the adjacent marrow to leave only struts of calcified cartilage. The cartilage undergoes osteoclastic resorption followed by osteoblastic bone deposition. In effect, the calcified cartilage columns undergo remodelling and modelling to form bone trabeculae, some of which, close to the epiphyseal plate, still contain calcified cartilage cores.

The factors controlling the alterations in chondrocyte morphology and physiology that result in cartilage calcification and epiphyseal growth are poorly understood. 1,25-dihydroxycholecalciferol plays a central role in this process. One of its actions is to induce the synthesis of type X collagen by the 'maturing' chondrocytes (Kwan *et al.*, 1986). In the absence of type

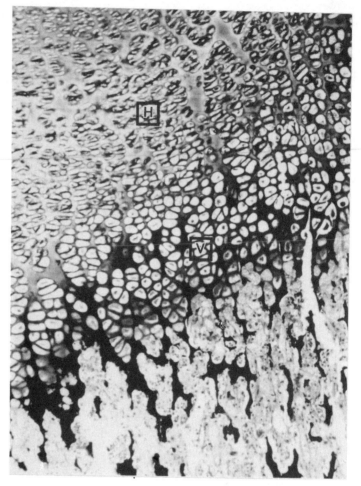

Figure 2.10   An epiphyseal growth plate. (H) Hypertrophic zone. (V) vertical columns of chondrocytes.

X collagen, mineralisation will not occur. There is also some evidence that the synthesis of angiogenesis factors, i.e., substances that stimulate blood vessel growth, is central to the process of epiphyseal growth; but how and where they act is still a matter of some discussion (Brown *et al.*, 1987).

Calcified articular cartilage

The interface between articular cartilage and subchondral bone is said to function as a very slowly growing epiphyseal plate, but its structure is totally different (figure 2.11). Chondrocytes in articular cartilage appear to be randomly distributed; there is no equivalent of the hypertrophic zone or

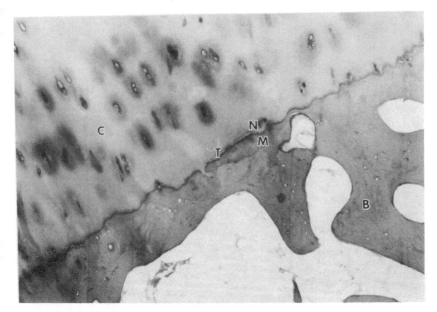

Figure 2.11 Subarticular bone (B) and articular cartilage (C). Note the differences between this and the epiphyseal plate in figure 2.10. The 'tidemark' (T) can be seen at the junction of mineralised (M) and non-mineralised (N) cartilage.

of column formation. The zone of calcification, which occupies the lower 2–5 per cent of the articular cartilage, is sharply demarcated from the non-calcified cartilage by a line known as the tidemark. The tidemark runs generally parallel to the articular surface and in conventionally stained decalcified tissue sections is a different colour from both the adjacent cartilage and bone, indicating it to contain different matrix components. The nature of this alteration in the matrix and its importance to cartilage mineralisation has never been investigated.

PATHOLOGICAL MINERALISATION

Abnormal (pathological) calcification is a frequent accompaniment of disease in a wide variety of organs. In some, excessive mineral deposition represents an abnormal extension of a normal process. For instance, in the non-inflammatory joint disease osteoarthritis there is reduplication of the tidemark (figure 2.12) and thickening of the zone of calcification in articular cartilage. It follows from the observations made above that this represents some change in the cartilage matrix which promotes calcification deeper within cartilage than occurs normally.

In other diseases, there is an abnormal synthesis of a naturally mineralised matrix (osteoid and cartilage), and in a third group mineralisation occurs within a matrix not usually associated with calcification.

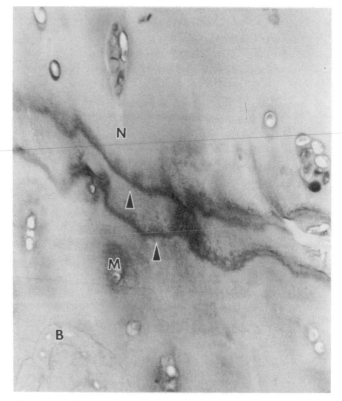

Figure 2.12 Osteoarthritis – reduplication of the tidemark (arrowed) between non-mineralised articular cartilage (N) and mineralised cartilage (M). A small area of bone (B) is included in the photograph.

Disorders associated with the abnormal formation of osteoid and cartilage

Diseases of connective tissues sometimes result in the formation of osteoid and chondroid matrix which may undergo calcification. Archetypal among such disorders are bone fractures and tumours (Collins, 1966). In these conditions, matrix of a type which conventionally undergoes mineralisation (i.e., osteoid and cartilage) is synthesised, either, as in the case of fracture, as a physiological event following stimulation of normal uncommitted connective-tissue precursor cells, in response to the pathological process or (figure 2.13), as is the case in tumours, from abnormal connective tissue cells which synthesise osteoid or cartilage in an uncontrolled fashion.

Calcification in these sites could therefore be considered to be a natural consequence of the abnormal synthesis of a specific connective tissue matrix.

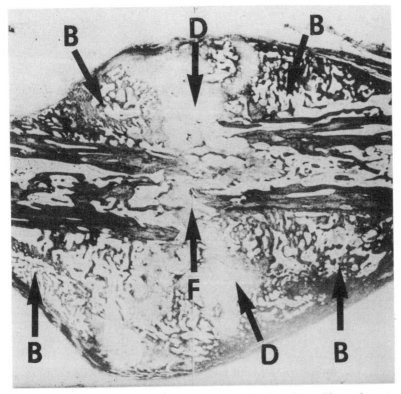

Figure 2.13 A microradiograph of a fracture site (F) in a long bone. The exuberant new bone (B) shows up because it is radiodense. Within the bone are areas of cartilage (D).

Calcification unrelated to deposition of a specific matrix

Calcification may occur in other circumstances without the synthesis of a specific matrix. Pathological calcification of this type is conventionally divided into two types – dystrophic and metastatic (Robbins *et al.*, 1984).

Dystrophic calcification
In dystrophic calcification, the level of plasma calcium is normal and calcification occurs secondary to local changes in the affected tissue. It is found predominantly in the following:

(1) Areas of abnormal extracellular protein synthesis, such as the changes seen in the walls of arteries in ageing, hypertension and diabetes; in damage to dense connective tissues, e.g. tendon; and in some tumours, e.g. uterine smooth-muscle tumours (leiomyomas or 'fibroids').

(2) Tissue death, such as the necrotic lipid debris of atheromatous

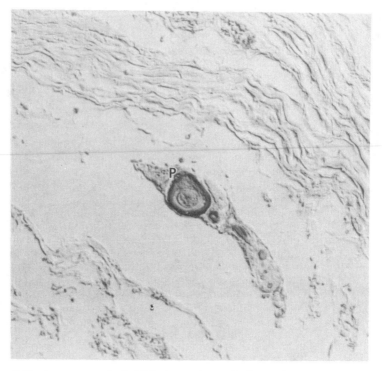

Figure 2.14   A psammoma body (P) in the meninges of a damaged nerve root.

plaques, fat necrosis, old tissue infarcts, the areas of caseous necrosis characteristic of tuberculosis and dead parasites, e.g. tapeworm cysts.

(3)   Inspissated pus and organic material within hollow structures (e.g. ducts etc.). Pus, unless discharged, may be dehydrated allowing calcification to occur. Calcification may also occur in organic material accumulating in, for instance, the ducts of salivary glands or the appendix, ultimately resulting in the formation of loose crumbly calcific 'stones'.

(4)   Thrombi. Calcification occurs in old blood clots in veins and may come to resemble stones – so-called phleboliths.

Histologically, the calcium salts have a basophilic, amorphous, granular, sometimes clumped appearance and are electron dense. The first signs of mineral deposition may be intracellular (often in mitochondria) or extracellular (in matrix vesicles).

On occasion, single necrotic cells may constitute a nidus that becomes encrusted by the mineral deposits. Progressive accumulation of calcium salts sometimes leads to the production of concentrically lamellated calcific bodies known as psammoma bodies (figure 2.14). These structures are characteristic of certain tumours, in particular tumours of the investments of the brain (meningiomas) and papillary carcinoma of the thyroid.

Sometimes, extracellular deposits of calcium salts can undergo ossification by a process of modelling and remodelling to form heterotopic bone.

On occasion, other metals are recruited into the mineral, deposited in this way. One example is the golden-brown, dumbell-shaped 'asbestos bodies' seen in the lungs of patients with asbestosis, in which mixed salts of calcium and iron precipitate on asbestos fibres.

The pathogenetic mechanisms underlying calcification are slowly coming to light. Extracellular calcification is essentially very similar to that occurring during mineralisation of bone. Electron microscopy shows that membrane-bound calcium and phosphate-rich vesicles, similar to matrix vesicles, are produced by certain dividing, degenerating, or ageing cells, and it is thought that these form the basis on which a crystal lattice is deposited (Anderson, 1983; Kim, 1983). Crystal formation is dependent upon the serum calcium and phosphate, and the presence of mineralisation inhibitors and collagen fibres. The dependence on collagen may explain why calcification frequently occurs in a linear fashion, at least initially.

Intracellular calcification shares many features with extracellular calcification. Instead of involving a membrane-bound vescicle, calcification is initiated by calcium deposition within mitochondria, but the propagation phase of crystal lattice formation would appear to be much the same morphologically and ultrastructurally as that occurring extracellularly.

Metastatic calcification
Metastatic calcification occurs in normal tissues whenever there is hypercalcaemia (high serum calcium ion concentration). The causes of hypercalcaemia include: hyperparathyroidism (increased circulating levels of the hormone parathormone – which causes bone breakdown and consequent liberation of calcium); vitamin D intoxication, where hypercalcaemia is multifactorial with increased bowel absorption, increased bone breakdown and decreased renal excretion of calcium; systemic sarcoidosis – a disease characterised by a proliferation of specialised macrophages which have the ability to synthesise excessive amounts of 1,25-dihydroxycholecalciferol in an uncontrolled way (Adams *et al.*, 1983); and increased bone breakdown associated with disseminated bone tumours and immobilisation (Potts, 1983).

Metastatic calcification can occur in almost every organ, but principally affects the interstitial tissues of the blood vessels, kidneys, lungs and bowel. Calcification appears to start in mitochondria and results in fine calcification throughout the tissue.

Metastatic calcification tends to cause little tissue dysfunction except in the kidneys, where long-standing severe calcium deposition (nephrocalcinosis) may lead to renal dysfunction. Dystrophic calcification, by contrast, is not only evidence of tissue injury, but may lead to dysfunction of the organ. Possibly one of the best examples of this is the heart valve abnormalities that result from calcification secondary to rheumatic fever or congenital valvular disease. These may be too severe for the heart to compensate, resulting ultimately in heart failure and even death.

Non-tissue calcification

Sometimes, calcification does not occur in tissues but inside hollow viscera. This has already been alluded to in the renal tubules and appendix, but occurs most frequently in the renal pelvis and gall bladder. In these sites, stones form (renal stones and gallstones; figure 2.15). Stones are, in

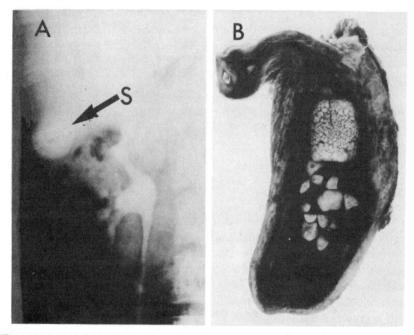

Figure 2.15   (A) Radiograph of the gall bladder region showing a lamellated stone (S). (B) A gall bladder showing two types of gallstone. The largest consists predominantly of cholesterol, the others of calcium salts.

chemical terms, heterogenous structures, but many types have in common the presence of calcium as a constituent. Stone formation in both sites is believed to be due primarily to excessive quantities of the stone-forming substance (including calcium) in the secretion handled by the organ (bile or urine), although other factors, such as altered pH, change in glycoprotein secretion, infection and reduced production of inhibitors of crystal formation, may all play a role in the production of stones (Anderson, 1980).

SUMMARY

Mineralisation, both pathological and physiological, is a complex and still poorly understood process. Histological studies give important clues to this process. In particular, they show how and where mineralisation occurs, both at the tissue and at the cellular level. New techniques, including immunohistochemistry, lectin histochemistry, ultrastructural histochemistry and *in-situ* DNA and RNA hybridisation, offer ways of probing the structure and localised composition of mineralised tissues, and of studying the complex processes that result in mineralisation of tissues.

REFERENCES

Adams, J. S., Sharma, O. P., Gacad, M. A. and Singer, F. R. (1983). Metabolism of 25-hydroxyvitamin D3 by cultured pulmonary alveolar macrophages in sercoidosis. *J. Clin. Invest.*, **72**, 1856–60

Anderson, J. R. (1980). *Muir's Textbook of Pathology*, Edward Arnold, London

Anderson, C. (1982). *Manual for the Examination of Bone*, CRC press, Boca Raton, FL

Anderson, H. C. (1983). Calcific disease: a concept. *Arch. Pathol. Lab. Med.*, **107**, 341–52

Boyde, A. (1981). Evidence against 'osteocytic osteolysis'. *Metab. Bone Dis. Rel. Res.*, **2S**, 483–6

Brown, R. A., Taylor, C., McLaughlin, B., McFarlane, C. D., Weiss, J. B. and Ali, S. Y. (1987). Epiphyseal growth plate cartilage and chondrocytes in mineralising cultures produce a low molecular mass angiogenic procollagenase activator. *Bone and Mineral*, **3**, 143–8

Chambers, T. J. (1980). The cellular basis of bone resorption. *Clin. Orthop.*, **151**, 283–93

Chambers, T. J. (1985). The pathobiology of the osteoclast. *J. Clin. Pathol.*, **38**, 241–52

Collins, D. H. (1966). *The Pathology of Bone*, Butterworths, London

Courpron, P., Meunier, P., Bressot, C. and Giroux, J. M. (1977). Amount of bone in iliac crest biopsy. In *Bone Histomorphometry, Second International Workshop* (ed. P. J. Meunier), Société de la Nouvelle Imprimerie Fournie, Toulouse

Deftos, L. J. and Catherwood, B. D. (1983). BGP and bone metabolism. In *Clinical Disorders of Bone and Mineral Metabolism* (eds B. Frame and J. T. Potts), Excerpta Medica, Amsterdam, pp. 112–15

Dent, C. E. and Stamp, T. C. B. (1977). Vitamin D, rickets and osteomalacia. In *Metabolic Bone Disease* (eds L. V. Alvioli and S. M. Krane), Academic Press, New York, pp. 237–305

Denton, J., Freemont, A. J. and Ball, J. (1984). The detection and distribution of aluminium within bone. *J. Clin. Pathol.*, **37**, 136–42

Ellis, H. A. (1981). Metabolic bone disease. In *Recent Advances in Histopathology*, Vol. **11** (eds P. P. Anthony and R. N. M. MacSween), Churchill Livingstone, Edinburgh

Kim, K. M. (1983). Pathological calcification. In *Pathobiology of Cell Membranes*, Vol. **3** (eds B. Trump and A. Arstilla), Churchill Livingstone, Edinburgh, pp. 185–202

Kwan, A. P. L., Freemont, A. J. and Grant, M. E. (1986). Immunoperoxidase localisation of type X collagen. *Bioscience Rep.*, **6**, 155–62

Melsen, F., Melsen, B. and Mosekilde, L. (1978). An evaluation of the quantitative parameters applied in bone histology. *Acta Path. Microbiol. Scand.*, **86**, 63–9

Merz, W. A. and Schenk, R. K. (1970). Quantitative structural analysis of human cancellous bone. *Acta Anat.*, **75**, 54–66

Owen, M. (1980). The origin of bone cells in the postnatal organism. *Arthr. Rheum.*, **23**, 1073–9

Parfitt, A. M. (1982). The coupling of bone formation to bone resorption: a critical analysis of the concept and of its relevance to the pathogenesis of osteoporosis. *Metab. Bone Dis. Rel. Res.*, **4**, 1–6

Peck, W. A., Shen, V. and Rifas, L. (1983). Locally elaborated factors in the co-ordination of bone cell activity. In *Clinical Disorders of Bone and Mineral Metabolism* (eds B. Frame and J. T. Potts), Excerpta Medica, Amsterdam, pp. 179–82

Pommer, G. (1925). Untersuchhung über Osteomalacia und Rachitis nebst Beitragen zur Kenntis der Knochrenresorption und apposition im verschiedenen Altersperioden und der durchbohrenden Gefässe. *Deutsch Kliniken Chirugie*, **136**, 1–29

Potts, J. T. (1983). Non-parathyroid hypercalcaemia. In *Clinical Disorders of Bone and Mineral Metabolism* (eds B. Frame and J. T. Potts), Excerpta Medica, Amsterdam, pp. 281–3

Raisy, L. C. and Kream, B. E. (1983a). Regulation of bone formation. *N. Engl. J. Med.*, **309**, 29–35

Raisy, L. G. and Kream, B. E. (1983b). Regulation of bone formation. *N. Engl. J. Med.*, **309**, 83–9

Revell, P. A. (1983). Histomorphometry of bone. *J. Clin. Pathol.*, **36**, 1323–31

Revell, P. A. (1986). *Pathology of Bone*, Springer, Berlin, pp. 13–15

Robbins, S. L., Cotran, R. S. and Kumar, V. (1984). *The Pathologic Basis of Disease*. W. B. Saunders, Philadelphia

Russell, R. G. G., Kanis, J. A. and Gowan, M. (1983). Cellular control of bone formation and repair. In *Osteoporosis: A Multidisciplinary Problem* (eds A. St. J. Dixon, R. G. G. Russell and T. C. B. Stamp), Academic Press, London, pp. 31–42

Silve, C. M., Hradek, G. T., Jones, A. L. and Arnaud, C. D. (1982). Parathyroid hormone receptor in intact embryonic chick bones: characterisation and cellular localisation. *J. Cell Biol.*, **94**, 379–86

Vanderwiel, C. J. (1980). An ultrastructural study of the components which make up the resting surface of bone. *Metab. Bone Dis. Rel. Res.*, **25**, 109–16

3

Scanning X-ray microradiography and microtomography of calcified tissues

J. C. Elliott, P. Anderson, R. Boakes and S. D. Dover

INTRODUCTION

The rigidity of a calcified tissue derives almost entirely from its mineral content. This means that information about the mineral distribution is fundamental to the understanding of its mechanical properties. Changes in the mineral content can occur in diseases such as osteoporosis, a common condition of postmenopausal women where mineral loss from bones predisposes them to fracture. The changes that can occur in this and other conditions of bone can be due to volume changes in the amount of mineralised tissue and/or changes in the degree of mineralisation of that tissue. Thus changes in gross mineral density alone give a very incomplete picture. What is required is the complete three-dimensional distribution at a microscopic level.

The mineral is the major absorber of X-rays, so that microradiography is an important technique for studying the distribution of mineral in calcified tissues on a scale above a micron, the approximate resolution limit for this method. Backscattered electron imaging is a technique which gives higher resolution that is very sensitive to small changes in mineral content, but there are difficulties in putting the measurements on an absolute scale (Boyde and Jones, 1983).

The most common method of microradiography is to use a photographic emulsion to record and measure the intensity of the transmitted X-rays. This has the advantages of simplicity, speed, low cost and a large field of view, and does not require a very stable source of X-rays. To be offset against these formidable advantages is the fact that the accuracy of the intensity measurement is not very high. The purpose of this chapter is to compare these photographic methods with more recent X-ray absorption techniques that have a number of advantages. These derive from the use of counters to determine the intensity of the transmitted beam. The accuracy is then limited, at least in principle, only by the counting statistics, which can always be improved by an increase in the observational time or by a more intense beam.

Two systems will be considered. In the first, scanning X-ray micro-radiography (sometimes called scanning X-ray microscopy), a thin section is stepped through a narrow X-ray beam in one or two dimensions, and the transmitted intensity measured at each point with a suitable counter. In the second technique, X-ray microtomography, the specimen (preferably with an approximately cylindrical shape, so that the absorption across any diameter will be fairly constant) can also be rotated. As will be explained later, this technique enables the complete three-dimensional distribution of X-ray absorption to be determined on a microscopic scale. For both systems to be practical, the motion of the specimen and the X-ray counting have to be fully automated.

ABSORPTION OF X-RAYS BY CALCIFIED TISSUES

When a monochromatic X-ray beam passes through an absorbing medium, the transmitted intensity, I, obeys Beer's law accurately, so that

$$I = I_0 \exp\left(-\int_0^t \mu(z) \, dz\right) \tag{3.1}$$

where I_0 is the incident intensity, $\mu(z)$ the linear absorption coefficient at a distance z into the specimen and t the thickness. If t is measured in cm, μ has dimensions cm^{-1}. For a homogeneous specimen, this reduces to the more familiar form:

$$I = I_0 \exp(-\mu t) \tag{3.2}$$

The processes involved in the absorption of X-rays are well understood (Koch and MacGillavry, 1962), and the values of the linear absorption coefficient for a known elemental composition, wavelength and density is easily calculated from published mass absorption coefficients for the elements (McMaster *et al.*, 1969). This is sufficient information because the absorption of an element is very nearly independent of its form of chemical combination. (However, the dependence on chemical combination can provide useful information – see Chapter 4.)

In the wavelength range usually of interest for microradiography and microtomography of calcified tissues (0.2–2.0 Å; 62–6.2 keV), the principal mechanism of absorption is the photoelectric effect in which an X-ray photon is completely absorbed by an atom, and its energy used to eject an electron (the photoelectron) from an inner orbital. A less energetic electron from an outer orbital replaces this with the emission of a fluorescent X-ray quantum. The absorption is highly wavelength and atomic-number dependent. There are abrupt decreases in absorption (absorption edges) when the incident photons are no longer sufficiently energetic to eject electrons from the particular orbital, and eject electrons from a less energetic one instead. Between absorption edges, the photo-electric absorption coefficient is proportional to λ^3, where λ is the wavelength and the constant of proportionality contains the factor Z^m, where Z is the atomic number and m is approximately 4. This strong dependence on atomic number and wavelength can be either an advantage or a disadvantage in the experimental arrangements required for micro-radiography and microtomography, as will be discussed later.

There are two other ways in which energy can be lost from an X-ray beam. Both are scattering processes: one in which there is no change in wavelength (called coherent, elastic or Rayleigh scattering); and the other in which the scattered radiation has a longer wavelength (incoherent, inelastic or Compton scattering). Table 3.1 gives the photoelectric, coherent, incoherent and total cross-sections for the elements of interest in calcified tissues for a range of energies of the incident X-ray quanta, and allows the relative importance of these three processes to be judged. In the lower energy range, which is of interest for microradiography, the photo-electric effect is by far the most important mechanism for the loss of X-ray intensity, but at 80 keV, the kind of energy that would be required for tomography of a fully formed tooth, incoherent scattering is as important as the photoelectric effect. The cross-section for incoherent scattering is approximately proportional to the atomic number and changes much more slowly with wavelength than either the photoelectron cross-section or the coherent cross-section. Coherent scattering is never the dominant process, but as phase relationships are preserved between the scattered radiation from different atoms, interference effects can occur, and it is this co-herently scattered radiation that is responsible for the X-ray diffraction phenomena that are observed from crystals. Before leaving this discussion of the basic physics of the interaction between X-rays and atoms, it should be noted that Beer's law as given above is obeyed exactly only if none of the scattered or fluorescent radiation is recorded with the transmitted beam.

In the following, consideration will be given to the information that can

Table 3.1   X-ray cross-sections for some elements in calcified tissues, $cm^2 \, g^{-1}$ at 6, 30, and 80 keV (2.07, 0.413 and 0.155 Å)

Photoelectric			Coherent			Incoherent			Total		
keV 6	30	80	6	30	80	6	30	80	6	30	80
O 26.5	0.148	0.006	0.521	0.055	0.009	0.096	0.161	0.152	27.1	0.363	0.168
P 176.1	1.36	0.060	1.10	0.139	0.025	0.077	0.150	0.144	177.2	1.64	0.228
Ca 378.6	3.63	0.180	1.51	0.211	0.037	0.077	0.144	0.146	380.2	4.00	0.363

be obtained from measurements of the X-ray absorption in calcified tissues. Particular emphasis will be given to the assumptions that have to be made, and to the possible errors that can occur. Equation 3.1 above expresses the attenuation of the X-ray beam in terms of the linear absorption coefficient. However, it is equally valid, and often more convenient, to express the attenuation in terms of the mass absorption coefficient μ_m (usually measured in $cm^2\,g^{-1}$), so that

$$I = I_0 \exp\left(-\mu_m m\right) \tag{3.3}$$

where m is the projected mass of the absorbing material/unit area. The relation between μ and μ_m is

$$\mu_m = \mu/\rho \tag{3.4}$$

where ρ is the density. The value of μ_m can be calculated from the values of the mass absorption coefficients of the n individual elemental constituents of the calcified tissue

$$\mu_m = \sum_1^n p_i \mu_i \tag{3.5}$$

where p_i is the mass fraction of the ith element with mass absorption coefficient μ_i. It is clear that the above relationship relies on the fact that the individual elemental constituents absorb X-radiation independently of each other, so that the absorption is determined only by the total number of atoms in the X-ray beam. If it is assumed that the calcified tissue is made up of only two phases, an inorganic phase A comprising j elements, and an organic phase B comprising k elements, the mass absorption coefficient can be split up so that

$$\mu_m = \sum_1^j p_i \mu_i + \sum_1^k p_i \mu_i \tag{3.6}$$

$$= p\mu_A + (1-p)\mu_B \tag{3.7}$$

where p is the mass fraction of A. The calculated values of μ_m, μ_A and μ_B for a range of wavelengths for bone together with the individual contributions from calcium and phosphorus are plotted in figure 3.1. From this, it is clear that calcium is the major contributor to the X-ray absorption by bone and other calcified tissues in the wavelength region of interest for microradiography and microtomography.

Equations 3.3 and 3.7 can be combined to give

$$\log_e(I_0/I) = mp\mu_A + m(1-p)\mu_B \tag{3.8}$$

where m is the projected mass/unit area of bone in the section. I and I_0 can be measured experimentally, and μ_A and μ_B can be calculated from an assumed composition of the bone. This leaves two unknowns, m and p. If

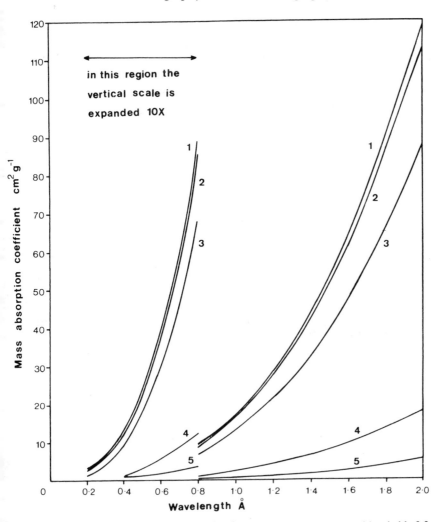

Figure 3.1 Mass absorption coefficient (cm² g⁻¹) for bone of typical composition (table 3.2, column 1) and the contributions to it from its major constituents in the wavelength range 0.2–2.0 Å. (1) total, (2) inorganic, (3) calcium, (4) phosphorus, and (5) organic. The values of the coefficients in the range 0.2–0.8 Å have been multiplied by 10.

$\mu_B \ll \mu_A$, which is the case for most mineralised tissues, the second term on the right-hand side of equation 3.8 will be very small compared with the first term, so that an approximate value for $m(1-p)$ will suffice. This term is the projected mass/unit area of the organic fraction M_B, which can be estimated from the section thickness and approximate values of p and ρ, where ρ is the bulk density of the bone. mp is equal to M_A, the projected mass of mineral/unit area, so that:

$$M_A = (\log_e I_0/I - M_B\mu_B)/\mu_A \qquad (3.9)$$

μ_A can be calculated from typical analyses of the tissue concerned, but this cannot be exactly correct for the sample in question because, as is well known, apatitic calcium phosphates have a wide compositional range. By contrast, calcified tissues containing calcium carbonates will be subject to much less variation (mainly from the substitution of Mg for Ca). The presence of different calcium carbonate polymorphs will not affect the result, as this is expressed in terms of projected mass per unit area.

The effect of errors in the value of the mass absorption coefficient can be determined by ignoring the term containing M_B in equation 3.9 and differentiating so that

$$\frac{dM_A}{M_A} = -\frac{d\mu_A}{\mu_A} \tag{3.10}$$

which shows that the fractional error in projected mineral mass/unit area is equal to the fractional error in the mass absorption coefficient. For apatitic calcified tissues, this can be estimated from the calculated mass absorption coefficients for the inorganic fraction and possible synthetic analogues. This shows (table 3.2) that differences of 9 per cent in M_A could occur, depending on the assumed composition of the inorganic fraction, but this could be reduced were μ_A to be calculated from analyses of the bulk tissue.

From a biological point of view, it is often more useful to know m_A, the mass of mineral/unit volume, p_A the mass fraction of mineral, and q_A, the volume fraction of mineral. These are given by

$$m_A = (\log_e I_0/I - M_B\mu_B)/\mu_A t \tag{3.11}$$

$$p_A = (\log_e I_0/I - M_B\mu_B)/\mu_A \rho t \tag{3.12}$$

and $$q_A = (\log_e I_0/I - M_B\mu_B)/\mu_A \rho_A t \tag{3.13}$$

where t is the section thickness and ρ_A the density of the inorganic component.

Typical sections for microradiography of calcified tissues are 50–200 μm thick and therefore present some difficulty in their precise measurement. In a recent careful study of the mineral content of enamel, Wilson and Beynon (1989) stated that the 95 per cent confidence limits for the prediction of the thickness of 80 μm sections of enamel were ± 0.59 per cent when measured with an accurate micrometer dial gauge. If two different tissues are present, say dentine and enamel, the errors are likely to be greater, because it will be harder to make plane parallel sections. To the errors in the thickness measurement must be added the errors from shrinkage during preparation that arise as a result of loss of water from the tissue. Both these difficulties can be avoided by the use of microtomography, for which, as will be described later, there is no requirement for the physical cutting of sections.

The average bulk density of the tissue will probably be known, but this

Table 3.2 Weight percentage compositions and mass absorption coefficients ($cm^2\ g^{-1}$) for various inorganic fractions

Element	1	2	3	4	5	6
H	0.3	0.3	0.3	0.2	0.2	0.2
C	1.0	1.0	1.0	0.7	0.7	—
O	29.8	28.1	27.2	42.0	44.2	41.4
P	11.1	10.4	10.0	17.4	18.5	18.5
Ca	25.0	23.2	22.8	36.4	35.0	39.9
Total	67.3	63.1	61.4	98.0	99.8	100.0
$\mu_A\lambda = 0.18$ Å	0.306	0.305	0.306	0.302	0.302	0.316
$\mu_A\lambda = 0.56$ Å	4.47	4.43	4.47	4.45	4.37	4.78
$\mu_A\lambda = 0.71$ Å	8.83	8.76	8.83	8.79	8.64	9.47
$\mu_A\lambda = 1.54$ Å	81.0	80.4	81.0	80.8	79.5	86.9
$\mu_A\lambda = 1.79$ Å	122	121	122	122	120	131

Columns 1–3, skull, rib and ilium (after Agna *et al.*, 1958). Columns 4 and 5, permanent and deciduous enamel (after Table 4/II, Nikiforuk, 1985; the minor elements in this table are not listed above, but were included in the calculation of μ_A); and column 6, hydroxyapatite respectively. The collagen content for the bone was calculated from the reported N-analysis, and the required balance (about 6 per cent) to make the total to 100 per cent was taken as the water content, which was arbitrarily allocated equally to the inorganic and organic fractions. The inorganic oxygen content was calculated from the carbon and phosphorus contents on the assumption they were present as PO_4^{3-} and CO_3^{2-} with an addition for the assumed water content. The organic analysis for column 1 was H 2.47, C 11.68, N 4.81 and O 13.77 per cent.

will almost certainly be significantly different from ρ, the local bulk density, which is required in equation 3.12. An idea of the variations that might occur in enamel can be seen from density flotation studies, which show variations from 2.84 to 3.00 g cm^{-3} (Weidmann *et al.*, 1967), and for bone from centrifuge density fractionation studies of particles below 20 μm, which had a density range of 1.9–2.2 g cm^{-3} (Grynpas *et al.*, 1986).

The appropriate value of ρ_A to calculate the volume fraction of mineral presents a problem. The value calculated from the lattice constants of well-crystallised hydroxyapatite (3.15 g cm^{-3}) could be used, but this would be incorrect because of the likelihood of disorder and vacancies from the presence of water, carbonate, hydrogen phosphate and other extraneous species in the lattice or adsorbed on the surface of the crystals. There have been few attempts at the direct determination by pyknometric methods of the density of sub-micron-sized precipitated calcium phosphate analogues of the mineral in calcified tissues. Difficulties could be anticipated with this type of measurement, because finely divided particles often give erratic results with a density several per cent different from that obtained from well-crystallised material. Smales (1975) determined the densities of two finely divided apatites, one with a Ca/P molar ratio of 1.60 and the other a stoichiometric sample (molar ratio 1.67), and found that the measured density for both depended on the immersion liquid used. He proposed a theory for this effect which gave corrected densities of 3.09 ± 0.03 and 3.14 ± 0.09 g cm^{-3} respectively (the correction of about

$+0.16 \text{ g cm}^{-3}$ was largest for the stoichiometric hydroxyapatite). This work illustrates the uncertainties in this type of measurement, even before an attempt is made to isolate the mineral from the tissue in an unaltered state, a prerequisite for measuring its density.

The above discussion shows that the calculation of the mass of mineral per unit volume involves the least approximations and likelihood of error, because the only significant uncertainties are in the chemical composition required to calculate the mass absorption coefficient, and in the thickness of the section.

PHOTOGRAPHIC CONTACT AND POINT PROJECTION MICRORADIOGRAPHY

Microradiography (also known as X-ray contact microscopy) is a well-established technique first used soon after the discovery of X-rays. An extensive bibliography has been compiled by Cheng and Jan (1987). General references of interest include Cosslett and Nixon (1960) and Ely (1980).

The image is usually recorded on a silver halide photographic emulsion that has a resolution limit of a fraction of a micron. However, in the last few years, contact microradiography has been developed in which photoresists are used. These materials are virtually grainless and allow a resolution of at least 500 Å if examined in the scanning electron microscope. They are relatively insensitive to X-rays used for conventional microradiography and are normally used with very much softer radiation from a synchrotron or plasma source, particularly in the 'water window' from 23 to 44 Å, where there is an order of magnitude less absorption by water compared with protein. As far as the authors know, photoresists have not so far been used to study calcified tissues. This technique is at present not very quantitative, so will not be mentioned further; more details can be found in Cheng and Jan (1987) and Schmahl and Rudolph (1984).

In contact microradiography, a thin section is placed in direct contact with the emulsion. Although this may have a resolution of less than a micron, this is degraded by superposition of detail from different depths because, for calcified tissues, the section is usually from 50 to 200 μm thick. Sometimes detail can be seen at a resolution of a micron or so, such as the cross-striations on enamel prisms, which probably arise from calcium fluorescence radiation from the layer of enamel in immediate contact with the emulsion.

Greater magnification can in principle be obtained from point projection microradiography, in which the section is placed over a fine X-ray source (about 1 μm), with the emulsion some distance away to give geometrical magnification. The resolution is now no longer limited by the photographic emulsion, but the finite wavelength of the X-rays can cause Fresnel diffraction fringes around the edges of objects (Cosslett and Nixon, 1960; Hobdell and Braden, 1971). X-ray image magnification in microradiographs of calcified tissues can also be obtained by using a parallel X-ray beam from a synchrotron source and two asymmetrically cut, perfect silicon crystals mounted so that two-dimensional magnification is produced (Takagi *et al.*, 1984; Boettinger *et al.*, 1979).

Both contact and point projection microradiography are subject to other artefacts from the silver halide emulsion, collectively known as 'adjacency effects' (Barrows and Wolfe, 1971). These can cause the appearance of false detail at the edges of objects if there is an abrupt change in X-ray intensity, which is not uncommon with calcified tissues.

Quantitative studies are possible with photographic emulsions, but the range of intensities that can be measured is limited (this could be extended by the use of multiple film packs, as in X-ray crystallography, but this would not be suitable for microradiography). The emulsion also limits the accuracy of intensity measurements to ± 0.5 per cent, even if great care is taken (Rose and Jeffery, 1964). Because the response of the emulsion is non-linear and subject to variation with processing, it is usual to calibrate it for every exposure with an aluminium step wedge adjacent to the specimen so that both are exposed simultaneously. The value of $\log_e(I_0/I)$ can be calculated from equation 3.3 for every step from the mass absorption coefficient of aluminium and the mass/unit area for the particular step. This enables the value of $\log_e(I_0/I)$ to be determined for any part of the image by a comparison of its optical density with that of the step wedge after suitable interpolation. There is a potential complication because the emulsion's response and the absorption coefficients are all highly wavelength dependent: this is significant because polychromatic radiation is usually used. The method can therefore work only if the ratio of the mass absorption coefficient of aluminium to the mass absorption coefficient of the calcified tissue is the same for all incident wavelengths. This will be nearly true because the atomic number of aluminium ($Z = 13$) is fairly close to that of calcium ($Z = 20$) and phosphorus ($Z = 15$), and, more particularly, none of these elements has an absorption edge in the relevant wavelength range. The constancy of this ratio can be judged from its calculated values for bone (table 3.2, column 1) at 0.18, 0.56, 0.71, 1.54 and 1.79 Å, which are 0.768, 0.567, 0.570, 0.618, and 0.633 respectively.

The use of an appropriate calibrating foil neatly overcomes a number of difficulties, but there is still the problem that the X-ray intensity will not be uniform over the field of view. This could be overcome partly by having several calibrating foils around the specimen, but a better method, applicable only to contact microradiography, is to move the cassette across the beam so that a uniform exposure is obtained.

Quantitative aspects of photographic microradiography of calcified tissues are considered by Angmar *et al.* (1963), Boivin and Baud (1984), de

Josselin de Jong and ten Bosch (1985) and de Josselin de Jong *et al.* (1987a, b).

SCANNING X-RAY MICRORADIOGRAPHY AND X-RAY MICROTOMOGRAPHY

These techniques have several features in common which distinguish them from contact and point projection microradiography. Two of these are that the requirements of the X-ray source are much more critical, and both use X-ray counters instead of film, so these will be considered first.

Generation of X-rays

Both techniques take many hours for a set of measurements whose purpose is to obtain accurate information about the mineral content of calcified tissues and synthetic analogues, so that particular attention has to be paid to the short- and long-term stability of the X-ray source. As a consequence, the Hilger and Watts (now Rank Precision Industries Ltd, Margate, Kent) Y-33 microfocus X-ray generator that was used was modified so that the vacuum was improved, the previously unstabilised filament and high-voltage supplies were replaced by stabilised ones, and the resistors that determine the bias voltage on the electron gun were replaced by high-stability types. The quoted stability of the high-voltage supply (Hunting Hivolt Ltd, Shoreham-by-Sea, Sussex, UK; Type 250R) was ±0.02 per cent for ±10 per cent supply fluctuation, and less than 0.02 per cent per degree centrigrade.

The usual operating conditions for the X-ray generator were 2 mA at 35 kV. With a molybdenum target, this gave a total flux through a 10 μm aperture 30 mm from the source of about 10^5 counts per second, which was about the maximum that the counting system could cope with. The maximum rating for the tube with a molybdenum target was 3 mA at 50 kV, so the total experimental time was determined by the counting system rather than the power of the X-ray tube.

X-ray intensity measurement with counters

The principal advantage of counter methods over photographic emulsions for measuring the intensity of an X-ray beam is that individual photons are counted, usually with little loss. This means that intensities can be measured very accurately because, in principle, the accuracy is limited only by counting statistics. Assume that N counts are observed in a time t and that the average of a large number of determinations is L. N will have a Gaussian distribution if L is large, with a standard deviation of $L^{1/2}$. It follows then that an estimate of the intensity is given by $N/t \pm N^{1/2}/t$.

Therefore, if the X-ray generator output is sufficiently stable, the longer the counting time, the better the estimate. Photon counting also allows a very wide range of X-ray intensities to be measured. The lower limit is set by extraneous counts from a variety of sources, but this is very much lower than the limit for a photographic emulsion, where there is always appreciable darkening even if the emulsion has not been exposed to an X-ray beam. The upper limit is set by the ability of the system to cope with high count rates. This may be due to the processes involved in the conversion of X-ray quanta to electrical pulses in the detector, or in the electronics required to process these pulses. In either case, the upper limit can be 10^5–10^6 counts per second in the counters of interest for microtomography and microradiography. However, at high count rates, dead time corrections have to be applied, as will be described shortly, otherwise the system will be very non-linear.

Another advantage of counters, compared with photographic emulsions, is that it is often possible to arrange to count only those quanta that fall within a given energy range. This means a degree of monochromatisation is achieved, so that the absorption measurements are made with a narrow wavelength range. Different types of counters differ in their ability to achieve this (Knoll, 1979). Also, scattered and fluorescent radiation can easily be excluded from the counter with a guard aperture after the specimen, which is not possible with contact or point projection microradiography.

Two types of counters were used, an NaI (thallium-activated) scintillation detector and an HPGe (high-purity germanium) detector (GLP series with preamplifier feedback resistor selected for high count rates, followed by a 673 spectroscopy amplifier and gated integrator, EG & G ORTEC, Oak Ridge, Tn., USA). A single-channel pulse height analyser was used in both systems for energy discrimination, which is rather poor with low-energy X-rays for a scintillation counter (about 45 per cent full-width distribution at half height), but much better for the HPGe detector (about 4 per cent full-width distribution at half-height). With the flux of 10^5 counts per second of white radiation from the molybdenum target, about one-fifth passed through the analyser as Mo K_α radiation. Dead time for the HPGe detector system was corrected for by gating the oscillator that determined the counting time by the 'busy' output of the 673 amplifier, so that amplifier dead time was excluded. This system was usually used for microtomography because of the need for accurate intensity measurements with monochromatic radiation, so that correct values of the linear absorption coefficients are given by the tomographic reconstruction (see later). However, it might be possible to calibrate a system with poor wavelength discrimination with aluminium, as described earlier for photographic intensity determinations.

Nickel (15 μm) or zirconium (75 μm) filters were used to reduce Cu K_β or

Mo K_β radiation respectively for the scintillation counter, but not the HPGe detector. The combined stability of the X-ray generator and the HPGe detector was better than ±0.25 per cent over 32 hours.

Scanning microradiography

The details of the method (Elliott *et al.*, 1981) are illustrated in figure 3.2. A platinum electron microscope aperture (typically 10 μm) is positioned as close as possible (30 mm) to the source to maximise the X-ray flux, and the specimen mounted on a stepper-motor-driven XY stage as close as possible behind it (about 1 mm) to minimise the effects of beam divergence. The motion of the stage and X-ray counter used to measure the transmitted intensity are under automatic control (Digital Equipment Corporation 11/23 computer and CAMAC system), so that sequential measurements can be made by step scanning along a line to give a single scan, or a series of lines to give a two-dimensional image. The intensity and time for each measurement are recorded, and corrections made for drift in the X-ray output and counter system instability from timed measurements of the direct beam taken approximately every 15 minutes. The results can then be displayed in a variety of formats as will be shown.

In scanning microradiography, the specimen can be mounted in an environmental chamber (figure 3.2), so the technique is ideally suited to real-time experiments in which the rate of loss or gain of mineral is studied as reactants are pumped past it. Such experiments are not practical with contact microradiography, but can be done with point projection methods (Langdon *et al.*, 1980), but the photographic emulsion limits its usefulness. A system in which only one specimen at a time can be mounted does not make very efficient use of a sophisticated and expensive piece of equipment, because the changes in the specimen are often so slow that it is only necessary to spend 1 in every 12 hours in scanning it. A more efficient system is illustrated in figure 3.3, in which up to 20 specimens can be positioned on a kinematically mounted carriage, so that any one can be scanned across the X-ray beam in two dimensions. The mechanical design is such that a particular specimen can be relocated to within ±5 μm after another one has been examined. The software is written so that the specimens can be examined in any order, with independent scan parameters that can be changed while the system is running.

Examples of applications
Figures 3.4 and 3.5 demonstrate the application of scanning microradiography to the study of demineralisation processes in permeable apatite sinters. This is a one-dimensional process, so that line scans (figure 3.4) are usually sufficient. However, it is sometimes necessary to check the specimen for uniformity and the presence of defects, which can best be

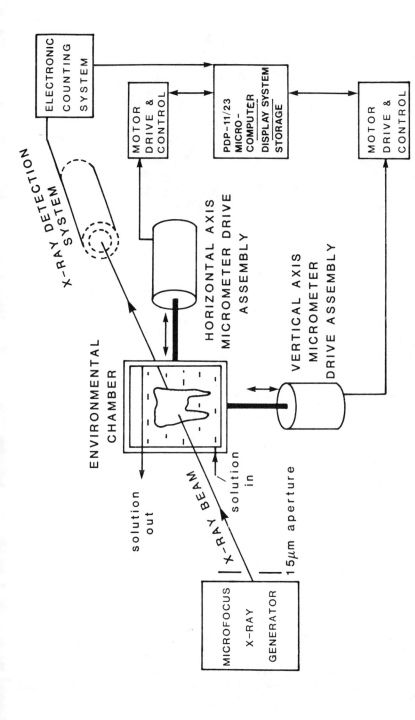

Figure 3.2 Experimental arrangement for scanning microradiography. A sample in an environmental chamber for the study of mineral loss or gain is shown.

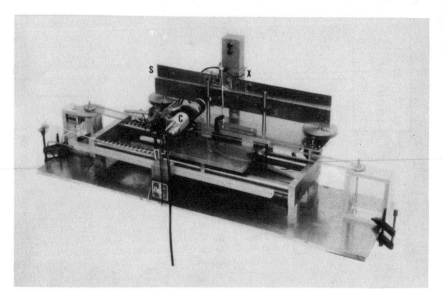

Figure 3.3   Multiple specimen arrangement for scanning microradiography. (X) X-ray source, (S) specimen holder, and (C) counter.

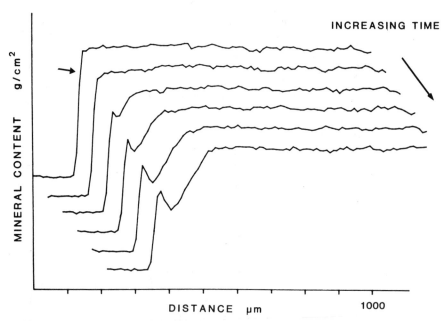

Figure 3.4   Time series of mineral profiles in a 200 μm section of permeable hydroxyapatite sinter dissolving in acid which flowed through the environmental chamber past its front edge (arrowed). The top scan shows the initial state, with subsequent scans taken at 5-hour intervals beneath (displaced for clarity). The progression of subsurface demineralisation that occurs in these systems can be clearly seen. Mo K_α radiation, 10 μm step size, 10 s at each point.

done with area scans (figure 3.5), but these take very much longer.

An area scan of a section of a tooth with a small carious lesion is shown in figure 3.6. This form of presentation gives a good visualisation of the different mineral contents of the various tissues, but more of the quantitative information present can be shown by labelled contour lines of constant mineral content (Elliott *et al.*, 1981).

Microtomography

Computerised axial tomography (also called 'CAT or CT scanning', 'transaxial tomography' and 'reconstruction from projections') is a well-established method for the study of the internal structure of an object without physically cutting sections (Herman, 1980). Literature on the more recent microscopic developments and applications has been cited by Elliott *et al.* (1988), including some on calcified tissues (Bowen *et al.*, 1986; Elliott *et al.*, 1987; Elliott and Dover 1984, 1985).

Theory
In tomographic methods, the three-dimensional internal structure of the object is normally built up from a series of consecutive parallel 'sections', each one being determined individually. In order to do this, the object has to be mounted so that it can be rotated about an axis perpendicular to the plane of the 'section'. The projection of the X-ray absorption in this plane onto a line is then measured for a large number of orientations over the angular range 0–180°. Each projection is measured by stepping the object (and its axis of rotation) across a narrow monochromatic X-ray beam (the diameter of this determines the 'section' thickness), in a direction in the plane of the 'section' and at right angles to the beam, and recording the transmitted X-ray intensity at all points (usually 128). This set of projections contains all the information that is required for the reconstruction of the 'section', provided enough projections and points on each projection have been measured. A number of algorithms has been devised for this calculation, which results in the pixel-by-pixel distribution of the linear absorption coefficient. The one we use is based on Fourier methods. An origin, usually taken as the mechanical axis of rotation, has to be defined for the reconstruction algorithm, but this is not very suitable for microscopic systems, where the position of the axis is not immediately known and changes between specimens. The centre of gravity of the 'section' is much more suitable, because its position can be calculated from its projected positions in each projection, a calculation that is independent of changes in the position of the axis of rotation between projections (Dover *et al.*, 1988). This procedure introduces shifts between consecutive 'sections' because their centres of gravity are not on a consistent axis, so that they cannot be immediately assembled to form a complete three-dimensional

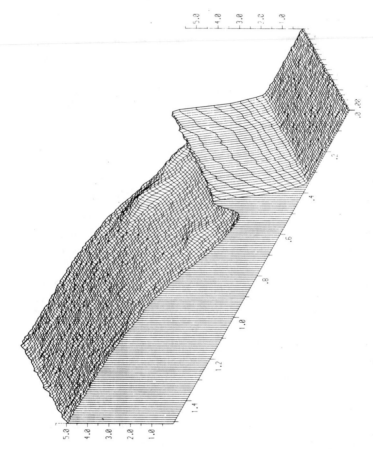

Figure 3.5   Similar experiment to that in figure 3.4, but 1 mm × 2.5 mm area scan after 137 hours. Mo K_α radiation, 10 μm × 25 μm step size, 10 s at each point. X and Y scales are different.

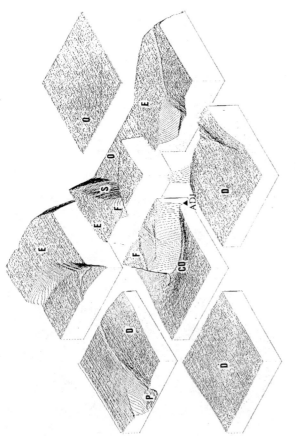

Figure 3.6 A montage of 2 mm × 2 mm surface plots of the mineral in a 250 μm section of a maxillary first permanent molar. (E) enamel, (S) enamel surface, (O) outside section, (D) dentine, (P) pulp horn, (F) fissure, (CD) carious dentine, (ADJ) amelodentinal junction. Mo K_α radiation, step size 20 μm, 5 s at each point.

Calcified Tissue

image. This difficulty is overcome, provided the axis of rotation is reasonably well defined, by shifting the individually reconstructed 'sections' so that they have this axis as a common origin.

It is important to note that tomographic reconstructions will give correct values of the linear absorption coefficient only if equation 3.1 is strictly obeyed, so there are critical requirements on the X-ray measurement system (see above). Monochromatisation is particularly important if the measurements are made at a wavelength at which the photoelectric effect dominates, because of its very strong wavelength dependence; this is less critical for harder (longer-wavelength) radiation, when the incoherent scattering becomes comparable to the photoelectric absorption.

Experimental

It is very important in microtomography that the motion of the specimen should be accurate and reproducible to within a fraction of a pixel, in this case usually 10 μm. In order to meet this requirement, a special stage designed on kinematic principles has been built (Bowen *et al.*, 1986; Elliott *et al.*, 1987) which is shown in figure 3.7. In this stage, the axis of rotation is

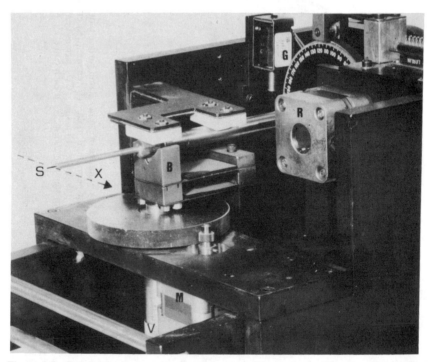

Figure 3.7 Detail of microtomography apparatus. (S) specimen, (X) transmitted X-ray beam, (B) 'V' block surfaced with sapphire in which one of the tungsten carbide balls rotates, (V) vertical micrometer driven by motor (M), (G) gear on spindle driven by motor (R) to provide rotation between projections.

provided by two accurately ground tungsten carbide balls cemented to each end of a 15 cm steel rod. A further short rod on which to mount the specimen (S) is cemented to one of the balls, so that the two rods are colinear. Each ball rests in a sapphire-faced 'V' block, one of which (B) is mounted on a beryllium–copper parallelogram spring so that it can be driven in a vertical direction by a micrometer (V) to provide the motion to measure a projection. A spur gear (G) on the spindle is driven by the motor (R) to rotate the specimen between projections. The whole spindle assembly is spring loaded against a horizontal micrometer, which bears against the ball farthest from the specimen (not shown). The motion of this micrometer moves different parts of the specimen into the X-ray beam (X) for examination. A computer control system similar to that described earlier for the scanning microradiography is used.

Some consideration has to be given to the approximate dimensions of the specimen and the wavelength to be used. If the X-ray attenuation is too low then the intensity with the specimen in the beam will be indistinguishable from that when it is out, and if it is too thick then insufficient counts will be recorded to determine the intensity accurately. The X-ray attenuation will depend on the wavelength used, hence the specimen and wavelength should be matched so that the maximum reduction in intensity is about 50 per cent (table 3.3).

Table 3.3   Thickness in μm of bone and enamel (columns 1 and 4, table 3.2) to halve the X-ray intensity at various wavelengths. The densities were taken as 2.15 and 2.95 g cm^{-3} respectively

Radiation	Wavelength (Å)	Bone	Enamel
Au K_α	0.18	11 800	7 440
Ag K_α	0.56	967	502
Mo K_α	0.71	501	258
C K_α	1.54	56.4	28.9
Co K_α	1.79	36.2	18.6

Examples of applications

A reconstruction of a 'section' through a rat rib is shown in figure 3.8, which clearly shows cortical bone and detail of the trabeculae. The information available is greater than can be presented in one photograph, because the eye can only distinguish about 32 grey levels, whereas there are more than 150 meaningful levels in the reconstruction. As a result, scale expansion has been used so that only part of the information is shown. As with scanning microradiography, more detailed analysis is possible. One of the most useful of these is likely to be the calculation of histograms of the X-ray absorption distribution (Elliott and Dover, 1984; Elliott *et al.*, 1988).

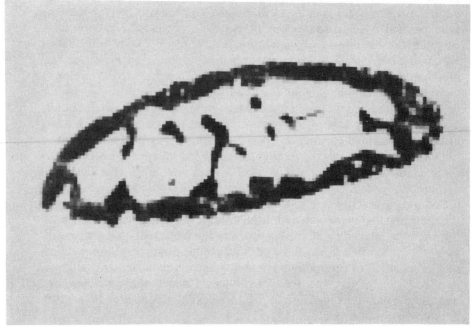

Figure 3.8   Reconstruction of a 'section' through a rat rib. 128 points per projection, step size 12 μm, 120 projections and 5 s counts at each point. The width of the photograph represents 1535 μm.

Comparison with microradiography

As was mentioned earlier, microtomography very substantially reduces the uncertainties in the determination of the section thickness that is required in equation 3.11 for the calculation of the mass of mineral per unit volume. The reason for this is that the accuracy of the volume element part of the measurement is now defined by the accuracy with which the mean size of the individual steps in the projections can be determined. This is very high, because the step motion is controlled by an accurate screw micrometer over a distance of 1000–1500 μm. Microtomography also eliminates uncertainties in section thickness and other problems from water loss and disturbances during section preparation because the tissue being studied is left undisturbed in the middle of the specimen. Because physical sections of brittle calcified tissues do not have to be cut, much thinner 'sections' can be examined, so that the resolution is, at least in one dimension, higher than for microradiography. The method is also non-destructive, so that the specimen is preserved for further study.

FUTURE DEVELOPMENTS AND APPLICATIONS FOR SCANNING MICRORADIOGRAPHY AND MICROTOMOGRAPHY

One of the major drawbacks of the systems that have been described is that they take many hours to examine a single specimen. The obvious reason for this is that the specimen is examined only point by point. Much faster systems would result from the use of linear or two-dimensional arrays of counters (Arndt, 1986), although further development is required to realise their maximum potential. Microtomography with a two-dimensional counter and synchrotron radiation has recently been described by Flannery *et al.* (1987). Because synchrotrons are very powerful X-ray sources of continuous wavelength, they provide greater potential for X-ray microscopy than laboratory sources. Work with these new sources is only at the beginning of its development, but it should be possible to obtain results in a much shorter time, at higher resolution, and with the possibility of elemental analysis from observations on either side of absorption edges. For example, Kenney *et al.* (1985) used a scanning microscope in which X-rays were focused with a zone plate to produce a 140×140 0.19 μm pixel map of the calcium distribution in a chip of human skull bone. The measurements were made at 35.5 and 35.8 Å at the calcium L absorption edge. Bowen *et al.* (1986) have used synchrotron radiation for microtomography at a resolution of 4 μm.

Scanning microradiography can be used to obtain information about the mineral content of calcified tissues, but perhaps more interesting applications will be to the real-time study of *in vitro* changes that can be made in them and in their synthetic analogues. Reference has already been made to the study of de- and remineralisation processes as they actually occur; this should lead to a better general understanding of precipitation and dissolution processes in permeable ionic solids, including a better evaluation of the various regimes that have been proposed for the *in vivo* repair of early carious lesions. Another interesting application is the study of transport phenomena in calcified tissues by X-ray absorption studies of the uptake of heavy ions (say, I^-) or of iodinated organic molecules of various molecular sizes. Similar experiments could be used to study the accessibility of different chemical species to the various zones that have been described in polarised light microscopy of carious lesions.

Microtomography gives accurate mineral distributions at a resolution of at least 10 μm, and could be used to make detailed studies of the mineral distribution in bones from individuals of different ages, and possibly to study changes in disease and response to therapy from biopsy samples. It could also be used to measure any small changes in mineral content of enamel that might be correlated to caries susceptibility, and to study mineral density changes associated with developmental features. With larger specimens and more energetic radiation, the three-dimensional pattern of mineral loss in carious lesions could be determined, as well as the accurate mapping of the internal geometry of the enamel–dentine junction.

ACKNOWLEDGEMENTS

The authors' research reported here has been supported by the Medical Research Council and the Special Trustees of the London Hospital. The design of the microtomography stage and synchrotron work was done in collaboration with Dr D. K. Bowen and was supported by the Science and Engineering Research Council. Mr Tim Davies is thanked for writing the original CAMAC control programs, and Mr Alan Lewis of UKAEA, Harwell, for the Industrial Real Time Basic in which they were written.

REFERENCES

Agna, J. W., Knowles, H. C. and Alverson, G. (1958). The mineral content of normal human bone. *J. Clin. Invest.*, **37**, 1357–61

Angmar, B., Carlström, D. and Glas, J. E. (1963). The mineralization of normal human enamel. *J. Ultrastruct. Res.*, **8**, 12–23

Arndt, U. W. (1986). X-ray position-sensitive detectors. *J. Appl. Crystallogr.*, **19**, 145–63

Barrows, R. S. and Wolfe, R. N. (1971). A review of adjacency effects in silver photographic images. *Photogr. Sci. Eng.*, **15**, 472–9

Boettinger, W. J., Burdette, H. E. and Kuriyama, M. (1979). X-ray magnifier. *Rev. Sci. Instrum.*, **50**, 26–30

Boivin, G. and Baud, C. A. (1984). Microradiographic methods for calcified tissues. *Methods of Calcified Tissue Preparation* (ed. G. R. Dickson), Elsevier, Amsterdam, pp. 391–412

Bowen, D. K., Elliott, J. C., Stock, S. R. and Dover, S. D. (1986). X-ray microtomography with synchrotron radiation. *SPIE Proc.*, **691**, 94–8

Boyde, A. and Jones, S. J. (1983). Backscattered electron imaging of dental tissues. *Anat. Embryol.*, **168**, 211–26

Cheng, P. and Jan, G. (1987). *X-ray Microscopy, Instrumentation and Biological Applications*, Springer, New York

Cosslett, V. E. and Nixon, W. C. (1960). *X-ray Microscopy*, Cambridge University Press, Cambridge

de Josselin de Jong, E. and ten Bosch, J. J. (1985). Measurement and optimization of the MTF's of the microradiographic method and its subsystems. *SPIE Proc.*, **492**, 486–92

de Josselin de Jong, E., ten Bosch, J. J. and Noordmans, J. (1987a). Optimised microcomputer-guided quantitative microradiography on dental mineralised tissue slices. *Phys. Med. Biol.*, **32**, 887–99

de Josselin de Jong, E., van der Linden, A. H. I. M. and ten Bosch, J. J. (1987b). Longitudinal microradiography: a non-destructive automated quantitative method to follow changes in mineralised tissue slices. *Phys. Med. Biol.*, **32**, 1209–20

Dover, S. D., Elliott, J. C., Boakes, R. and Bowen, D. K. (1989). Three-dimensional X-ray microscopy with accurate registrations of tomographic sections. *J. Microsc.* **153**, 187–91

Elliott, J. C. and Dover, S. D. (1984). Three-dimensional distribution of mineral in bone at a resolution of 15 μm determined by x-ray microtomography. *Metab. Bone Dis. Rel. Res.*, **5**, 219–21

Elliott, J. C. and Dover, S. D. (1985). X-ray microscopy using computerized axial tomography. *J. Microsc.*, **138**, 329–31

Elliott, J. C., Boakes, R., Dover, S. D. and Bowen, D. K. (1988). Biological applications of microtomography. In *X-ray Microscopy II* (eds D. Sayre, M. Howells, J. Kirz and H. Rarback), Springer, Berlin, pp. 349–55

Elliott, J. C., Bowen, D. K., and Dover, S. D. and Davies, S. T. (1987). X-ray microtomography of biological tissues using laboratory and synchrotron sources. *Biol. Trace Elem. Res.*, **13**, 219–27

Elliott, J. C., Dowker, S. E. P. and Knight, R. D. (1981). Scanning microradiography of a section of a carious lesion in dental enamel. *J. Microsc.*, **123**, 89–92

Ely, R. V. (1980). *Microfocal Radiography*, Academic Press, London

Flannery, B. P., Deckman, H. W., Roberge, W. G. and D'Amico, K. L. (1987). Three-dimensional X-ray microtomography. *Science*, **237**, 1439–44

Grynpas, M. D., Patterson-Allen, P. and Simons, D. J. (1986). The changes in quality of mandibular bone mineral in otherwise totally immobilized Rhesus monkeys. *Calcif. Tiss. Int.*, **39**, 57–62

Herman, G. T. (1980). *Image Reconstruction from Projections: the Fundamentals of Computerized Tomography*, Academic Press, New York

Hobdell, M. H. and Braden, M. (1971). An investigation into some diffraction effects observed in microradiographic images of bone sections. *Calcif. Tiss. Res.*, **7**, 1–11

Kenney, J. M., Jacobsen, C., Kirz, J. and Rarback, H. (1985). Absorption microanalysis with a scanning soft X-ray microscope: mapping the distribution of calcium in bone. *J. Microscop.*, **138**, 321–8

Knoll, G. L. (1979). *Radiation Detection and Measurement*, John Wiley, New York

Koch, B. and MacGillavry, C. H. (1962). X-ray absorption. In *International Tables for X-ray Crystallography*, Vol. **3**, International Union of Crystallography, Birmingham, pp. 157–61

Langdon, D. J., Elliott, J. C. and Fearnhead, R. W. (1980). Microradiographic observation of acidic subsurface decalcification in synthetic apatite aggregates. *Caries Res.*, **14**, 359–66

McMaster, W. H., Kerr del Grande, N., Mallett, J. H. and Hubbell, J. H. (1969). *Compilation of X-ray Cross Sections*, Report UCRL-50174, Sec. II, Rev. 1, Lawrence Radiation Laboratory, University of California, Livermore

Nikiforuk, G. (1985). *Understanding Dental Caries*, Vol. **1**, Karger, Basel

Rose, K. M. and Jeffery, J. W. (1964). Errors arising from the photographic recording of X-ray intensities. *Acta Crystallogr.*, **17**, 21–4

Schmahl, G. and Rudolph, D. (eds) (1984). *X-ray Microscopy*, Springer, Berlin

Smales, F. C. (1975). Pyknometric density determinations on finely-divided calcium phosphates. In *Physico-chimie et Cristallographie des Apatites d'Intérêt Biologique*, Colloques Intern. CNRS, No. 230, Paris, pp. 131–3

Takagi, S., Chow, L. C., Brown, W. E., Dobbyn, R. C. and Kuriyama, M. (1984). Parallel beam microradiography of dental hard tissue using synchrotron radiation and X-ray image magnification. *Nucl. Instr. Meth.*, **222**, 256–8

Weidmann, S. M., Weatherell, J. A. and Hamm, S. M. (1967). Variations of enamel density in sections of human teeth. *Arch. Oral Biol.*, **12**, 85–97

Wilson, P. R. and Beynon, A. D. (1989). Mineralization differences between human deciduous and permanent enamel measured by quantitative microradiography. *Archs. Oral Biol.*, **34**, 85–8

4

X-ray absorption spectroscopy of mineral deposits

D. W. L. Hukins, S. S. Hasnain and J. E. Harries

INTRODUCTION

X-ray absorption spectroscopy (XAS) can be used to investigate the environment of atoms or ions of selected elements in solids, which need not be crystalline, or liquids. In practice, some elements are more easy to investigate than others – for reasons which will be explained when the principles of the technique are discussed below. As a result, calcium environments in biological calcium phosphates have been extensively studied and some preliminary experiments on phosphorus environments have been performed. XAS requires a continuously tunable source of X-rays. The difficulty of obtaining sufficient intensity, over a range of wavelengths, from conventional X-ray sources was one important reason why the technique was not widely used until the availability of synchrotron radiation. Synchrotron radiation is produced by accelerators, called synchrotrons and storage rings, in which electrons or positrons move in a circular path with a typical diameter of 30 m (Catlow and Greaves, 1986). There are less than a dozen laboratories in the world with the facilities for XAS using synchrotron radiation, and, indeed, all the results described in this chapter have been obtained at three of them: LURE at Orsay (France), the Stanford Synchrotron Radiation Laboratory (USA) and the SERC Daresbury Laboratory (UK).

A spectrum is conventionally divided into two regions: the X-ray absorption near edge spectrum (XANES), and the extended X-ray absorption fine structure (EXAFS) spectrum. These terms will be defined below, but the exact definition is somewhat arbitrary, as there is no sharp boundary between the two regions. EXAFS was first described by Kronig (1931, 1932a, b) and is sometimes referred to as 'Kronig structure', although it is only relatively recently that it was realised that it was capable of providing structural information (Sayers *et al.*, 1971). The theory of EXAFS is now well established (Ashley and Doniach, 1975; Lee and Pendry, 1975) and it has been widely applied to a variety of systems; several reviews have been published – for example, those by Eisenberger and Kincaid (1978), Lee *et al.* (1981), Bordas (1982), Gurman (1982) and Hasnain (1987). The analysis of XANES is more recent (Durham *et al.*, 1982).

XAS appears well suited to investigating the structures of calcified deposits from biological tissues, since they are so frequently structurally disordered and/or associated with other materials, e.g. in micelles. Furthermore, the synthetic compounds prepared in order to obtain further information on biological calcification processes are often amorphous solids (see Chapter 1). Indeed, the highly variable coordination geometry of calcium may be implicated in the frequency with which it forms disordered solids (Taylor *et al.*, 1986), and may explain why it is so widely involved in biological processes (Williams, 1976). Although some spectra have been recorded which provide empirical information on the phosphorus environments in biological calcium phosphates and model compounds (Hukins *et al.*, 1986a; Hukins and Harries, 1987), most investigations have been concerned with the environment of calcium – the subject of this chapter. Systems which have been investigated are: bone (Eanes *et al.*, 1981; Miller *et al.*, 1981; Binsted *et al.*, 1982; Harries *et al.*, 1988), micellar calcium phosphate of milk (Holt *et al.*, 1982, 1989a; Irlam *et al.*, 1985), secretory granules of snails (Greaves *et al.*, 1984; Taylor *et al.*, 1986), arthropathic deposits (Harries *et al.*, 1984) and deposits formed in urinary catheters (Cox *et al.*, 1987a; Hukins *et al.*, 1986b, 1989). In order to understand the results of these investigations, it has been necessary to record and analyse spectra from a range of model compounds: fully crystalline hydroxyapatite ($Ca_5(PO_4)_3OH$; Harries *et al.*, 1986a), partially crystalline hydroxyapatite and a related amorphous calcium phosphate prepared under alkaline conditions (Harries *et al.*, 1987a), carbonated hydroxyapatite (Harries *et al.*, 1987b), brushite ($CaHPO_4 . 2H_2O$; Harries *et al.*, 1987c), monetite ($CaHPO_4$; Harries *et al.*, 1987c) and amorphous calcium phosphate prepared under neutral (Holt *et al.*, 1988) and slightly acid (Holt *et al.*, 1989b) conditions. Structures of calcium phosphates precipitated in the presence of phosphoproteins have also been investigated (Irlam *et al.*, 1984). Periodic reviews of the investigation of biological calcium phosphates and model compounds have been published (Hasnain, 1984; Hukins *et al.*, 1986a, c; Hukins and Harries, 1987). Some of the investigations, especially the earlier ones, simply involve comparison of spectra from different substances, whilst others involve detailed analyses of the spectra. Before these applications are described, it will be necessary to summarise the experimental techniques and to describe the principles involved.

EXPERIMENTAL TECHNIQUES

So far, all X-ray absorption spectra of biological calcium phosphates and synthetic model compounds have been recorded from solid samples. These samples have usually been in the form of a thin, even layer (thickness about 30 μm) mounted on adhesive tape, although spectra have also been recorded from powders secured to polycarbonate filter discs (Eanes *et al.*, 1980, 1981).

Figure 4.1 is a schematic diagram of the apparatus required to record an absorption spectrum in the 'transmission mode'. Although there are other methods of recording spectra (reviewed by Lee *et al.*, 1981), this is the most suitable technique at present for investigating the calcium environment in biological deposits. Polychromatic radiation from the synchrotron is incident on a monochromator, which allows each wavelength in the required range to be selected; the most successful type of monochromator for obtaining the kind of spectra described here has proved to be one which consists of two separate silicon crystals (Greaves *et al.*, 1983). The resulting monochromatic beam passes through the first detector (an ion chamber), which absorbs only about 20 per cent of the beam and records the intensity, I_0, of the X-rays for each wavelength incident on the sample. The second detector (also an ion chamber), which absorbs about 60 per cent of the emerging beam, records the intensity I_t, transmitted by the sample at each wavelength.

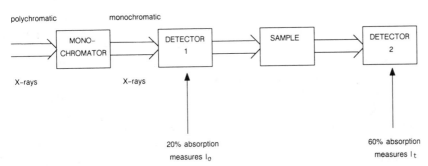

Figure 4.1 Schematic diagram of the apparatus used to record X-ray absorption spectra.

PRINCIPLES

Origin of the absorption spectrum

Monochromatic X-rays can be considered as waves with a single wavelength, λ, or as a stream of photons whose energy, E, is given by

$$E = hc/\lambda, \tag{4.1}$$

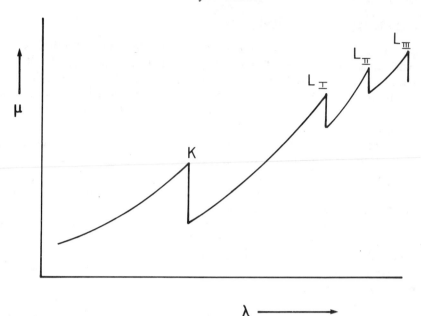

Figure 4.2   Schematic diagram of the dependence of X-ray absorbance, μ, of an element on wavelength, λ, which is related to photon energy by equation 4.1. The diagram shows K, L_I, L_{II}, and L_{III} absorption edges.

where c is their velocity of propagation and h is Planck's constant. The greater the value of E, the more easily the photons pass through matter; i.e., the absorption of X-rays by a given sample decreases with E and increases with λ. However, a photon whose energy is equal to the binding energy of an electron in an atom will have a high probability of being absorbed, so that the electron is emitted by the photoelectric effect. Therefore, elements exhibit discontinuities in their X-ray absorbance which correspond to the binding energies of their electrons. These discontinuities are known as 'absorption edges' and are conventionally designated K, L_I, L_{II}, L_{III}, ..., as shown in figure 4.2. Each absorption edge corresponds to a binding energy, E_0, for an electron in an isolated atom of an element. Energies associated with the K edges for calcium, phosphorus and oxygen are listed in table 4.1 (based on data from Bearden, 1974), together with corresponding values of the X-ray wavelength.

Figure 4.3 shows a photon leading to emission of a photoelectron from a calcium ion in a schematic calcium phosphate structure. This electron may be considered as a particle or as a spherical wave propagated by the calcium ion – in a way which resembles the propagation of a radio wave by an antenna. As the electron wavefront spreads out, it encounters an oxygen atom in direction 1, a phosphorus atom in direction 2 and no other

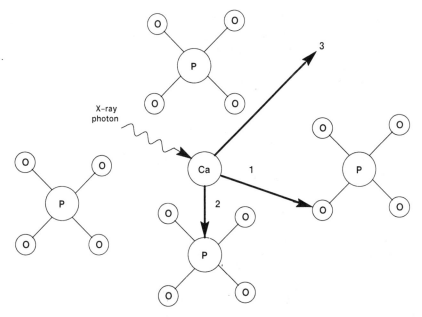

Figure 4.3 A calcium ion in a hypothetical calcium phosphate structure absorbs an X-ray photon of the correct energy to emit a photoelectron (see text).

atoms in direction 3. Thus the electron wave is capable of providing information on the surroundings of the calcium ion which is similar to the detection of objects, on a much larger scale, by radar. Since the mean free path of a photoelectron emitted from calcium, in an insulator, is around 1 nm, we need not consider atoms beyond this distance when analysing EXAFS spectra (Teo, 1981). Oxygen and phosphorus atoms, in directions 1 and 2, respectively, are detected because they scatter the electron back – towards the emitting calcium ion (Stern, 1974). As a result of interference between back-scattered and emitted photoelectrons, atoms in a solid or liquid have subsidiary absorption bands on the high-energy side of their absorption edges, as shown in figure 4.4 (Sayers *et al.*, 1971; Stern, 1974). The XANES region of an XAS spectrum is difficult to interpret because the photoelectron wave can undergo 'multiple scattering' effects (Durham *et al.*, 1982).

The EXAFS region of the absorption spectrum is conventionally considered to begin about 50 eV above the absorption edge. It is generally supposed that complications like multiple scattering are not so important in this region (Lee *et al.*, 1981). However, multiple scattering has to be invoked to explain why some of the atoms surrounding calcium do not contribute to EXAFS spectra recorded above the calcium K edge of crystalline calcium phosphates (Harries *et al.*, 1986a, b; 1987c.).

The type of atom or ion whose environment is to be investigated is selected simply by choosing the appropriate range of X-ray wavelengths. For example, an absorption spectrum measured with X-rays whose photons have an energy of around 4 keV (see table 4.1) provides information on the environment of the calcium ions in a sample. X-Rays of this energy are appreciably attenuated by a few centimetres of air and by the thin beryllium foils used to maintain the vacuum around the accelerator. In order to record spectra around the lower energy phosphorus K edge, samples have to be surrounded by a vacuum, and considerable attention has to be given to attenuation by the apparatus, including the monochromator (MacDowell *et al.*, 1986). Although some preliminary results have been obtained on biological calcium phosphates (Hukins, *et al.*, 1986a; Hukins and Harries, 1987), it has not yet been satisfactorily demonstrated that reproducible spectra can be recorded above the phosphorus K edge from these systems. It seems unlikely that any attempt to record spectra above the oxygen K edge from such specimens would yield results which were worth the effort of overcoming the technical difficulties.

Table 4.1 Positions of the K absorption edges for calcium, phosphorus and oxygen

	Wavelength (nm)	Energy (keV)
Ca	0.307	4.038
P	0.578	2.144
O	2.332	0.532

Most investigations of biological calcium phosphates have concentrated on the EXAFS region of the spectrum. The reason is that this region is much easier to interpret than the XANES. Although the XANES region might provide qualitative structural information, by comparison of spectra from unknown samples with the spectra of well-characterised model compounds, we concentrate on EXAFS in this chapter. There are three reasons for neglecting XANES: (1) that insufficient results are available on calcium phosphates to draw general conclusions, (2) that the XANES of calcium phosphate have not been analysed and (3) that little, if any, difference is observed in the XANES of different calcium phosphates. We shall see later that it was not until EXAFS spectra from well-characterised calcium phosphates had been properly analysed that their limitations for investigating the corresponding biological systems were fully appreciated. In order to discuss the EXAFS spectra further, it is necessary to outline how they are obtained from the values of I_0 and I_t measured for a series of X-ray wavelengths, in an experiment.

Extraction of an EXAFS spectrum

The X-ray absorbance, μ, of a material depends on the energy, E, of the

X-ray photons and is defined by

$$\mu(E) = (1/t) \log_e[I_0(E)/I_t(E)] \tag{4.2}$$

where $I_0(E)$ and $I_t(E)$ are the incident and transmitted intensities measured at that energy (Koch and MacGillavry, 1968); t is the thickness of the sample. Sample thickness is usually adjusted so that μt is of the order of 2 at the absorption edge.

The value of $\mu(E)$ depends on absorption by atoms of the type whose environment is being investigated (calcium in this chapter) and on the absorption by all the other atoms in the material. We define the first contribution as $\mu_A(E)$ and the absorption by the others as $\mu_B(E)$. Since the spectrum is to be recorded above the absorption edge of atoms of type A, it is only the $\mu_A(E)$ term which exhibits the oscillatory features of the EXAFS spectrum. Thus $\mu_A(E)$ can be expressed as the sum of a function $\bar{\mu}_A(E)$, which decreases smoothly with increasing E, and an oscillatory function, $\tilde{\mu}_A(E)$. Hence we can write

$$\mu(E) = \mu_A(E) + \mu_B(E)$$
$$= \bar{\mu}_A(E) + \tilde{\mu}_A(E) + \mu_B(E) \tag{4.3}$$

The EXAFS spectrum, $\chi(E)$, is then defined by

$$\chi(E) = \tilde{\mu}_A(E)/\bar{\mu}_A(E)$$
$$= \{[\mu(E) - \mu_B(E) - \bar{\mu}_A(E)]/\bar{\mu}_A(E)\} - 1 \tag{4.4}$$

Figure 4.4 indicates how $\chi(E)$ is obtained from $\mu(E)$ in practice. A smooth curve is fitted through the $\mu(E)$ values for $E < E_0$ and extrapolated to the region $E > E_0$. A second curve is calculated which passes smoothly through the $\mu(E)$ values for $E > E_0$, so that the EXAFS spectrum appears as oscillations about it. For a given photon energy, E', say, values for $\mu_B(E')$ and $\bar{\mu}_A(E')$ may be extracted from the first and second curves, as indicated in figure 4.4, provided $E' > E_0$. These results may be combined with the observed absorbance, $\mu(E')$, at this energy to calculate a single point, $\chi(E')$ in the EXAFS spectrum from equation 4.4. Details of a procedure for extracting an EXAFS spectrum in this way have been reported by Diakun *et al.* (1984).

It is conventional to plot the EXAFS spectrum as a function of k, the modulus of the scattering vector for the photoelectron, which is defined by

$$k = 2\pi/\lambda = 2\pi p/h \tag{4.5}$$

Here λ is the wavelength of the photoelectron and p is its momentum. The energy of the photoelectron emitted as the result of absorption of an X-ray photon of energy E is simply $(E - E_0)$. Therefore,

$$p^2 = 2m(E - E_0) \tag{4.6}$$

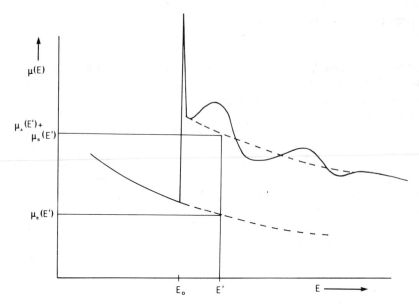

Figure 4.4   Schematic diagram of the X-ray absorbance, $\mu(E)$, of a material plotted against photon energy, E. There is fine structure on the high-energy side of the absorption edge whose position defines the energy E_0. A smooth curve through $\mu(E)$ values for $E < E_0$ has been extrapolated to allow $\mu_B(E')$ to be determined at an energy $E' > E_o$, as described in the text.

where m is the rest mass of an electron. Hence, from equations 4.5 and 4.6, k can be calculated from E using the relationship

$$k = (2\pi/h)[2m(E - E_0)]^{1/2} \qquad (4.7)$$

where π, h and m are all constants.

Relationship between $\chi(k)$ and structure

In this section we shall describe the relationship between $\chi(k)$ and structure, in terms of the simple 'plane wave' approximation used by Sayers *et al.* (1971). The exact 'curved-wave' theory of EXAFS is more complicated but depends on exactly the same parameters; for high values of $(E - E_0)$, the exact theory reduces to the approximate form (Ashley and Doniach 1975; Lee and Pendry, 1975). Although we explain the theory in terms of an approximation, we have used the exact formulation to calculate the theoretical spectra presented later in this chapter.

The environment of the atom which emits a photoelectron is considered to consist of a series of concentric spherical coordination shells of atoms; the shells are centered at the emitting atom. Each shell contains N atoms of the same type and is characterised by its radius r_j. According to the approximate theory,

$$\chi(k) = \sum_j (N_j/kr_j^2) f_j \exp(-2\sigma_j^2 k^2) \exp(-2r_j/\Lambda) \sin[2kr_j + \alpha_j(k)], \quad (4.8)$$

where the summation is over all shells with r_j not much greater than Λ, the mean free path of a photoelectron. Here $f_j(k)$ and $\alpha_j(k)$ are, respectively, the amplitude and phase with which the photoelectron is scattered back by the atoms of the jth shell. The Debye–Waller factor, $\exp(-2\sigma_j^2 k^2)$, accounts for static and thermal variation in the value of r_j; $2\sigma_j$ is the root-mean-square displacement of the atoms in the jth shell.

It is usual to present EXAFS spectra as $\chi(k)$ multiplied by k^3. The reason is to enhance the amplitude of the peaks at high k values, but the disadvantage of this procedure is that the noise levels associated with these peaks are amplified by the same factor.

The shell structure surrounding the atom which emits the photoelectron can be calculated from $\chi(k)$ by calculating

$$g(r) = \left| \int_0^\infty \chi(k) \exp\{i[2kr + \alpha(k)]\} \, dk \right| \quad (4.9)$$

(Sayers *et al.*, 1971; Gurman and Pendry, 1976). Strictly, $g(r)$ is the radial distribution of back-scattering amplitude around the emitting atom. An integral of the form of that in equation 4.9 is known as the Fourier transform of $\chi(k)$ and is complex; $g(r)$ is defined to be its modulus. The major problem associated with evaluating the integral is that $\alpha(k)$ is unknown, unless the shell structure is known already. An empirical method for overcoming this problem is simply to calculate $\alpha_1(k)$ from a suitable model for $g(r)$, as described later in this chapter. The result of this procedure is not then a true representation of $g(r)$, but provides a representation of the structural data conveyed by $\chi(k)$. In this chapter $g(r)$ will always be computed by this empirical method. A further problem is that $\chi(k)$ cannot be recorded over an infinite range of k values. Ripples appear in $g(r)$ as a result of using a finite range of values, although they can be suppressed to some extent (Gurman, 1980). Hence, some knowledge of the true structure is required to interpret $g(r)$ sensibly.

Structures cannot, therefore, be deduced directly from EXAFS spectra; models have to be developed for the environment of the emitting atom and their predictions compared with the experimental data. If the model is reasonably satisfactory, it can then be adjusted to minimise the discrepancy between theory and experiment. This procedure is identical to the trial-and-error method of interpreting X-ray diffraction patterns and suffers from the same disadvantage: 'The unsatisfactory feature of trial-and-error solution is that one cannot be sure that all possible models have been considered. Thus the true structure may have been overlooked. In consequence, the resulting models cannot be established with the same degree of certainty as can deductive models.' (Hukins, 1981.)

The features of an EXAFS spectrum arise from diffraction effects involving electrons generated from within the sample by the photoelectric effect. Therefore, there are similarities in the analysis of EXAFS and X-ray diffraction data to obtain structural information.

Reliability of structural determination

The precision with which distances can be determined by EXAFS depends on how far the experimental data extend above the absorption edge, i.e. on the range of k values over which the spectrum extends. By analogy with other diffraction/scattering experiments, and as in the Abbe theory of the microscope, the smallest distance in the structure to which the technique is sensitive is of the order of the wavelength of, in this case, the photo-electrons (see, for example, Hukins, 1981; Lipson and Lipson, 1966). More specifically, the smallest separation between points which can be resolved is 0.61λ. Typically, EXAFS spectra are recorded for $k \leqslant 120$ nm^{-1}, implying, from equation 4.5, a minimum wavelength for the photoelectrons of 0.05 nm. This wavelength suggests, at best, a value of 0.03 nm for the lower limit to the precision with which distances between shells can be resolved.

Smaller standard deviations than this resolution limit are achieved for the shell radii of calcium phosphates. The reason is that the interpretation of their spectra assumes a model; the standard deviations are then determined as a result of using the parameters defined by this model to fit the spectrum with a precision of better than 0.002 nm.

However, the model should not be used to introduce more variable parameters than the number which can have their values defined by the experimental data. Typically, 200 measurements of $I_0(E)$ and $I_t(E)$ are made in an EXAFS experiment. The number of parameters that can be sensibly varied depends on the signal-to-noise ratio, as well as on the data-to-parameter ratio (Shannon, 1948). Unfortunately, many of the absorption spectra published in the literature are smoothed to remove the noise, so that the quality of the data cannot be assessed. Considerations of this kind are implicit in explaining the results from biological calcium phosphates in the remainder of the chapter.

MODEL COMPOUNDS

Appearance of spectra

Figure 4.5 compares the EXAFS spectra of three crystalline compounds which might be used as models for biological calcium phosphates: (a) hydroxyapatite, abbreviated to HAP, (b) brushite, and (c) monetite. Differences between these spectra are also revealed by the moduli of their Fourier transforms, $g(r)$, as defined by equation 4.9, in figures 4.5(d), (e) and (f); these curves were computed from the spectra by exactly the same procedures as described previously and provide a representation of those features of the calcium ion environment which give rise to EXAFS. However, the peaks at distances of less than 0.2 nm do not correspond to structural features (since the closest atoms to the calcium ion in all these crystals structures are oxygen at around 0.24 nm) but to difficulties in extracting the spectrum. The results presented in figure 4.5 for HAP correspond to a highly crystalline form of this compound (Harries *et al.*, 1986a). However, poorly crystalline forms of HAP can also be precipitated from solution.

Figure 4.6 shows the effect of degree of crystallinity on the EXAFS spectrum of HAP. An amorphous calcium phosphate (ACP) can be prepared under alkaline conditions which matures into poorly crystalline HAP in about 20 h, unless it is carefully dried or chemically stabilised (Harris *et al.*, 1987a). The EXAFS spectrum of ACP consists of four peaks as shown in figure 4.6(a). (There is the hint of a shoulder on the leading edge of the first peak.) Further structure appears on these peaks when the EXAFS spectrum is recorded from poorly crystalline HAP (figure 4.6(b)) produced by maturation of the ACP. In particular, subsidiary peaks appear on the leading edges of the two major peaks and on the trailing edge of the third. These subsidiary peaks are even better defined in the EXAFS spectrum of fully crystalline HAP repeated, for comparison, in figure 4.6(c). A simple example of the same kind of effect is provided by EXAFs spectra recorded from elemental germanium above its *K* edge (Sayers *et al.*, 1971). The spectrum of the crystalline germanium shows considerably more detail than that of the amorphous material, although the major peaks of both coincide.

Figure 4.6 also shows that the moduli of the Fourier transforms, $g(r)$, of these spectra exhibit some of the differences which might be expected for similar materials with differing degrees of crystallinity. The result for ACP (figure 4.6(d)) shows no evidence for clearly defined shells of atoms corresponding to distances of greater than 0.4 nm from the emitting calcium ion, whereas figures 4.6(e) and (f) show that the EXAFS of crystalline HAP is sensitive to the arrangement of atoms up to at least 0.6 nm from calcium.

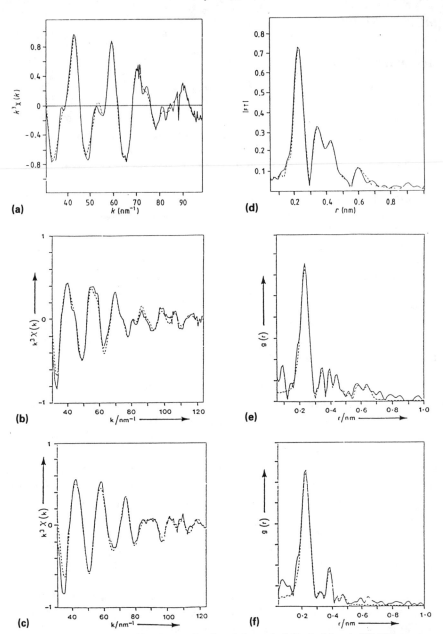

Figure 4.5   Experimental (continuous lines) and theoretical (dashed lines), EXAFS spectra, recorded above the calcium K edge, from: (a) hydroxyapatite, (b) brushite and (c) monetite. Spectra are presented as $k^3\chi(k)$ plotted against k, as described in the text. Moduli of the Fourier transforms, $g(r)$, of the experimental (continuous lines) and theoretical (dashed lines) spectra are shown for: (d) hydroxyapatite, (e) brushite and (f) monetite. These curves represent the distribution of back-scattering amplitude as a function of distance, r, from a calcium ion in an averaged environment in the structure.

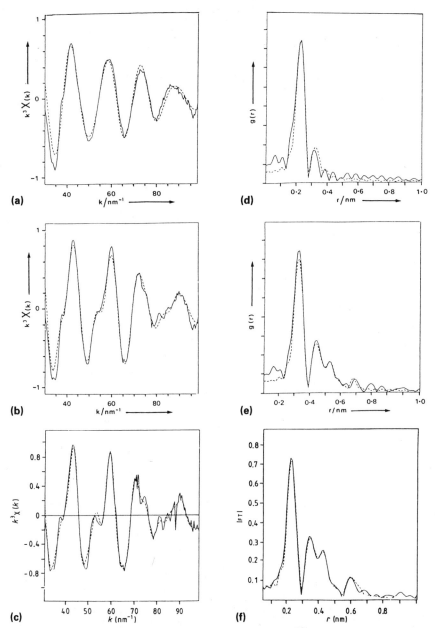

Figure 4.6 Experimental (continuous lines) and theoretical (dashed lines) EXAFS spectra, recorded above the calcium K edge, from: (a) amorphous calcium phosphate (prepared at pH 10), (b) poorly crystalline hydroxyapatite (prepared by maturation of the amorphous calcium phosphate), and (c) fully crystalline hydroxyapatite (repeated from figure 4.5(a)) for comparison.) Spectra are presented as $k^3\chi(k)$ plotted against k. Moduli of the Fourier transforms, $g(r)$, of the experimental (continuous lines) and theoretical (dashed lines) spectra are shown for: (d) amorphous calcium phosphate, (e) poorly crystalline hydroxyapatite and (f) fully crystalline hydroxyapatite (repeated from figure 4.5(d)). These curves represent the radial distribution of back-scattering amplitude for an average calcium ion environment.

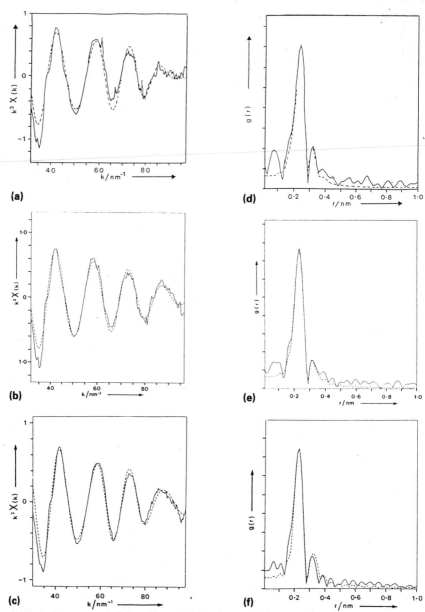

Figure 4.7   Experimental (continuous lines) and theoretical (dashed lines) EXAFS spectra, recorded above the calcium K edge, from amorphous calcium phosphate prepared at pH values of: (a) 7, (b) 6, and (c) 10 (repeated from figure 4.6(a) for comparison). Spectra are presented as $k^3\chi(k)$ plotted against k. Moduli of the Fourier transforms, $g(r)$, of the experimental (continous lines) and theoretical (dashed lines) spectra are shown for amorphous calcium phosphates prepared at pH values of: (d) 7, (e) 6, and (f) 10 (repeated from figure 4.6(d) for comparison). These curves represent the radial distribution of backscattering amplitude for an average calcium ion environment.

However, forms of ACP can be prepared which are chemically distinct from that described by Harries *et al.* (1987a), yet which have virtually identical EXAFS spectra (Holt *et al.*, 1988b, c). Figures 4.7(a) and (b) show EXAFS spectra obtained from ACP prepared at pH7 and pH6, respectively. Unlike the ACP formed under alkaline conditions, in which all the phosphate groups are present as PO_4^{3-}, many of the phosphate groups in these new forms of ACP are protonated, i.e. they contain HPO_4^{2-} as well as PO_4^{3-} ions. Nevertheless, their EXAFS spectra, in figures 4.7(a) and (b), are not distinguishable from the spectrum of ACP prepared under alkaline conditions, repeated in figure 4.7(c) for comparison. Moduli of the Fourier transforms of these spectra, $g(r)$, shown in figures 4.7(d)–(f), are also unable to distinguish these chemical differences. Thus it appears that EXAFS spectra alone cannot be used to reliably distinguish between different amorphous forms of calcium phosphate because the average environment of the calcium ions is almost the same in all of them.

Analysis of spectra from crystalline model compounds

The known crystal structures of HAP, brushite and monetite have been used to analyse the EXAFS spectra of figure 4.5 (Harries *et al.*, 1986a, 1987c). These analyses were performed in order to interpret spectra from related compounds whose structures are not so well defined. Thus they formed a necessary first stage in the application of EXAFS to investigating the structures of poorly crystalline and amorphous model compounds, as well as for determining the structures of biological calcium phosphates.

The first step in the analysis of the EXAFS spectrum of HAP was to describe the environment of a calcium ion as a series of shells, each containing atoms of the same kind. Calcium ions occur in two distinct environments in the crystal structure of HAP (Kay *et al.*, 1964). A single unit cell of HAP contains two formula units of $Ca_5(PO_4)_3OH$. Four of the ten calcium ions occupy one kind of environment in the unit cell; the remaining six occupy another kind of site. This crystal structure could be used to calculate a mean calcium ion environment which consisted of shells of the same kind of atom. Each shell was then characterised by its radius, r_j, and an occupancy, N_j, which need not be integral, as defined in the explanation of equation 4.8. Shells whose r_j values were not sufficiently different to be resolved by the experimental data were combined and reasonable values were assigned to σ_j, of equation 4.8, as described by Harries *et al.* (1986a).

Values of $f_j(k)$ and $\alpha_j(k)$, in equation 4.8, were also calculated from the known crystal structure of HAP. These calculations involved estimating the electron density around each atom in the crystal structure by the methods conventionally used to analyse low-energy electron diffraction

(Pendry, 1974). A reasonable value was assigned to the mean free path, Λ, of a photoelectron. Further details are given by Harries *et al.* (1986a).

These shells were then used to calculate a theoretical EXAFS spectrum, $\chi(k)$, using the exact 'curved wave' theory for a polycrystalline sample (Gurman *et al.*, 1984) rather than the approximate form of equation 4.8. Values of r_j, and of σ_j, were adjusted so that the theoretical spectrum agreed as closely as possible with that observed experimentally. Final values for r_j were very similar to those calculated from the known crystal structure of HAP and reasonable values were obtained for σ_j (Harries *et al.*, 1986a). It was found that no shells with r_j greater than 0.622 nm were required to explain the features of the EXAFS spectrum of HAP. However, the agreement between theory and experiment was insensitive to the radii of four shells within this range. Three of the shells back-scattered photoelectrons almost exactly in phase or antiphase with the photoelectrons scattered by other shells – so that their positions cannot be determined. The remaining shell whose position had little influence on the features of the theoretical spectrum contained calcium ions 0.545 nm from the emitting atom. This shell back-scatters photoelectrons which interfere destructively with photoelectrons which have undergone forward multiple scattering by oxygen atoms. The multiple scattering calculations required to reach this conclusion were performed by the method of Gurman *et al.* (1986), as described by Harries *et al.* (1986a, b).

Table 4.2 gives the final form of a shell model for HAP, which may be used to explain the features of its EXAFS spectrum. Figure 4.5(a) compares the theoretical spectrum (dashed line), calculated from these shells, with that observed experimentally (continuous line). Similarly, figure 4.5(d) shows that the modulus of the Fourier transform, $g(r)$, calculated from the theoretical spectrum by exactly the same method as that from the experimental spectrum with which it is compared.

It is clear that we would not have been able to analyse the EXAFS spectrum of HAP if its crystal structure had not been known already; a

Table 4.2 Shell model developed for the analysis of the EXAFS spectrum of fully crystalline hydroxyapatite

Atom type	Shell occupancy, N_j	Shell radius, r_j (nm)	RMS displacement, $2\sigma_j$ (nm)
O	5.4	0.237	0.015
O	1.0	0.256	0.016
P	2.4	0.311	0.021
Ca	0.8	0.346	0.021
Ca	8.4	0.395	0.032
O	4.8	0.445	0.018
O	6.5	0.469	0.029
Ca	2.0	0.574	0.024
Ca	6.0	0.622	0.029

Table 4.3 Shell model developed for the analysis of the EXAFS spectrum of brushite

Atom type	Shell occupancy, N_j	Shell radius, r_j (nm)	r.m.s. displacement, $2\sigma_j$ (nm)
O	8	0.238	0.023
P	1	0.302	0.019
P	1	0.320	0.022
P	2	0.362	0.018
O	4	0.406	0.017
O	5	0.428	0.018
O	3	0.492	0.024
O	2	0.520	0.014
Ca	2	0.608	0.026
Ca	4	0.641	0.022

similar knowledge of crystal structures was required to interpret EXAFS spectra of brushite and monetite (Harries *et al.*, 1987c). In order to explain the features of the brushite spectrum satisfactory, we had to use atomic coordinates from the crystal structure as described by Curry and Jones (1971), rather than that determined previously by Jones and Smith (1962). Thus the EXAFS spectrum of brushite was capable of determining which of these two models for its crystal structure was the better. Nevertheless, the spectrum was insensitive to back-scattering contributions from some shells and the model finally used to analyse the EXAFS spectrum is listed in table 4.3. Omission of some of the shells in the brushite crystal structure can be explained by constructive and destructive interference of their back-scattered photoelectrons with those scattered by other shells (Harries *et al.*, 1986b, 1987c). Theoretical spectra, and the moduli of their Fourier transforms (dashed lines) are compared with those observed experimentally (continuous lines) in figures 4.5(b) and (e), respectively, for brushite and in figures 4.5(c) and (f), respectively, for monetite.

Analysis of spectra from poorly crystalline and amorphous model compounds

EXAFS spectra from ACP and poorly crystalline HAP have been analysed using the inner shells of the HAP model of table 4.2 (Harries *et al.*, 1987a). The minimum number of shells was used to calculate a theoretical spectrum which reproduced the features observed experimentally, using the exact theory for a polycrystalline sample (Gurman *et al.*, 1984). Values of r_j and σ_j for these shells were then adjusted to obtain the best fit between theoretical and experimental spectra. The theoretical spectrum (dashed line) of ACP required only the three inner shells ($r_j < 0.32$ nm) of the HAP model to reproduce the features of the observed spectrum (continuous line) shown in figure 4.6(a). Final values of the three shell radii, r_j, differed from their starting values, derived from the HAP model, by no more than

0.004 nm; values of σ_j increased slightly to account for the expected increase in static disorder in ACP as compared with fully crystalline HAP. However, only the outer shell in table 4.2 ($r_j = 0.622$ nm) could be omitted if the features of the spectrum of poorly crystalline HAP were to be reproduced satisfactorily. Once again, final values of r_j differed from their starting values by no more than 0.004 nm. As expected, values of σ_j for the three inner shells were intermediate between those for ACP and fully crystalline HAP. Figure 4.6(b) shows the level of agreement between theoretical (dashed line) and experimental (continuous line) spectra.

Thus the analysis of EXAFS spectra can be used to develop reasonable structural models for disordered calcium phosphates, provided crystal structures of appropriate model compounds are known. The structural models which result from this analysis of the spectra have the form of tables 4.2 and 4.3; i.e., they consist of values for the radii of shells of atoms surrounding a calcium ion together with a measure of the root-mean-square displacement of atoms about this radius. Thus these models do not consist of three-dimensional coordinates, but are equivalent to a radial distribution function which is a conventional description for the structure of disordered systems (see, for example, Hukins, 1981; Kittel, 1986), but in this case the radial distribution is specific to the environment of calcium.

Analysis of the EXAFS spectrum of a disordered phase may be ambiguous when the choice of an appropriate crystalline model compound is not clear. For example, in the ACP samples whose spectra are shown in figures 4.7(a) and (b), about half of the phosphate groups appear to be in the form of HPO_4^{2-} rather than PO_4^{3-} (Holt *et al.*, 1988, 1989b). It is not then clear whether to use HAP (which contains PO_4^{3-}) or brushite (which contains HPO_4^{2-}) as the model compound. Both models provide theoretical spectra which agree equally well with that observed experimentally. The level of agreement is illustrated using the two inner shells of brushite (table 4.3) as the basis for the theoretical calculation in figures 4.7(a) and (b). A satisfactory alternative model is based on the three inner shells of HAP (table 4.2). It is clear that the EXAFS spectra alone cannot distinguish between the two kinds of model, which in any case are very similar, and so cannot provide direct evidence as to the degree of protonation of the phosphate groups in related amorphous samples of unknown structure.

BIOLOGICAL DEPOSITS

Appearance of spectra

Bone has been investigated more thoroughly than any other calcified biological system by EXAFS (Eanes *et al.*, 1981; Miller *et al.*, 1981;

Binsted *et al.*, 1982; Harries *et al.*, 1988). Earlier spectra had much higher noise levels than shown in figure 4.8(a), but were clearly very similar to the spectrum of poorly crystalline HAP. Even in figure 4.8(a), the shape of the third main EXAFS peak is obscured by noise; nevertheless, this spectrum and the modulus of its Fourier transform, $g(r)$, shown in figure 4.8(d), are closely similar to the corresponding results for poorly crystalline HAP in figures 4.6(b) and (e). This similarity is consistent with the accepted view of the structure of bone mineral (Boskey, 1981) and demonstrates very clearly its poor crystallinity when compared with fully crystalline HAP whose EXAFS spectrum is shown in figure 4.6(c).

Figure 4.8(b) shows the EXAFS spectrum recorded from casein micelles extracted from cow's milk. Casein is a phosphoprotein whose micelles contain calcium phosphate. EXAFS spectra show that the calcium ion environment in this micellar calcium phosphate (MCP) is the same in cow, pig, goat, rabbit, rat and human micelles, despite their having very different concentrations of calcium as well as their containing different types of casein (Irlam *et al.*, 1985). Initially, this spectrum was considered to resemble that of brushite, shown in figure 4.5(d), more closely than that of any other model compound then available (Holt *et al.*, 1982). Since X-ray diffraction patterns recorded from MCP showed no evidence for an extended crystal lattice, even after the removal of the casein, it was supposed that the MCP consisted of microcrystalline brushite, only a few unit cells in extent, or of an amorphous phase in which the calcium ion environment was similar to that in brushite (Holt *et al.*, 1982). As more spectra with lower noise levels have been recorded from a wider range of model compounds, this interpretation has appeared less reliable – although the conclusion that many of the phosphate groups of MCP are protonated, as in brushite, still appears valid (Holt *et al.*, 1989a). The spectra originally recorded from ACP were rather different from those of figure 4.7, and the details of many of the other early spectra were obscured by high noise levels. Thus it was originally supposed that the EXAFS spectrum of MCP more closely resembled that of brushite than that of ACP prepared under alkaline conditions. Comparison of figure 4.8(b) and figures 4.5(b) and 4.7(a) does not support this conclusion; indeed it appears that MCP resembles ACP very closely. However, the ACP samples prepared under neutral and acid conditions, in which about half of the phosphate groups are protonated (Holt *et al.*, 1988, 1989b) have EXAFS spectra, shown in figures 4.7(b) and (c), which are equally similar to the spectrum of MCP. It also appears, on chemical grounds, that these forms of ACP, which contain HPO_4^{3-} ions, provide a good model for the MCP structure (Holt *et al.*, 1989a).

EXAFS has also been used to investigate the structures of calcium phosphates precipitated in association with phosphoproteins *in vitro* (Irlam *et al.*, 1984). In these experiments, calcium phosphates were precipitated

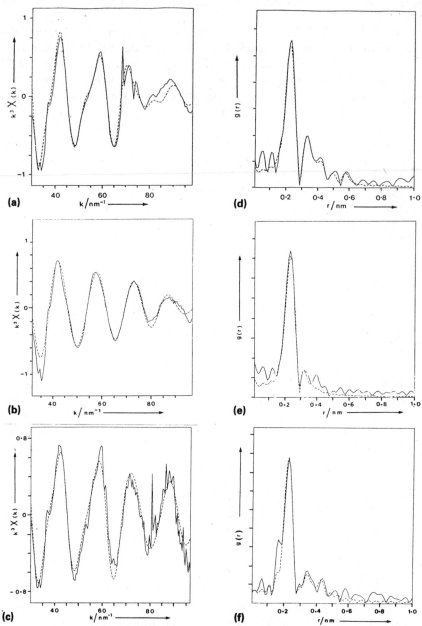

Figure 4.8 Experimental (continuous lines) and theoretical (dashed lines) EXAFS spectra, recorded above the calcium K edge, from: (a) bone mineral, (b) micellar calcium phosphate (from cow's milk), and (c) an encrusting deposit from an in-dwelling urinary catheter. Spectra are presented as $k^3\chi(k)$ plotted against k. Moduli of the Fourier transforms, $g(r)$, of the experimental (continuous lines) and theoretical (dashed lines) spectra are shown for: (d) bone mineral, (e) micellar calcium phosphate, and (f) the encrusting deposit. These curves represent the radial distribution of back-scattering amplitude for an average calcium ion environment.

under appropriate conditions for the formation of HAP or brushite, both in the presence and in the absence of phosphoproteins. Two different phosphoproteins, casein and phosvitin, were used in these experiments. When no phosphoprotein was present, the expected crystalline calcium phosphate was formed and could be identified by X-ray powder diffraction. However, the X-ray diffraction patterns of calcium phosphates bound to phosphoproteins showed no evidence for any long-range order. Nevertheless, the EXAFS spectra of these calcium phosphates were very similar to those of the corresponding crystalline deposits. Thus it was concluded that the local environment of the calcium ions in calcium phosphates incorporated in phosphoprotein micelles is similar to that in model compounds, but that they do not develop long-range order.

Figure 4.8(c) shows the EXAFS spectrum of an encrusting deposit formed on an in-dwelling urinary catheter. These deposits form when urease, secreted by bacteria, converts urea into ammonia – so raising the pH of the urine (Cox *et al.*, 1987b). Usually, the only crystalline component of the deposits which can be identified by X-ray powder diffraction is ammonium magnesium phosphate hexahydrate ($NH_4MgPO_4.6H_2O$), which occurs naturally as the mineral struvite (Hukins *et al.*, 1983). However, atomic absorption spectroscopy invariably demonstrates the presence of appreciable concentrations of calcium in the deposits (Cox *et al.*, 1987a). Furthermore, a few deposits yield X-ray powder diffraction patterns characteristic of poorly crystalline HAP (Hukins *et al.*, 1986b). EXAFS spectra, like figure 4.8(c), clearly indicate the presence of calcium in the deposits and are closely similar to the spectra of the amorphous calcium phosphates in figure 4.7. Figure 4.8(f) shows that, as expected, $g(r)$, the modulus of the Fourier transform of the spectrum, is also very similar to the corresponding results from amorphous calcium phosphates in figures 4.7(d)–(f). The evidence summarised in the remainder of this paragraph indicates that the form of amorphous calcium phosphate prepared at high pH (spectrum in figure 4.7(a)), whose phosphate groups are not protonated, is the appropriate model for the catheter deposits. Urine from patients who have been infected has a pH value in the range 6.5–10 (Norberg *et al.*, 1980), at which crystalline calcium phosphates would be precipitated as hydroxyapatite; i.e., with their phosphate groups unprotonated (Elliot *et al.*, 1958). Furthermore, in an *in vitro* system for encrusting catheters, the pH rises rapidly to a value of 9.2 (Cox *et al.*, 1987b). Finally, struvite dissolves at pH values of less than 7; i.e., when phosphate groups would be protonated (Elliot *et al.*, 1958).

Analysis of spectra

The EXAFS spectrum of bone has been analysed in exactly the same way as that of poorly crystalline HAP (Harries *et al.*, 1988). Shells from the

HAP model of table 4.2 were used to explain the features of the spectrum in figure 4.8(a). This model was considered appropriate because it is well established that bone mineral resembles a poorly crystalline form of HAP which contains other ions, especially carbonate (Termine, 1972; Boskey, 1981). Of course, had the HAP model proved incapable of explaining the features of the EXAFS spectrum in figure 8(a), this established view of the structure of bone mineral would have had to be examined more critically. The eight inner shells of the HAP model in table 4.2 were required to calculate the theoretical spectrum (dashed line), which is compared with that observed experimentally (continuous line) in figure 4.8(a). Figure 4.8(d) compares the moduli of the Fourier transforms of the experimental (continuous line) and theoretical (dashed line) spectra. In order to obtain the theoretical spectrum, values of r_j and σ_j were systematically varied to obtain the best agreement between theory and experiment. Final values for r_j differed from those of poorly crystalline HAP, used to compute the theoretical spectrum (dashed line) of figure 4.6(b), by less than 1 per cent; these values are very close to those listed for the eight inner shells of table 4.2. Values of σ_j tended to be slightly higher than those for the poorly crystalline HAP, presumably reflecting greater disorder within the structure of bone mineral because of, for example, the carbonate ions which it contains (Harries *et al.*, 1988). Indeed, EXAFS has shown that carbonate induces structural disorder in synthetic HAP (Harries *et al.*, 1987b).

The EXAFS spectrum of MCP from milk, shown in figure 4.8(b), closely resembles the spectra of the amorphous calcium phosphates of figures 4.7(d)–(f). Since about half the phosphate groups in the MCP are protonated (i.e., it contains both PO_4^{3-} and HPO_4^{2-} ions), it is not clear whether to use the shell model of HAP (table 4.2) or of brushite (table 4.3) to analyse the spectrum – exactly the same problem as occurred in understanding the spectra of ACP samples with a similar composition. Not surprisingly, the same conclusion was reached for both systems – the inner shells of both starting models were capable of providing theoretical spectra which agreed perfectly well with those observed experimentally (Holt *et al.*, 1989a). Dashed lines in figure 4.8(b) and (e) show the theoretical spectrum and its Fourier transform, respectively, compared with the corresponding experimental data (continuous lines). In this example, the three inner shells of the HAP model (table 4.2) were used and the values of r_j and σ_j adjusted to obtain the best agreement between theory and experiment. Starting with the inner three shells of the brushite model (table 4.3) produces an equally acceptable fit, and, indeed, a very similar final model for MCP.

There is no such doubt as to the model compound to be used in the analysis of EXAFS spectra, like figure 4.8(d), from catheter deposits. The five inner shells of the HAP model provide a theoretical spectrum (dashed line) which agrees well with that observed experimentally (continuous line) after slight variations of r_j and σ_j values. Final values of r_j and σ_j were very similar to those obtained in interpreting the spectrum of poorly crystalline HAP shown in figure 4.6(e). Figure 4.8(f) shows good agreement between the modulus of the Fourier transforms, $g(r)$, of experimental (continuous line) and theoretical (dashed line) spectra.

CONCLUSIONS

The EXAFS regions of the absorption spectra of biological calcium phosphates have been used to provide information about their structures in two different ways: (1) to provide qualitative information by comparing spectra with those of known model compounds, and (2) to develop quantitative models for their structures in the form of the radial distribution of atoms around their calcium ions.

Simple comparison of spectra can be used to indicate the degree of crystallinity of a sample, and, in favourable cases, to provide some information about its chemical nature. Thus many EXAFS spectra lack the detailed subsidiary peaks characteristic of those recorded from highly crystalline model compounds, and so can be seen to be amorphous. This effect is illustrated, for synthetic model compounds, by comparing the spectrum of amorphous calcium phosphate (figure 4.6(a)) with that of fully crystalline hydroxyapatite (HAP; figure 4.6(c)), to which it is chemically very similar. It can be seen that the spectrum of figure 4.8(b) indicates that micellar calcium phosphate does not have an extended crystalline lattice. Also, the spectrum of bone mineral, in figure 4.8(a), clearly shows that it is a poorly crystalline form of HAP (whose spectrum is shown in figure 4.6(b)), rather than the highly crystalline form (spectrum in figure 4.6(c)).

Comparison of spectra might also be expected to identify the chemical nature of biological calcium phosphates – given the differences between the spectra of HAP, brushite and monetite in figure 4.5. Thus, for example, the spectrum of bone mineral (figure 4.8(a)) clearly resembles that of HAP (figure 4.5(a)) more closely than those of brushite (figure 4.5(b)) or monetite (figure 4.5(c)). However, it has never been seriously proposed that brushite or monetite provide models for the structure of mature bone mineral. Furthermore, the EXAFS spectrum of tricalcium phosphate ($Ca_3(PO_4)_2$) is very similar to that of HAP. Consequently, such qualitative comparisons, although they have proved useful in the past, are of limited value for defining the structures of biological calcium phosphates.

Analysis of EXAFS spectra is capable of providing useful structural information, provided there is independent evidence for the chemical nature of the calcium phosphate present. When the kind of starting model to be used is well defined, a theoretical spectrum can be very sensitive to the values of its structural parameters. For example, analysis of the

EXAFS spectrum of brushite was sensitive to which of two competing modes for its crystal structure was the better (Harries *et al.*, 1987c). Thus precise structural models for biological calcium phosphates can be developed by analysis of their EXAFS spectra, provided the appropriate model compound can be identified. This approach has provided useful structural information on bone mineral (Harries *et al.*, 1988) and on the poorly crystalline form of HAP encrusting urinary catheters (Hukins *et al.*, 1989). In both these cases, the calcium phosphate present resembles a poorly crystalline form of HAP. Since HAP has two different calcium ion sites within a unit cell, these models represent the environment of an averaged calcium ion site. Furthermore, these models consist of a radial distribution of atoms around this calcium ion, rather than the kind of stereochemical model provided by X-ray crystallography. Such radial distribution functions are a conventional method of describing the structures of disordered systems.

It has been more difficult to develop a model for the micellar calcium phosphate of milk because of the difficulty of choosing an appropriate model compound to use for the analysis of its EXAFS spectrum. Indeed, it was necessary to synthesise new forms of amorphous calcium phosphate, in which some of the phosphate groups are protonated, before any progress could be made (Holt *et al.*, 1988, 1989a, b). Thus X-ray absorption spectroscopy can provide precise quantitative structural information on biological calcium phosphates – provided that other chemical and spectroscopic techniques can provide information on their compositions.

ACKNOWLEDGEMENTS

We thank Dr C. Holt for collaboration in many aspects of the research reported here, and Professor J. Bordas for his encouragement and interest.

REFERENCES

Ashley, C. A. and Doniarch, S. (1975). Theory of extended X-ray absorption fine structure (EXAFS) in crystalline solids. *Phys. Rev.*, **B11**, 1279–88

Bearden, J. A. (1974). In *International Tables for X-Ray Crystallography* (eds J. A. Ibers and W. C. Hamilton), Vol. **4**, Kynoch Press, Birmingham, pp. 5–43

Binsted, N., Hasnain, S. S. and Hukins, D. W. L. (1982). Developmental changes in bone mineral structure demonstrated by extended X-ray absorption fine structure (EXAFS) spectroscopy. *Biochem. Biophys. Res. Commun.*, **107**, 89–92

Bordas, J. (1982). In *Uses of Synchrotron Radiation in Biology* (ed. H. B. Stuhrmann), Academic Press, New York, pp. 107–14

Boskey, A. L. (1981). Current concepts of the physiology and biochemistry of calcification. *Clin. Orthop. Rel. Res.* **157**, 225–57

Catlow, C. R. A. and Greaves, G. N. (1986). Synchrotron radiation – characteristics and techniques. *Chemy. Brit.*, **22**, 805–11

Cox, A. J., Harries, J. E., Hukins, D. W. L., Kennedy, A. P. and Sutton, T. M. (1987a). Calcium phosphate in catheter encrustation. *Brit. J. Urol.*, **59**, 159–63

Cox, A. J., Hukins, D. W. L., Davies, K. E., Irlam, J. C. and Sutton, T. M. (1987b). An automated technique for *in vitro* assessment of the susceptibility of urinary catheter materials to encrustation. *Eng. Med.*, **16**, 37–41

Curry, N. A. and Jones, D. W. (1971). Crystal structure of brushite, calcium hydrogen orthophosphate dihydrate: a neutron-diffraction investigation. *J. Chem. Soc. A.*, 3725–9

Diakun, G. P., Greaves. G. N., Hasnain, S. S. and Quinn, P. D. (1984). X-Ray absorption spectroscopy. SERC Daresbury Laboratory, Warrington, UK, Technical Memorandum DL/SCI/TM38E

Durham, P. J., Pendry, J. B. and Hodges, C. H. (1982). Calculation of X-ray absorption near edge structure, XANES. *Comput. Phys. Commun.*, **25**, 193–205

Eanes, E. D., Costa, J. L., MacKenzie, A. and Warburton, W. K. (1980). Technique for the preparation of solid specimens for X-ray absorption studies. *Rev. Sci. Inst.*, **51**, 1579–80

Eanes, E. D., Powers, L. and Costa, J. C. (1981). Extended X-ray absorption fine structure (EXAFS) studies on calcium in crystalline and amorphous solids of biological interest. *Cell Calcium*, **2**, 251–62

Eisenberger, P. and Kincaid, B. M. (1978) EXAFS: new horizons in structure determinations, *Science*, **200**, 1441–7

Elliot, J. S., Quaide, W. L., Sharp, R. F. and Lewis, L. (1958). Mineralogical studies of urine: the relationship of apatite, brushite and struvite to urinary pH. *J. Urol.*, **80**, 269–71

Greaves, G. N., Diakun, G. P., Quinn, P. D., Hart, M. and Siddons, D. P. (1983). An order-sorting monochromator for synchrotron radiation. *Nucl. Instr. Methods.*, **208**, 335–9

Greaves, G. N., Simkiss, K., Taylor, M. and Binsted, N. (1984). The local environment of metal sites in intracellular granules investigated by using X-ray absorption spectroscopy. *Biochem J.*, **221**, 855–68

Gurman, S. J. (1980). Notes on the EXAFS programs at the Daresbury Laboratory. SERC Daresbury Laboratory, Warrington, UK, Technical Memorandum DL/SCI/TM21T

Gurman, S. J. (1982). EXAFS studies in materials science. *J. Mater. Sci.*, **17**, 1541–70

Gurman, S. J. and Pendry J. B. (1976). Extraction of crystal parameters from EXAFS spectra. *Solid State Commun.*, **20**, 287–90

Gurman, S. J., Binsted, N. and Ross, I. (1984). A rapid, exact curved-wave theory for EXAFS calculations. *J. Phys. C: Solid State Phys.*, **17**, 143–51

Gurman, S. J., Binsted, N., and Ross, I. (1986). A rapid, exact, curved-wave theory for EXAFS calculations. II. The multiple scattering contributions. *J. Phys. C: Solid State Phys.*, **19**, 1845–61

Harries, J. E., Shah, J. S., and Hasnain, S. S. (1984). Structural study of arthropathic deposits. *Springer Proc. Phys.*, **2**, 142–4

Harries, J. E., Hukins, D. W. L. and Hasnain S. S. (1986a). Analysis of the EXAFS spectrum of hydroxyapatite. *J. Phys. C: Solid State Phys.*, **19**, 6859–72

Harries, J. E., Hukins, D. W. L. and Hasnain, S. S. (1986b). Multiple scattering in the EXAFS of calcium phosphates. *J. Physique*, **47**, C8.603–6

Harries, J. E., Hukins, D. W. L., Holt, C. and Hasnain, S. S. (1987a). Conversion of amorphous calcium phosphate into hydroxyapatite investigated by EXAFS spectroscopy. *J. Crystal Growth*, **84**, 563–70

Harries, J. E., Hasnain, S. S. and Shah, J. S. (1987b). EXAFS study of structural disorder in carbonate-containing apatites. *Calcif. Tiss. Intl.*, **41**, 346–50

Harries, J. E., Irlam, J. C., Holt, C., Hasnain, S. S. and Hukins, D. W. L. (1987c). Analysis of EXAFS spectra from the brushite and monetite forms of calcium phosphate. *Mater. Res. Bull.*, **22**, 1151–7

Harries, J. E., Hukins, D. W. L. and Hasnain, S. S. (1988). Calcium environment in bone mineral determined by EXAFS spectroscopy. *Calcif. Tiss. Intl.*, **43**, 250–3

Hasnain, S. S. (1984). Environment of calcium in biological calcium phosphates. *Springer Proc. Phys.* **2**, 145–80

Hasnain, S. S. (1987). Application of EXAFS and XANES to metalloproteins. *Life Chemistry Reports*, **4**, 273–331

Holt, C., Hasnain, S. S. and Hukins, D. W. L. (1982). Structure of bovine milk calcium phosphate determined by X-ray absorption spectroscopy. *Biochim. Biophys. Acta.*, **719**, 299–303

Holt, C., van Kemenade, M. J. J. M., Harries, J. E., Nelson, L. S., Bailey, R. T., Hukins,

D. W. L., Hasnain, S. S. and de Bruyn, P. L. (1988). Preparation of amorphous calcium and magnesium phosphates at pH 7 and characterisation by X-ray absorption and Fourier transform infrared spectroscopy. *J. Crystal Growth.*, **92**, 239–52

Holt, C., van Kemenade, M. J. J. M., Nelson, L. S., Sawyer, L., Harries, J. E., Bailey, R. T. and Hukins, D. W. L. (1989a). Composition and structure of micellar calcium phosphate. *J. Dairy Res.*, in press.

Holt, C., van Kemenade, M. J. J. M., Nelson, L. S., Hukins, D. W. L., Harries, J. E., Bailey, R. T., Hasnain, S. S. and de Bruyn, P. L. (1989b). Preparation and properties of amorphous calcium phosphates precipitated at pH 6.5 and 6.0. *Mater. Res. Bull.*, **23**, 55–62

Hukins, D. W. L. (1981). *X-Ray Diffraction by Disordered and Ordered Systems*, Pergamon, Oxford

Hukins, D. W. L. and Harries, J. E. (1987). Application of X-ray absorption spectroscopy to the investigation of biological calcification. In *Biophysics and Synchrotron Radiation* (eds A. Bianconi and A. Congiu Castellano), Springer, Berlin, pp. 238–45

Hukins, D. W. L., Hickey, D. S. and Kennedy, A. P. (1983). Catheter encrustation by struvite. *Br. J. Urol.*, **55**, 250–4

Hukins, D. W. L., Harries, J. E., Hasnain, S. S. and Holt, C. (1986a). Biological calcification: investigation by X-ray absorption spectroscopy, *J. Physique*, **47**, C8.1185–8

Hukins, D. W. L., Cox, A. J. and Harries, J. E. (1986b). EXAFS characterisation of poorly crystalline deposits from biological systems in the presence of highly crystalline mineral. *J. Physique*, **47**, C8.1181–4

Hukins, D. W. L., Harries, J. E. and Hasnain, S. S. (1986c). Extended X-ray absorption fine structure studies of calcification. *Biochem. Soc. Trans.*, **14**, 545–9

Hukins, D. W. L., Nelson, L. S., Harries, J. E., Cox, A. J. and Holt, C. (1989). Calcium environment in encrusting deposits from urinary catheters investigated by interpretation of EXAFS spectra. *J. Inorg. Biochem.*, in press

Irlam, J. C., Hukins, D. W. L., Holt, C. and Hasnain, S. S. (1984). Influence of phosphoproteins on calcification. *Springer Proc. Phys.*, **2**, 139–41

Irlam, J. C., Holt, C., Hasnain, S. S. and Hukins, D. W. L. (1985). Comparison of the structure of micellar calcium phosphate in milk from six species by extended X-ray absorption fine structure spectroscopy. *J. Dairy Res.*, **52**, 267–73

Jones, D. W. and Smith, J. A. S. (1962). The structure of brushite, $CaHPO_4 . 2H_2O$. *J. Chem. Soc.*, 1414–20

Kay, M. J., Young, R. A. and Posner, A. S. (1964). Crystal structure of hydroxyapatite. *Nature Lond.*, **204**, 1050–2

Kittel, C. (1986). *Introduction to Solid State Physics*, 6th edn, Wiley, New York

Koch, B. and MacGillavry, C. M. (1968). In *International Tables for X-Ray Crystallography* (eds C. H. MacGillavray and G. D. Rieck), Vol. 3, Kynoch Press, Birmingham, 157–200

Kronig, R. de L. (1931). Zur Theorie der Feinstruktur in den Röntgenabsorptionsspektren. *Zeitschrift Physik*, **70**, 317–23

Kronig, R. de L. (1932a). Zur Theorie der Feinstruktur in der Röntgenabsorptionsspektren. II. *Zeitschrift Physik*, **75**, 191–210

Kronig, P. de L. (1932b). Zur theorie der Feinstruktur in den Röntgenabsortionsspektren. III. *Zeitschrift Physik*, **75**, 468–75

Lee, P. A. and Pendry, J. B. (1975). Theory of the extended X-ray absorption fine structure. *Phys. Rev.*, **B11**, 2795–811

Lee, P. A., Citrin, P. H., Eisenberger, P. and Kincaid, B. M. (1981). Extended X-ray absorption fine structure – its strengths and limitations as a structural tool. *Rev. Mod. Phys.*, **53**, 769–806

Lipson, S. G. and Lipson, H. (1966). *Optical Physics*, Cambridge University Press, Cambridge

MacDowell, A. A., Norman, D. and West, J. B. (1986). Soft X-ray beam line for surface EXAFS studies in the energy range. $60 \leqslant h\nu \leqslant 11\,100$ eV at the Daresbury SRS. *Rev. Sci. Instrum.*, **57**, 2667–79

Miller, R. M., Hukins, D. W. L., Hasnain, S. S. and Lagarde, P. (1981). Extended x-ray absorption fine structure (EXAFS) studies of the calcium ion environment in bone mineral and related calcium phosphates. *Biochem. Biophys. Res. Commun.*, **99**, 102–6

Norberg, A., Norberg, B., Lundbeck, K. and Parkhede, U. (1980). Urinary pH and the indwelling catheter. *Uppsala J. Med. Sci.*, **85**, 143–50

Pendry, J. B. (1974). *Low Energy Electron Diffraction*, Academic Press, New York

Sayers, D. E., Stern, E. A. and Lytle, F. W. (1971). New technique for investigating noncrystalline structures: Fourier analysis of the extended X-ray absorption fine structure. *Phys. Rev. Lett.*, **27**, 1204–7

Shannon, C. E. (1948). A mathematical theory of communication. *Bell System Tech. J.*, **27**, 379–423

Stern, E. A. (1974). Theory of extended X-ray absorption fine structure. *Phys. Rev.*, **B10**, 3027–37

Taylor, M., Simkiss, K. and Greaves, G. N. (1986). Amorphous structure of intracellular mineral granules. *Biochem. Soc. Trans.*, **14**, 549–52

Termine, J. D. (1972). Mineral chemistry and skeletal biology. *Clin. Orthop. Rel. Res.*, **85**, 209–41

Teo, B. K. (1981). Novel method for angle determinations by EXAFS via a new multiple-scattering formalism. *J. Amer. Chem. Soc.*, **103**, 3990–4001

Williams, R. J. P. (1976). Calcium chemistry and its relation to biological function. *Symp. Soc. Exp. Biol.*, **30**, 1–17

5

Fourier transform infrared spectroscopy and characterisation of biological calcium phosphates

R. T. Bailey and C. Holt

INTRODUCTION

Biological calcium phosphates are, with few exceptions, poorly or partly crystalline and impure, and sometimes comprise a mixture of phases. Each component of a complex calcified deposit may be described with reference to some highly crystalline model compound of perfect stoichiometry such as the minerals hydroxyapatite (HAP, $Ca_{10}(OH)_2(PO_4)_6$), brushite (DCPD, $CaHPO_4 \cdot 2H_2O$) and monetite (DCPA, $CaHPO_4$), or octacalcium phosphate (OCP, $Ca_8H_2(PO_4)_6 \cdot 5H_2O$). The fascination of biological calcium phosphates arises from the deviations from these well-defined forms resulting in unique physical and chemical properties, some of which may reflect the history of the structure. Thus, the degree of static and dynamic disorder, the nature and location of substituents in a lattice, and larger-scale morphological differences such as crystal size, interlayering with non-calcium phosphate phases and crystal orientation, have all to be described. Infrared spectroscopy can and has played a part in the characterisation of biological calcium phosphates. Fourier transform instruments can do better what was done before and make possible some new types of measurements.

Infrared spectroscopy underwent a renaissance in the mid-1970s with the introduction of commercial Fourier transform infrared (FTIR) spectrometers. Subsequent rapid developments in minicomputers and associated hardware have resulted in the increased use of FTIR instruments covering a wide range, from low-cost, bench-top designs to high-cost, high-resolution research spectrometers covering the entire spectral range from the UV to the far infrared. In parallel with spectrometer development, accessories and sampling techniques have also evolved and can now cope with even the most intractable samples. Today, FTIR spectrometers are the instruments of choice, especially if extensive data manipulation is required, since the results are already stored in digital form and powerful computing hardware and software are available.

Analysis of complex systems such as biological calcium phosphates, showing broad and overlapping peaks, is particularly well suited to FTIR methods. Spectral deconvolution of broad peaks is essential in such cases if progress is to be made in interpreting the spectrum. The high wavelength accuracy of FT instruments also allows accurate spectral subtractions to be carried out, so that systems of closely related materials such as amorphous and crystalline calcium phosphates can be untangled.

In this review, a brief introduction is given to the theory of the Fourier transform method, the principles of instrument design, the accessories available and software. In the second part of the review, example spectra of various calcium phosphate systems of increasing complexity are presented and discussed.

THEORY

The most commonly employed interferometer used for infrared spectroscopy is that introduced by Michelson nearly a hundred years ago (figure 5.1). It consists, basically, of a fixed mirror, M_1, and a movable mirror, M_2. Bisecting the two mirrors at 45° is a beamsplitter B, which ideally

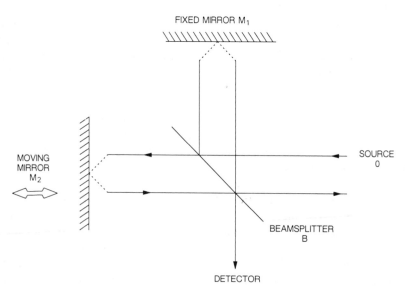

Figure 5.1   Schematic diagram of a Michelson interferometer.

transmits 50 per cent and reflects 50 per cent of the incident radiation. This is a critical and expensive component in any Michelson interferometer. The two reflected beams are recombined at the beamsplitter and are directed to a detector.

If M_1 and M_2 are positioned equal distances from B (zero retardation), the two beams are perfectly in phase and interfere constructively; the intensity passing to the detector is the sum of the intensities of the two interfering beams. If M_2 is moved by $x = \lambda/4$, where λ is the wavelength of the incident light, the beams will be 180° out of phase when recombined and will interfere destructively. At this point, all the light returns to the source and none passes to the detector. Thus, for a monochromatic light source, the signal generated at the detector is a cosine function of the mirror displacement. When a broad band light source is used, the output is a sum of all interferences produced by all the frequencies. The resulting signal is an interferogram, $I(x)$, which is related to the optical spectrum by the Fourier cosine transform:

$$I(x) = \int_{-\infty}^{\infty} \cos(2\pi x \nu) \cdot I(\nu)\, d\nu \qquad (5.1)$$

The optical spectrum, $I(\nu)$, is recovered by means of the inverse transform

$$I(\nu) = \int_{-\infty}^{\infty} \cos(2\pi x \nu) \cdot I(x)\, dx \qquad (5.2)$$

Practical application of equation (5.2) requires the use of a digital computer employing an algorithm similar to the Fast Fourier Transform (FFT) developed by Cooley and Tukey (1965) and applied to Fourier spectroscopy by Forman (1966). This algorithm extended the use of Fourier transform spectroscopy to encompass high-resolution data in all regions of the infrared spectrum.

Characteristics of FTIR spectroscopy

Since $I(\nu)$ in equation (5.2) is an even function, we can write

$$I(\nu) = \int_{0}^{\infty} \cos(2\pi x \nu) \cdot I(x)\, dx \qquad (5.3)$$

Thus, according to this expression, we could measure the complete spectrum from 0 to $+\infty$ (in cm^{-1}) at infinitely high resolution. However, to achieve this we would have to scan the moving mirror through an infinitely long distance, with x varying from 0 to $+\infty$ cm. Also, the Fourier transform would have to be digitised at infinitely small intervals of optical retardation. In practice, the signal is digitised at finite sampling intervals; the smaller the interval, the greater the spectral range that can be covered.

Also, the effect of moving the mirror through a limited distance causes the spectrum to have a finite resolution which is related to the retardation.

The Michelson interferometer measures all the frequencies simultaneously rather than one frequency at a time, as in a dispersion instrument. For the same output, therefore, FTIR spectroscopy is N times faster, where N is the number of elements in the spectrum. Alternatively, for the same measurement time, FTIR spectroscopy has a higher signal-to-noise ratio than that of a grating instrument. In addition, the use of mirrors in an interferometer, rather than narrow slits, results in an increase of 80–200 times greater energy throughput, depending on resolution. Other advantages of FTIR methods include high wavenumber precision, fast scanning options, lower stray light and multiple scanning capability.

A single-beam spectrum is recorded directly by an FTIR spectrometer, but usually either a transmittance or absorbance spectrum is required. The transmittance spectrum $\tau(\nu)$ is calculated by taking the ratio of single-beam spectra of a broad-band source with and without the sample present. The absorbance spectrum is subsequently calculated as $-\log_{10} \tau(\nu)$. In FT instruments, $\tau(\nu)$ cannot be obtained in real time, as with double-beam grating spectrometers, since its interferogram contains multiplexed information from all spectral elements.

Most of the present day mid-IR instruments are single-beam spectrometers and are purged with dry air to avoid atmospheric interference rather than being evacuated. This offers convenience where the small residual absorption due to water vapour is not important. However, if accurate spectral subtractions are to be carried out, interference from water vapour may pose a severe problem. The spectrum of atmospheric water and carbon dioxide is shown in figure 5.2. Double-beam instruments are available to reduce this potential problem.

Commercial FTIR instruments all have the sample compartment located between the interferometer and the detector. This is particularly important for the measurement of hot samples, since radiation from this source is not modulated and hence not detected by the electronics. The heating effect from the near IR radiation from the source is also reduced.

The optical throughput of commercial instruments varies considerably according to their design. If there is a choice, spectroscopists who deal mainly with small samples should choose an instrument which has low throughput optics or at least a small detector. However, if samples which absorb or scatter much of the incident light are to be examined, a higher throughput is preferred. Often a compromise is offered by manufacturers of medium-cost instruments.

For a given spectral range and resolution, there is a maximum solid angle, Ω_{max}, allowed:

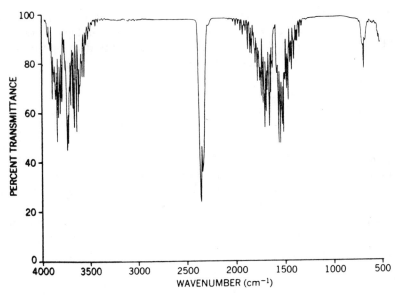

Figure 5.2 Transmittance spectrum of water vapour and carbon dioxide at the levels observed in a poorly purged FTIR spectrometer.

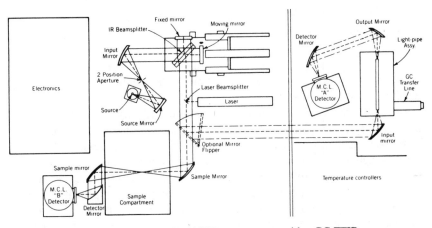

Figure 5.3 Optical layout of a Nicolet 20SXB spectrometer with a GC-FTIR accessory.

$$\Omega_{max} = 2\pi(\Delta\bar{\nu}/\bar{\nu}_{max})$$

where $\Delta\bar{\nu}$ is the desired resolution (in cm^{-1}) and $\bar{\nu}_{max}$ is the highest wavenumber in the spectrum. In medium- and high-resolution instruments, an aperture stop is installed in the source optics to control the solid angle. This aperture has the same effect as the entrance slit of a

·monochromator. In most spectrometers, the source is imaged at the aperture stop, at the focus in the sample compartment and at the detector.

Most middle-of-the-range instruments are configured to operate from about 5000 to 400 cm^{-1}, but some have alternative configurations which allow the near infrared up to 10 000 cm^{-1}, or the far infrared down to 50 cm^{-1} or below, to be employed. A typical mid-range instrument is the 20B series manufactured by Nicolet, the optical layout of which is shown in figure 5.3. The wavelength range is 5600 to 225 cm^{-1}, with a caesium iodide beamsplitter, and the maximum resolution is 0.5 cm^{-1}, continuously selectable down to 64 cm^{-1}. A maximum scan rate of 4 per second is available using an air bearing to move the mirror. An external collimated beam is available for use with remote detector experiments and accessories such as IR microscopes and GC-FTIR.

High-grade research instruments can cover the spectral range from 55 000 to 5 cm^{-1}; with suitable sources, beamsplitters and detectors and give very high resolution, in some cases better than 10^{-3} cm^{-1}.

ACCESSORIES

Absorption spectroscopy

Most cells have apertures of at least 10 mm in the shortest dimension, so that no significant fraction of the IR beam is blocked. Some accessories designed for grating spectrometers can also be used in FTIR instruments, but there will always be some loss of optical throughput, particularly with more optically complex accessories.

Beam condensers are available for examining small samples or small areas of larger samples. Often it is more convenient to use a microscope designed specifically for FTIR spectrometers. In these accessories, the size of the image at the sample is controlled by an aperture located at a focus in the microscope, where the solid angle of the beam is small, rather than at the sample focus, where it is large. The smallest sample that can be examined using an IR microscope is 10–20 μm diameter, limited by diffraction effects rather than by signal level. For greater efficiency, an MCT (mercury cadmium telluride) detector is preferred, fitted with a small element.

Reflection measurements

Specular reflectance spectra are easily recorded at incident angles of 15–75°, sometimes in conjunction with a beam condenser (4×–6×) for small samples. Smaller angles of incidence are more difficult to use with conventional optics, since the incident and reflected waves are difficult to separate. Measurements at normal incidence are easily made using a beamsplitter in the accessory.

Reflection–absorption (R–A) measurements of surface films, 1–20 μm thick, are generally made using standard specular reflectance accessories. For very thin layers (less than 1 μm thick), R–A measurements should be carried out using grazing incidence. A typical optical configuration used to achieve this is shown in figure 5.4 (Ishitari *et al.*, 1982). With this kind of arrangement, monolayers of the order of 1 nm thick have been measured using an incident radiation angle of 5° to the surface. A significant increase in sensitivity is achieved by the use of polarised radiation used at grazing angles of incidence. This enhancement arises from two factors. First, the grazing incidence increases the effective pathlength of the layer to $2d/\sin \theta$, where d is the thickness of the layer and θ the angle the beam makes with the surface. Second, the electric field (and, consequently, the absorption) is increased for light polarised perpendicular to the plane of incidence and hence parallel to the surface. Greenler (1966, 1969) has shown that if a beam polarised parallel to the surface is reflected at close to grazing incidence, interference between the incident and reflected rays can set up an intense standing wave at the surface. This can give an intensity enhancement for absorbing species on the surface by factors of up to 25 relative to the absorption of the perpendicularly polarised beam. Accessories have also been constructed that employ multiple reflections as well as grazing incidence.

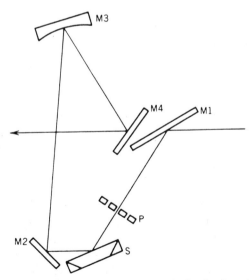

Figure 5.4   Optical configuration for measuring polarised reflection–absorption spectra at near-grazing incidence.

Attenuated total reflectance (ATR)

The principle of ATR is illustrated in figure 5.5. A beam of light entering the crystal undergoes total internal reflection when the angle of incidence at the interface of sample and crystal is greater than the critical angle for reflection, which is a function of the refractive indices of the crystal and sample. The beam penetrates a fraction of a wavelength (a few micrometres) beyond the reflecting surface into the sample. Selective absorption occurs and the resultant attenuated beam passes out through the exit face of the crystal. The depth of penetration is a function of the wavelength, of the refractive indices of the crystal and the sample, and of the angle of incidence. Generally, a high-refractive-index crystal such as KRS-5 is chosen. Depths of penetration for various angles of incidence for KRS-5 and germanium are included in figure 5.5.

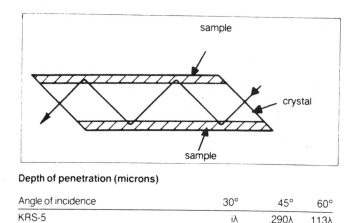

Depth of penetration (microns)

Angle of incidence	30°	45°	60°
KRS-5	iλ	.290λ	.113λ
Ge	.091λ	.041λ	.002λ

(i = total penetration. sample index = 1.5)

Figure 5.5   Optical transmission of an ATR (attenuated total reflection) crystal. The depth of penetration for various angles of incidence are also listed.

A spherical ATR (attenuated total reflection) cell specially designed for aqueous solutions is the Spectra-Tech Circle Cell shown schematically in figure 5.6. The energy transmitted by this cell is greater than 50 per cent when a zinc selenide crystal is used. A version of the cell with a crystal of square cross-section is also available. With such cells, good-quality spectra of the solute can be obtained in aqueous solutions of only 0.1 per cent concentration. These accessories have proved very useful for the study of FTIR spectra of biological molecules in an aqueous environment. Temperature-controlled and flow versions are available.

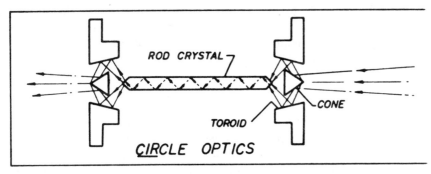

Figure 5.6 Optical alignment of the cylindrical internal reflection (CIRCLE) accessory.

Diffuse reflectance (DRIFT)

Diffuse reflectance infrared spectra of most powdered samples can now be recorded routinely. Even formerly intractable materials such as coal can now be analysed. Accessories for DRIFT measurements are available from several companies, most versions of which are based on two ellipsoidal mirrors. The first mirror condenses the beam and focuses it onto the sample and the second collects a high proportion of the diffuse reflectance while rejecting most of the specular component. In most designs, additional provision is made for rejecting specularly reflected light. One example of a DRIFT accessory is shown in figure 5.7. The sample is placed

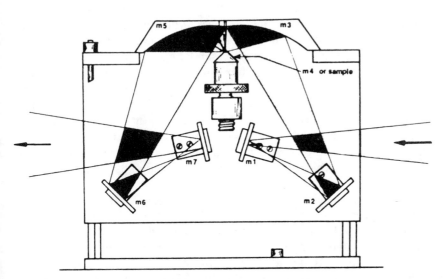

Figure 5.7 Optical diagram of the diffuse reflectance (DRIFT) accessory designed by Spectra-Tech.

in a small cup on which a knife edge can be placed to reduce the specular component. Specialist cells that can be used to study gas–solid reactions at high pressures and temperatures are also available. These cells are designed to be used in conjunction with the DRIFT accessory.

Software

Once interferograms have been collected and averaged, the next stage is usually Fourier transformation to yield the spectrum. Since all FTIR spectrometers are single-beam instruments, background and sample spectra are stored and collected independently. Once the data have been collected and transformed, the rest of the software performs other operations such as spectral comparisons, smoothing, interpolation, baseline subtraction, integration, differentiation, deconvolution and curve fitting.

Sometimes spectra have sloping baselines which can be removed by subtraction of a smoothly varying function. The simplest baseline to subtract is a straight line defined by its intercept parameter (tilt, t) and slope (curvature, c). At each point in the spectrum, the ordinate value $Y(\bar{v})$ is corrected to $Y'(\bar{v})$ by:

$$Y'(\bar{v}) = Y(\bar{v}) - (t + c\bar{v})$$

Curved baselines can be subtracted using quadratic or higher-order polynomials.

Smoothing the spectrum reduces the effect of noise but degrades spectral resolution. One of the simplest smoothing operations is boxcar integration, which is accomplished by taking each ordinate in the spectrum and calculating a new value from the mean of a small number ($\leqslant 4$) of values on either side. Other algorithms perform similar operations, but the surrounding data are weighted by various functions such as Lorentzian, Gaussian or triangular curves. When these functions are employed, the points farther from the central value are given less weight. Smoothing may also be accomplished in the Fourier domain by computing the Fourier transform of the spectrum, multiplying by a suitable apodisation function and then computing the inverse transform. Although smoothing may make the data more aesthetically pleasing, it may reduce resolution by a factor of two or more.

Spectral subtraction is widely used in FTIR spectroscopy, for example in subtracting the spectrum of the solvent from the solution to reveal the spectrum of the dissolved solute. Some spectral subtraction routines permit data to be scaled to account for concentration differences. The scaling factors are selected by monitoring deviations from the baseline. The technique can also be used to identify a component or components by subtracting a known spectrum. These are just examples of the constantly expanding range of standard software supplied with FTIR instruments. In addition, many high-level languages are now supported, which has led to the development of specific software packages distributed by the instrument manufacturers. Some examples are spectral deconvolution, quantitative analysis, spectral peak fitting and GC-FTIR software.

Two useful procedures for analysing complex overlapping peaks are derivative spectroscopy and Fourier self-deconvolution.

If a single-sided absorption interferogram is multiplied by a function of the form ax^n, computation of the forward transform gives the nth derivative of the spectrum. Second-derivative FTIR spectra are most commonly used. The effect is to sharpen up the bands, giving apparently increased resolution, but at the expense of artificially distorting the peak shape. It should be noted, however, that taking the derivative of a spectrum increases the noise; increasing the order of a derivative by two degrades the signal-to-noise ratio of a spectrum by a factor of about 10.

Fourier self-deconvolution is a process whereby the apparent resolution of a spectrum is increased as overlapping bands are separated into their components. A selected part of the spectrum is Fourier transformed and the interferogram divided by an appropriate function (Kauppinen *et al.*, 1981a, b, c) before back-transforming the data. The reduction in the width of the peaks that can be achieved depends on the signal-to-noise ratio and also on the resolution at which the spectrum was originally recorded. It is theoretically impossible to create a linewidth less than the instrument resolution, even for noise-free spectra, unless severe side lobes can be tolerated. The selection of the parameters used in Fourier self-deconvolution is usually carried out empirically, so it is necessary to watch out for the appearance of side lobes which indicate that the spectrum has been 'overdeconvolved'. To check if all the features in a deconvolved spectrum are genuine, it is best to repeat the measurement at higher resolution and signal-to-noise ratio. If a feature varies when this is done then it is probably an artefact.

VIBRATIONAL SPECTRA OF CRYSTALLINE CALCIUM PHOSPHATES

The PO_4^{3-} ion has T_d symmetry (table 5.1). Consequently, the isolated ion is expected to have a symmetric stretch, v_1, not infrared active but observed in Raman spectra at about $936 \, cm^{-1}$, and a triply degenerate asymmetric stretch, v_3, at about $1004 \, cm^{-1}$. In addition, there is a doubly degenerate symmetric OPO bending mode, v_2, at about $420 \, cm^{-1}$ and a triply degenerate asymmetric OPO bend, v_4, at about $573 \, cm^{-1}$. Protonation of the phosphate group effectively reduces the symmetry to C_{3v} giving eight vibrational modes. These are the symmetric stretch, v_2, which is increased in frequency to about $988 \, cm^{-1}$, and the doubly degenerate OPO

Table 5.1   Vibrational modes of PO_4^{3-} and HPO_4^{2-}

PO_4^{3-} (T_d)		HPO_4^{2-} (C_{3v})	
P–O stretch	$\nu_1 A_1$ 936	P–O stretch	$\nu_2 A$ 988
O–P–O bend	$\nu_2 E$ 420	O–P–O bend	$\nu_8 E$ 394
		P–O(H) stretch	$\nu_3 A$ 862
P–O stretch	$\nu_3 F_2$ 1004 $\left\{\vphantom{\begin{array}{c}a\\b\end{array}}\right.$	P–O stretch	$\nu_6 E$ 1076
		O–P–O bend	$\nu_4 A$ 537
O–P–O bend	$\nu_4 F_2$ 573 $\left\{\vphantom{\begin{array}{c}a\\b\end{array}}\right.$	O–P–O bend	$\nu_7 E$ 537
		(P–)O–H stretch	$\nu_1 A$ 2900
		P–O–H bend	$\nu_5 E$ 1230

bend, ν_8, at the reduced frequency of 394 cm^{-1}, compared with 420 cm^{-1} for ν_2 (PO_4^{3-}). The triply degenerate asymmetric stretch, ν_3, is split into a doubly degenerate mode, ν_6, at about 1076 cm^{-1} and a P–O(H) stretch, ν_3, at 862 cm^{-1}. Although the ν_4 (PO_4^{3-}) mode is also split into doubly degenerate (ν_7) and non-degenerate (ν_4) OPO bends, these occur at the same frequency of about 537 cm^{-1}. Two new vibrational modes are introduced by protonation: ν_1, the PO–H stretch at about 2900 cm^{-1} and the doubly degenerate POH bend, ν_5, at about 1230 cm^{-1}.

The degenerate modes can be split in a crystal lattice by the effect of the symmetry of the site. Splitting of degenerate and non-degenerate modes can also occur through the correlated motions of phosphate groups in the primitive lattice (factor group splitting). In general, a site symmetry analysis is sufficient to predict the number of modes seen in spectra of powdered samples. However, evidence of the effects of factor group splitting has come from Raman studies on single crystals and from differences in frequencies observed in infrared and Raman spectra (Griffith, 1970; Kravitz *et al.*, 1968). A notable exception is monetite, where a factor group analysis has proved essential for the interpretation of its spectrum (Casciani and Condrate, 1980).

In crystalline hydrated calcium phosphates, vibrational bands due to water molecules are seen, and librational modes can also be expected in the range 700–300 cm^{-1}. In water vapour, the molecular (symmetry C_{2v}) gives rise to three internal modes: the asymmetric (ν_3) and totally symmetric (ν_1) stretches and the HOH deformation, ν_2. In crystalline hydrates, the stretching modes are found at 3550–3200 cm^{-1} and the bending mode at 1630–1600 cm^{-1}. The infrared spectra of the crystalline calcium phosphates are highly characteristic of the different phases and can be used with confidence for the purpose of identification.

Hydroxyapatite

Baddiel and Berry (1966) gave a detailed analysis of the infrared spectrum of HAP, but their sample was not very crystalline and the spectrum obtained was not of the same quality as can now be recorded routinely using an FTIR spectrometer (figure 5.8). The salient distinguishing features of the spectrum are as follows. A sharp band of low intensity at 3566 cm^{-1} is due to the OH stretch of the hydroxide ions. Three bands are seen in this HAP specimen in the region where the three components of ν_3 are expected; the peak positions are 1093.2, 1057.2 and 1034.0 cm^{-1}. The nominally forbidden, totally symmetric stretch is seen as a sharp band of low intensity at 962.6 cm^{-1}. In the region where the components of ν_4 are expected there are, indeed, three bands clearly resolved at 633.1, 604.0 and 565.2 cm^{-1}. However, Baddiel and Berry (1966) considered it possible

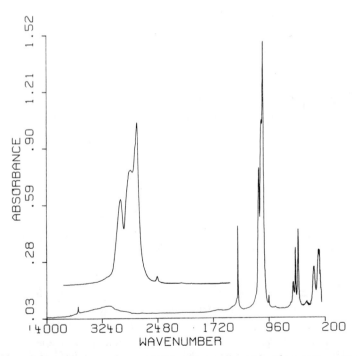

Figure 5.8 Infrared spectrum of crystalline hydroxyapatite at 2 cm^{-1} resolution with (inset) an expansion of the phosphate stretching region, 1300–700 cm^{-1}.

that the degeneracy of this mode was not completely lifted and that the band at the highest frequency in this triplet is not a component of v_4 but is either a librational mode of the hydroxide ion or a combination band formed by Fermi resonance of the two components of v_2 at 353.0 and 283.3 cm^{-1}. That the band at 633.1 cm^{-1} is not a component of v_4 is supported by Raman and IR spectra on single crystals of fluorapatite (Adams and Gardner, 1974), where IR bands at 580 (E_{1u}), 582 (A_u) and 614 (E_{1u}) cm^{-1} were assigned to the v_4 mode. The very sharp band at 1384.4 cm^{-1}, shown in figure 5.8, is due to nitrate ions trapped in the hydroxyapatite sample during its synthesis and not removed by subsequent washing.

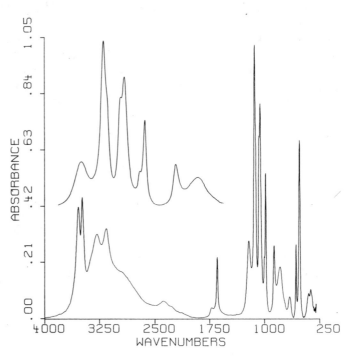

Figure 5.9   Spectrum of brushite, $CaHPO_4 . 2H_2O$, at 2 cm^{-1} resolution, with (inset) an expansion of the phosphate stretching region 1300–700 cm^{-1}.

Close inspection of the phosphate stretching region (figure 5.10b) reveals a shoulder on the most intense peak at 1034.0 cm^{-1} and Fourier self-deconvolution reveals a component at about 1041.9 cm^{-1}, which possibly arises by factor group splitting, though in fluorapatite there is incomplete site splitting of v_3, with two resonances at 1030 and 1034 cm^{-1} (Adams and Gardner, 1974).

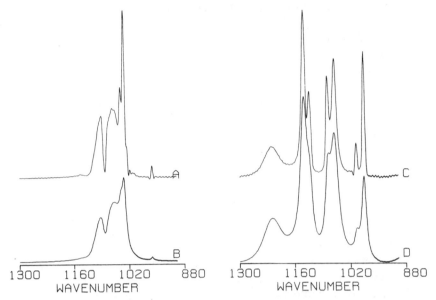

Figure 5.10 Spectra of brushite (D) and hydroxyapatite (B) at 2 cm^{-1} resolution in the phosphate stretching region and the same spectra after Fourier self-deconvolution. (A) hydroxyapatite deconvolved with a peak width of 10 cm^{-1} and resolution efficiency of 1.8. (B) Brushite deconvolved with a peak width of 10 cm^{-1} and a resolution efficiency of 2.0. In both cases a cosine apodisation was applied.

Brushite

The spectrum of brushite is more complicated than that of hydroxyapatite (figures 5.9 and 5.10), principally because of the presence of water molecules in two crystallographically distinct sets of sites. Casciani and Condrate (1979) have given a detailed interpretation of the Raman spectrum and reassessed the earlier infrared work. The main features of the spectrum at high frequency are a pair of doublets (3542.2 + 3489.1 cm^{-1} and 3285.7 + 3159.4 cm^{-1}), belonging to the stretching modes of water, and a broad resonance at about 3000 cm^{-1}, belonging to the OH stretch of the phosphate groups. The water bending mode, ν_2, occurs at 1649.3 cm^{-1}, with a subsidiary peak at 1729.5 cm^{-1}, which, in other work, has been identified only as a shoulder. This latter feature appears to be a combination band rather than a second bending mode of the two distinct water molecules.

The internal modes of the HPO$_4^{2-}$ ion are shown in greater detail in (figure 5.10). The totally symmetric stretch, ν_2, is shown here to be a doublet produced by factor group splitting, with the main component of symmetry A' at 986.7 cm^{-1} and a less intense resonance at 1004.5 cm^{-1} of symmetry A″. Previously recorded spectra showed only a shoulder in this region. Likewise, one of the components of v_6 is resolved as a doublet, whereas the other component appears as a peak with an unresolved shoulder. Fourier self-deconvolution in conjunction with Raman studies on single crystals allows the bands of A′ symmetry (1136.7 and 1059.8 cm⁻¹) and A″ symmetry (1122.8 and 1059.8 cm⁻¹) to be assigned. These results illustrate the high quality of spectra obtainable by Fourier transform spectroscopy.

The in-plane bending mode of POH occurs at 1219.4 cm⁻¹, whereas the other component of v_5, which involves rotation of the O–H bond about the P–O axis, occurs at 792.5 cm⁻¹. Neither these bands nor the P–O(H) stretch at 878.9 cm⁻¹ show evidence of factor group splitting in the infrared (figure 5.10).

Whereas the v_4 and v_7 OPO bending modes of the free HPO_4^{2-} are unresolved, in brushite these appear as a peak of medium intensity at 577.0 cm⁻¹ and a strong band with a shoulder at 528.0 cm⁻¹ respectively. In poorly crystalline calcium phosphates, the resolution of v_4 and v_7 bands is often seen, while degenerate modes remain unresolved.

The final point of interest in the brushite spectrum is a broad peak of low intensity at 661.0 cm⁻¹, having a shoulder at 673.0 cm⁻¹. Berry and Baddiel (1967) asign these to librations of the two water molecules.

Monetite

The infrared spectrum of monetite is shown in figure 5.11. Again, the high quality of the spectrum can be judged by comparison with the spectrum recorded using a conventional spectrometer (Petrov *et al.*, 1967). In the unit cell of monetite there are two sets of pairs of phosphate groups, and in each primitive cell the phosphate groups are related by a centre of symmetry. Coupled vibrational modes cause factor group splitting of site group bands and further splitting occurs because of the two sites present. Catti *et al.* (1977) have shown by neutron diffraction that three different hydrogen bonds occur within its structure and that disorder is introduced because one of the O–H---O bonds has two positions for the hydrogen atom. The number of OH stretches seen in the infrared (Petrov *et al.*, 1967) and Raman (Casciani and Condrate, 1980) spectra are consistent with the crystal structure, but as yet there have been no assignments of bands to the individual hydrogen bonds. The bands assigned to the in-plane POH bending mode cover an unusually wide spectral range (1410–1356 cm⁻¹ with a weak band at 1265 cm⁻¹). These, and the other phosphate internal vibrational modes, show a considerable degree of narrowing on cooling to 77 °K, to reveal the factor groups and site group splittings mentioned above (Petrov *et al.*, 1967). For example, the P–O(H) stretch at 900 cm⁻¹ is split at 77 K into three distinct bands of medium intensity at 910, 890 and 868

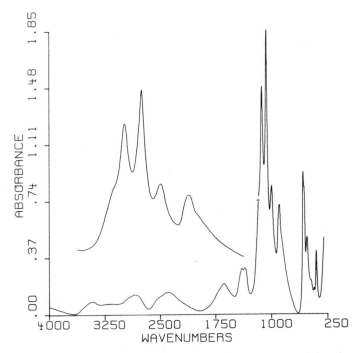

Figure 5.11 Spectrum of monetite, $CaHPO_4$, at $2\,cm^{-1}$ resolution, with (inset) an expansion of the phosphate stretching region $1200-700\,cm^{-1}$.

cm^{-1}, with a shoulder at $849\,cm^{-1}$. Moreover, the POH out-of-plane bend is not resolved at 300 K, but appears as a weak band at $790\,cm^{-1}$, with possibly two shoulders at 760 and $700\,cm^{-1}$ (Petrov *et al.*, 1967).

Octacalcium phosphate

The infrared spectrum of OCP is more complex than the other calcium phosphates considered so far. This compound usually occurs in association with hydroxyapatite and is usually prepared in the laboratory by hydrolysis of brushite (Brown *et al.*, 1957). The infrared spectrum of OCP was interpreted by Fowler *et al.* (1966), but because of its complexity many of the assignments are uncertain. A spectrum very similar to that obtained by Fowler *et al.* (1966) is shown in figure 5.12; the sample was prepared by precipitation from solution at pH 6.1 in the presence of a very low concentration of the milk protein κ-casein (van Kemenade, 1988). There is a broad and relatively featureless OH stretching band due to the hydrogen-bonded water molecules and HPO_4^{2-} ions, and the water bending mode appears as a band at $1630\,cm^{-1}$. The weak bands at 910 and $865\,cm^{-1}$ are assigned to the out-of-plane POH deformations of the two distinct HPO_4^{2-}

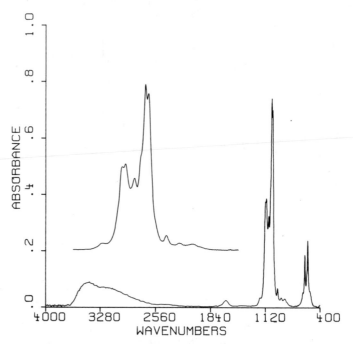

Figure 5.12 Spectrum of octacalcium phosphate, $Ca_8H_2(PO_4)_6 \cdot 5\,H_2O$, at 2 cm^{-1} resolution, with (inset) an expansion of the phosphate stretching region 1300–700 cm^{-1}.

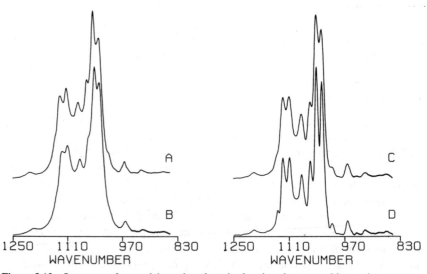

Figure 5.13 Spectrum of octacalcium phosphate in the phosphate stretching region at room temperature (B) and 10 K (A). Spectrum C is the room temperature spectrum after Fourier self-deconvolution using a peak width of 12 cm^{-1} and resolution efficiency of 1.1. Spectrum D employed a higher-resolution efficiency (1.3) and a peak width of 11 cm^{-1}.

groups in the unit cell of OCP, and are characteristic features of this phase. In the phosphate stretching region, the bands are relatively broad and show a considerable degree of overlap, but, in contrast to the observation with monetite, cooling to 10 K produces only a small degree of narrowing of the bands and only a shoulder at about 1050 cm^{-1} is resolved by cooling, as a distinct maximum at 1058.9 cm^{-1}. Shoulders at about 1004 and 1140 cm^{-1} are, however, more distinct at 10 K than at room temperature (figure 5.13). This possibly indicates that there is a significant contribution to the peak widths from static disorder in at least this preparation of OCP.

The effects of Fourier self-deconvolution on the spectrum of OCP at room temperature in the range 1250–850 cm^{-1} are illustrated by spectra C and D in figure 5.13. Qualitatively, the reduction of peak widths by 10 per cent (figure 5.13C) produces a similar effect on the spectrum, as does cooling to 10 K, though, of course, frequency shifts are not introduced by Fourier self-deconvolution. A reduction in peak widths of approximately a third was required to resolve the shoulders on either side of the main group of absorption bands (figure 5.13D). These examples illustrate the value of Fourier self-deconvolution in providing additional quantitative information about the spectra of calcium phosphates.

AMORPHOUS CALCIUM PHOSPHATES

The generic term amorphous calcium phosphate is applied to a wide range of materials. A hydrated ACP with the stoichiometry of a tricalcium phosphate ($Ca_3(PO_4)_2.xH_2O$) can be prepared by precipitation from solution at alkaline pH, and has been well studied. At lower pH, HPO_4^{2-} ions can be incorporated in the structure, but, below pH 6.6, OCP or brushite tends to form rather than an ACP. Nevertheless, ACPs can be produced at lower pH by incorporating a stabilising agent such as Mg^{2+} or citrate. Infrared spectroscopy provides a sensitive means of distinguishing between these different ACPs (Holt *et al.*, 1988; 1989).

The spectrum of an amorphous calcium phosphate prepared at pH 7 is shown in figure 5.14. It exhibits only broad phosphate stretching and bending modes and a broad, relatively featureless hydroxyl stretching region, characteristic of disordered hydrogen-bonded water molecules and phosphate hydroxyl groups. The phosphate stretching regions of various ACP preparations are shown in figure 5.15 and show that, while the spectra are superficially similar, there are clear differences of detail. The sample prepared at pH 10 contains few, if any, protonated phosphate groups, so the main absorption band and a shoulder at about 950 cm^{-1} can be assigned to the asymmetric and symmetric stretching modes of PO_4^{3-} species, respectively; there is very little absorption at about 890 cm^{-1}. The ACPs prepared at pH 7, 6.5 and 6.0 all show a broad band at 890 cm^{-1}, which can be assigned to the P–O(H) stretching mode of HPO_4^{2-} groups,

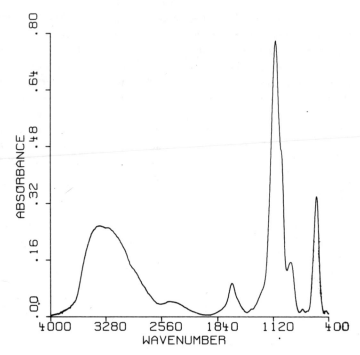

Figure 5.14 Spectrum of an amorphous calcium phosphate prepared at pH 7.0 in the presence of Mg^{2+}. The peak at 890 cm^{-1} is mainly due to the P–O(H) stretch, indicating an appreciable content of protonated phosphate groups.

but it overlaps the resonance at 950 cm^{-1}. The more acidic ACPs also differ from the basic ACP in having a prominent shoulder at about 1010 cm^{-1} and the main absorption bands are broadened on the high-frequency side of the peaks. In some acidic ACPs, a very broad shoulder at about 1200 cm^{-1} can be discerned which may be due to the in-plane bending mode of POH (Holt *et al.*, 1988; 1989). This latter feature, together with the more consistently observed differences between acidic and basic ACPs, can be revealed more clearly by Fourier self-deconvolution. The average peak width of Lorentzian peaks giving rise to the peaks and shoulders shown in figure 5.15 is in the range 30–70 cm^{-1}. Moreover, when the sample shown in figure 5.14 was cooled to 10 K, there was no change in the shape of the phosphate stretching envelope, demonstrating that thermal motion makes a negligible contribution to the breadth of the bands and hence that these samples are amorphous because of static disorder.

Biological calcium phosphates frequently contain carbonate ions substituting either for the hydroxide ion of apatites or for phosphate groups in the lattice. Carboxyl groups may also be preferentially located on the

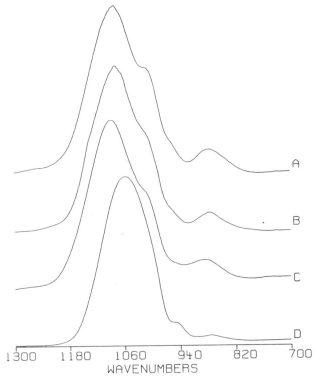

Figure 5.15 Spectra at 2 cm^{-1} resolution of amorphous calcium phosphates prepared at pH 6.0 in the presence of citrate (A); at pH 6.5 in the presence of Mg^{2+} (B); at pH 7.0 in the presence of Mg^{2+} (C, see figure 5.14), and at pH 10 (D). Note the change in relative amplitude of the peak at 890 cm^{-1}.

surface of crystallites (Elliot, 1963; LeGeros, 1965; Doi *et al.*, 1982). The spectrum of a carbonate-containing ACP is shown in figure 5.16, and shows the characteristic signature of carbonate groups with bands at about 1490, 1427 and 875 cm^{-1}. The latter band, due to the CO_3^{2-} out-of-plane vibration, can be confused, in the absence of other information, with the P–O(H) stretching mode of HPO_4^{2-}. In biological calcium phosphates formed near neutral pH, both types of resonance can be expected.

MICELLAR CALCIUM PHOSPHATE

Phosphoproteins and phosphopeptides are frequently found to be associated with mineralisation processes. One of the most easily studied phosphoprotein–calcium phosphate complexes is the casein micelle from milk. These colloidal particles comprise very many small clusters of calcium and phosphate ions, dispersed more or less uniformly throughout a matrix of

Calcified Tissue

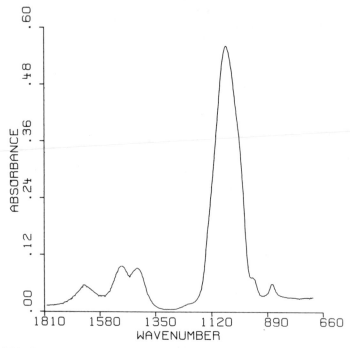

Figure 5.16 Spectrum of a carbonated amorphous calcium phosphate prepared at pH 10 and measured at 2 cm^{-1} resolution.

phosphoproteins. The phosphate moiety of phosphoseryl residues appears to be linked to the amorphous calcium phosphate clusters, so that a complex between phosphopeptides and calcium phosphate can be isolated for further study (Holt *et al.*, 1986). The spectrum of this micellar calcium phosphate is shown in figure 5.17; it shows major peaks at 1660.1 and 1565.6 cm^{-1} and a minor peak at 1248.8 cm^{-1}, which can be mainly assigned to the amide I, II and III modes of the peptide bonds of the phosphopeptides in the complex. A peak at 1410.4 cm^{-1} with a shoulder at 1441.6 cm^{-1} is due to the CH$_2$ groups of side-chains of amino acid residues, and citrate ions associated with the calcium phosphate. In the phosphate stretching region, there is a major peak at 1085.3 cm^{-1}, with a second peak at 997.0 cm^{-1}, but the lack of fine structure is consistent with an amorphous material. At the pH of milk (6.7), an amorphous calcium phosphate is expected to contain both PO$_4^{3-}$ and HPO$_4^{2-}$. Thus the peak at 997.0 cm^{-1} could be due to the symmetric stretch of the HPO$_4^{2-}$ and RPO$_4^{2-}$ (phosphoseryl) groups superimposed on the asymmetric stretching mode of all the phosphate groups. Notably absent from the spectrum of the isolated micellar calcium phosphate is the P–O(H) stretch at about 890 cm^{-1}, characteristic of the presence of protonated phosphate groups.

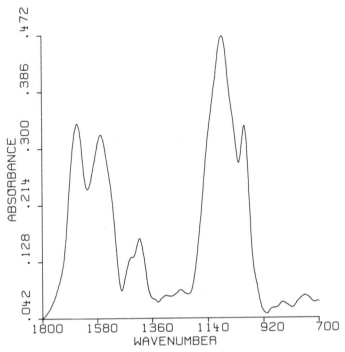

Figure 5.17 Spectrum at 2 cm^{-1} resolution of micellar calcium phosphate prepared from bovine casein micelles by the method of Holt *et al.* (1986).

However, in this region of the spectrum there are a number of other absorption peaks which could obscure the presence of this rather weak absorption band.

MIXED CALCIUM PHOSPHATE PHASES

Minerals provide many examples of non-interacting phases where the overall spectrum can be treated as a linear combination of the spectra of the individual components. The coefficients of the linear combination (i.e., the concentrations) can then be found by spectral fitting techniques.

The methodology for obtaining spectra suitable for a components analysis is not straightforward, because of the marked dependence of absorption on particle size for minerals dispersed in a potassium bromide matrix, but, with care, conditions can be found in which all components give a linear relation between absorption and concentration. Various curve-fitting programs are available for spectral analysis (Antoon *et al.*, 1977; Brown and Elliott, 1985; Brown *et al.*, 1982), and in simple cases spectral subtraction can be used.

Two examples of mixed systems will be considered, both of which are

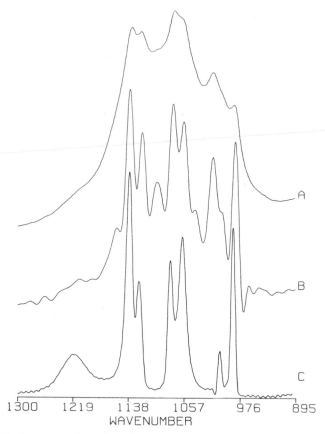

Figure 5.18 Spectrum at 2 cm^{-1} resolution of a maturing amorphous calcium phosphate at pH 7.0 (A) and after Fourier self-deconvolution with a peak width of 12 cm^{-1} resolution efficiency of 1.5 (B). Spectrum C is of brushite after Fourier self-deconvolution under the same conditions as B.

relevant to biological mineralisation processes. In the first, maturation of an ACP produced at pH 7 in the presence of Mg^{2+} results in a mixture of amorphous material and brushite; although the brushite nucleates and grows on the ACP, the degree of interaction of the two phases is small enough to be neglected and spectral subtraction can be used to establish the proportion of each phase. In the second example, maturation of an ACP prepared at pH 10 results in a poorly crystalline hydroxyapatite and at no stage is it appropriate to apply a components analysis for a non-interacting system. A components analysis is most likely to be appropriate in systems with clearly defined boundaries between microscopic phases, but even then there may be complications that are due to variations in the degree of crystalline order and/or the presence of impurities in one or more of the components.

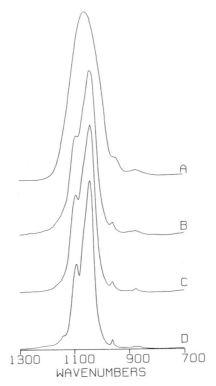

Figure 5.19   Spectra at 4 cm^{-1} resolution of maturing calcium phosphate, prepared at pH 10 and incubated in the same solution for periods of 6 (A), 14 (B), 19 (C) and 48 (D) hours.

The infrared spectrum of a maturing ACP/brushite mixture (Holt *et al.*, 1988) is shown in figure 5.18A, in the range 1300–900 cm^{-1}. Various sharper bands are superimposed on a broad band of degenerate phosphate stretching modes. Scanning electron microscopy showed plate-like crystals growing on the surface of an amorphous phase, indicating that a components analysis might be valid. Fourier self-deconvolution reveals the characteristic splitting pattern of brushite (figure 5.18B), and after subtraction of the spectrum of brushite a broad relatively featureless peak was recovered, very similar in shape to that of the original ACP. In this example, the proportion of phosphate groups in a brushite-like environment was 27 ± 3 per cent.

The spectra shown in figure 5.19 show a quite different process of maturation in which the original ACP, incubated at pH 10, in contact with the solution from which it was precipitated, matures to form poorly crystalline hydroxyapatite (Harries *et al.*, 1987). A careful analysis of the positions of features in the spectrum, aided by Fourier self-deconvolution, indicates that there are small frequency changes, as well as narrowing of the component peaks during maturation, such that the intermediate spectra (B and C in figure 5.19) cannot be represented as a weighted sum of the initial and final spectra (A and D in figure 5.19).

COMPLEX MINERALISED DEPOSITS

Infrared spectroscopy can be useful in identifying the components in complex biological calcified deposits, particularly in poorly crystalline materials where X-ray powder diffraction patterns may not be conclusive. Spectra A and C in figure 5.20 are of encrustations removed from urinary catheters and resemble, respectively, the spectra of struvite ($NH_4MgPO_4 . 6H_2O$, spectrum B) and a carbonate-containing ACP (spectrum D). Note, however, that spectrum C shows splitting of the OPO bending mode at about 570 cm^{-1}, whereas the main phosphate stretching peak is free of sharp bands.

The catheter encrustations whose spectra are shown in figure 5.20 are not typical, to the extent that most are mixtures of poorly crystalline carbonate–apatite and struvite (Cox *et al.*, 1987a). Both these phases tend to be formed at alkaline pH, probably as a result of urinary infections (Cox *et al.*, 1987b).

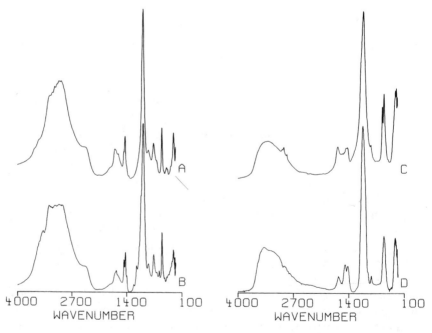

Figure 5.20 Spectra at 4 cm^{-1} resolution of some complex calcified deposits formed on urinary catheters (A and C); a commercial sample of struvite $NH_4MgPO_4 . 6H_2O$ (B); a carbonated amorphous calcium phosphate prepared at pH 10 (D).

CONCLUDING REMARKS

Fourier transform infrared spectroscopy allows spectra to be measured rapidly and with high signal-to-noise ratios. These advantages, combined with high wavenumber precision, allow subsequent manipulations of the spectrum to be made (e.g., Fourier self-deconvolution or spectral subtraction) more easily than with older instrumentation. Examples have been given of how the technique can be used in the characterisation of different amorphous calcium phosphates, in the identification of phases in non-interacting mixtures and to describe maturational changes in calcifying systems. Diffuse reflectance spectra can be measured, and, in conjunction with an infrared microscope, can be used to study layered deposits such as are found in some types of pathological stone-forming organs. The ability to subtract the spectrum of water from the spectra of aqueous solutions allows useful information to be obtained with minimum perturbation of biological specimens and offers the possibility of studying calcifying systems *in vivo*.

ACKNOWLEDGEMENTS

We thank Thea van Kemenade (who provided the OCP sample used to prepare figures 5.12 and 5.13), Averil Cox (who provided the urinary catheter encrustations), and Dr John Harries (who prepared the ACP samples at pH 10). We also thank Keith Hutton for help in recording the spectra of OCP and ACP at 10 K.

REFERENCES

Adams, D. M. and Gardner, I. R. (1974). Single crystal vibrational spectra of apatite, vanadinite and mimetite. *J. Chem. Soc. (Dalton)*, 1505–9

Antoon, M. K., Koenig, J. H. and Koenig, J. L. (1977). Least-squares curve-fitting of Fourier transform infrared spectra with applications to polymer systems. *Appl. Spectrosc.*, **31**, 518–24

Baddiel, C. B. and Berry, E. E. (1966). Spectra structure correlations in hydroxy and fluor-apatite. *Spectrochim. Acta*, **22**, 1407–16

Berry, E. E. and Baddiel, C. B. (1967). The infrared spectrum of dicalcium phosphate dihydrate (brushite). *Spectrochim. Acta*, **23A**, 2089–97

Brown, C. W., Lynch, P. F., Obremski, R. J. and Lavery, D. S. (1982). Matrix representations and criteria for selecting analytical wavelengths for multicomponent spectroscopic analysis. *Anal. Chem.*, **54**, 1472–9

Brown, J. M. and Elliot, J. J. (1985). In *Chemical Biological and Industrial Applications of Infrared Spectroscopy* (ed. J. R. Durig), Wiley Interscience, Chichester, 111–28

Brown, W. E., Lehr, J. R., Smith, J. P. and Frazier, A. W. (1957). Crystallography of octacalcium phosphate. *J. Amer. Chem. Soc.*, **79**, 5318–19

Casciani, F. and Condrate, R. A. (1979). The vibrational spectra of brushite, CaHPO₄.2H₂O. *Spectrosc. Lett.*, **12**, 699–713

Casciani, F. and Condrate, R. A. (1980). The Raman spectrum of monetite. *J. Solid State Chem.*, **34**, 385–8

Catti, M., Ferraris, G. and Filhol, A. (1977). Hydrogen bonding in the crystalline state. CaHPO₄ (monetite), P1 or P1̄? A novel neutron diffraction study. *Acta Crystallogr. Sect. B*, **33**, 1223–39

Cooley, J. W. and Tukey, J. W. (1965). An algorithm for the machine calculation of complex Fourier series. *Math. Comput.*, **19**, 297–301

Cox, A. J., Harries, J. E., Hukins, D. W. L., Kennedy, A. P. and Sutton, T. M. (1987a). Calcium phosphate in catheter encrustation. *Brit. J. Urol.*, **59**, 159–63

Cox, A. J., Hukins, D. W. L., Davies, K. E., Irlam, J. C. and Sutton, T. M. (1987b). An automatic technique for *in vitro* assessment of the susceptibility of urinary catheter materials to encrustation. *Eng. Med.*, **16**, 37–41

Doi, Y., Moriwaka, Y., Aoba, T., Takahashi, J. and Joshim, K. (1982). ESR and IR studies of carbonate containing hydroxyapatites. *Calcif. Tiss. Intl.*, **34**, 178–81

Elliott, J. C. (1963). Interpretation of carbonate bands in infrared spectrum of dental enamel. *J. Dent. Res.*, **42**, 1018 (Abstr.)

Forman, M. L. (1966). Fast Fourier transform technique and its application to Fourier spectroscopy. *J. Opt. Soc. Amer.*, **56**, 978–9

Fowler, B. O., Moreno, E. C. and Brown, W. E. (1966). Infra-red spectra of hydroxyapatite, octacalcium phosphate and pyrolysed octacalcium phosphate. *Arch. Oral Biol.*, **11**, 477–92

Greenler, R. G. (1966). Infrared study of adsorbed molecules on metal surfaces by reflection techniques. *J. Chem. Phys.*, **44**, 310–15

Greenler, R. G. (1969). Reflection method for obtaining the infrared spectrum of a thin layer on a metal surface. *J. Chem. Phys.*, **50**, 1963–8

Griffith, W. P. (1970). Raman studies on rock-forming minerals. Part II. Minerals containing MO_3, MO_4 and MO_6 groups. *J. Chem. Soc. A*, 286–91

Harries, J. E., Hukins, D. W. L., Holt, C. and Hasnain, S. S. (1987). Conversion of amorphous calcium phosphate into hydroxyapatite investigated by EXAFS spectroscopy. *J. Cryst. Growth*, **84**, 563–70

Holt, C., Davies, D. T. and Law, A. J. R. (1986). Effect of colloidal calcium phosphate content and free calcium ion concentration in the milk serum of the dissociation of bovine casein micelles. *J. Dairy Res.*, **53**, 557–72

Holt, C., van Kemenade, M. J. J. M., Harries, J. E., Nelson, L. S., Bailey, R. T., Hukins, D. W. L., Hasnain, S. S. and de Bruyn P. L. (1988). Preparation of amorphous calcium magnesium phosphates at pH 7 and characterization by X-ray absorption and Fourier transform infrared spectroscopy. *J. Cryst. Growth*, **92**, 239–52

Holt, C., van Kemenade, M. J. J. M., Nelson, L. S., Jr, Hukins, D. W. L., Bailey, R. T., Harries, J. E., Hasnain, S. S. and de Bruyn, P. L. (1989). Amorphous calcium phosphates prepared at pH 6.5 and 6.0, *Mat. Res. Bull.*, **25**, 55–62

Ishitari, A., Ishida, H., Soeda, F. and Nagasawa, Y. (1982). Fourier transform infrared reflection spectroscopy for chemical analysis for surface analysis. *Anal. Chem.*, **54**, 682–7

Kauppinen, J. K., Moffat, D. J., Cameron, D. G. and Mantsch, H. H. (1981a). Noise in Fourier self-deconvolution. *Appl. Optics*, **20**, 1866–79

Kauppinen, J. K., Moffat, D. J., Mantsch, H. H. and Cameron, D. G. (1981b). Fourier transforms in the computation of self-deconvoluted and first order derivative spectra of overlapped band contours. *Anal. Chem.*, **53**, 1454–57

Kauppinen, J. K., Moffat, D. J., Mantsch, H. H. and Cameron, D. G. (1981c). Fourier self-deconvolution: a method for resolving intrinsically overlapping bands. *Appl. Spectrosc.*, **35**, 271–6

Van Kemenade, M. J. J. M. (1988). Influence of casein on precipitation of calcium phosphates. Thesis, University of Utrecht, 54–75

Kravitz, L. C., Kingsley, J. D. and Elkin, E. L. (1968). Raman and infrared studies of coupled phosphate vibrations. *J. Chem. Phys.*, **49**, 4600–10

LeGeros, R. Z. (1965). Effect of carbonate on the lattice parameters of apatite. *Nature (Lond.)*, **206**, 403–4

Petrov, I. Soptrajanov, B., Fuson, N. and Lawson, J. R. (1967). Infrared investigation of dicalcium phosphates. *Spectrochim. Acta*, **23A**, 2637–46

6
Sonic velocity and the ultrastructure of mineralised tissues

Sidney Lees

INTRODUCTION

Bone and other normally mineralised tissues may be regarded as mineral-filled soft tissue (Currey, 1964, 1969a, b; Katz, 1971), resembling mineral-filled plastics. Chemical demineralisation leaves a rubbery material with the same shape and volume as the original mineralised tissue. Most remarkably, the mineralised substance can sustain a compressive load while the demineralised matrix cannot. The skeleton is characterised by its capability to support compressive loads, whereas similar connective tissues like tendons and ligaments are strong only in tension.

The soft organic part of bone is mainly type I collagen, which is the predominant component of much connective tissue. Presumably the high mineral content of bone is the source of the compressive stiffness, but the presumption is inaccurate. While the mineral component is important, it is the interaction between mineral and collagen that is the source of stiffness in calcified tissues. The details of the interaction between the mineral and organic phases are not well understood. Some recently acquired information concerning the properties of mineralised collagen tissues is given here, together with an interpretation of the intermolecular structure of fibrous type I collagen as a consequence of the new information.

There are two basic patterns for a mineral–organic composite. In the first, the mineral powder can be compacted and the organic matter infiltrated in the interstices. Alternatively, the mineral can be added to the organic phase, so that the mineral fills pores in the continuous organic medium. In the first, there are direct paths through the mineral solid, whereas in the second the organic phase separates and surrounds the mineral particles. At one time, Currey (1969b) suggested that the micro-crystals are fused together to make a hard fibrous structure. Weiner and

Price (1986a) produced transmission electron micrographs of clumped microcrystals extracted from very dense bone, which might be taken to verify Currey's suggestion. However, information presented here indicates that bone is the second type of material, where the principal paths are in the soft component and the mineral is dispersed inside the plastic. Clumped crystallites, seen by Weiner and Price, may be contained entirely within the softer matrix.

Formation of mineralised tissues proceeds in stages, where first an organic matrix is laid down, followed by mineralising processes from appropriate salts in the body fluids. The details of the process are not known. First, there is a purely extracellular organic medium, which may change composition and structure during the mineralising phase, and at the end there is the mineral-laden organic composite. The mineral particles in mammalian tissues have been identified as microscopic hexagonal calcium phosphate crystallites. The pure mineral is hydroxyapatite $(Ca_5OH(PO_4)_3)$, with density 3.17 g/cc. Biologically derived mineral crystallites are impure and imperfect and are designated as apatitic, rather than hydroxyapatite (HAP). The density is assumed to be about 3.0 g/cc and may be less.

Crystallites in compact mammalian long bone are frequently reported to be 40 to 70 nm long, with a lateral dimension of the order of 5 nm, although other dimensions have been described recently (Weiner and Price, 1986a; Weiner and Traub, 1986b). X-ray diffraction is said to show the c-axis of the crystallites predominately parallel to the collagen fibril axis (Termine, 1973). On the other hand, high-magnification electron micrographs showed extrafibrillar crystallites as thin hexagonal plates, with the c-axis perpendicular to the collagen fibril axis (Selvig, 1970; Voegel, 1977). The contradiction has not been resolved.

Anorganic bone can be made by destroying the organic material with a suitable reagent, leaving the mineral *in situ*. Frequently, the original bone shape is retained, but it is a very weak structure. It might be presumed that anorganic bone demonstrates the existence of purely mineral paths, but it is likely that traces of organic matter are retained, which cement the mineral particles together. Weiner and Price (1986a) disaggregated bone with sodium hypochlorite solution and reduced the mineral to powder. For very high density bone, the crystallites appear to be bonded in clusters. The clustering may well be due to the chemical process employed to destroy the organic phase. While it can be observed that the mineral is dispersed in the organic matrix, the detailed structural characteristics of mineralised tissue have not been resolved, particularly the interface between the mineral and organic components.

SONIC WAVE PROPAGATION

It should be possible to predict the elastic character of a composite from the values for the appropriate physical properties of the components, but the structure of the composite can influence the outcome. Values for longitudinal modulus and the density of a few plastics and minerals are given in table 6.1. If the plastic component dominates, the composite should be more compliant and less stiff than for the reverse situation, even though the composition is the same. Many models have been proposed for calculating the elastic moduli of composites from those of the components (Anderson, 1965; Hill, 1952; Curry, 1964; Katz, 1971). These are successful when the magnitudes of the component values are comparable, but not very good when there is a wide disparity.

Table 6.1 Properties of some representative materials

	Density (g/cc)	Longitudinal modulus (10^9 N/m^2)	Sonic velocity (km/sec)
Soft			
MMA	1.17	7.4	2.51
Epoxy	1.18	7.4	2.50
Vinyl chloride	1.26	5.0	1.99
Hard			
Tungsten	19.3	565	5.41
Crystabolite	2.32	85.7	6.08

Two early models are the Voigt and Reuss formalisms. The Voigt model assumes equal strain in the two constituents, and, according to Hill (1952), gives the upper bound for the elastic modulus. The Reuss model assumes equal stress and gives the lower bound. Other models, like Hill's, give intermediate values. While these various models are used to calculate the bulk and shear modulus, or Young's modulus and Poisson's ratio, Lees and Davidson (1977a, b) calculated the *longitudinal modulus*, which, as defined in table 6.2, is a combination of the bulk and shear moduli. The longitudinal sonic velocity is calculated from this modulus and the density.

Table 6.2 Some useful mathematical relationships

Longitudinal modulus: $K = k + \frac{4}{3}G = \rho c^2$
   (k = bulk modulus; G = shear modulus)
Longitudinal sonic velocity: $c = \sqrt{K/\rho}$
Density of composite: $\rho = vf_1\rho_1 + vf_2\rho_2$
The Voigt formalism: $K_V = vf_1 K_1 + vf_2 K_2$
The Reuss formalism: $1/K_R = vf_1/K_1 + vf_2 K_2$
vf_1 = volume fraction of constituent 1
vf_2 = volume fraction of constituent 2 = $1 - vf_1$

Sonic wave propagation through a solid composite depends in part on the structure. Sonic speeds should be high in a composite solid, in which there are many closely packed mineral paths. It should be much lower where the sonic path is mostly in the plastic. There may be striking differences where the shear wave is rapidly dissipated, as is frequently true in plastics.

Lees and Davidson (1977a, b) compared the experimentally determined sonic velocity for a few mineral-filled plastic composite systems with the values calculated by using both the Voigt and Reuss formalisms. The results are seen plotted in figures 6.1, 6.2 and 6.3. The wide difference between the Voigt and Reuss bounds is quite obvious. The Voigt curve is convex where the Reuss is concave. The experimental points fall on the Reuss curve in every instance. The low velocity indicates that the composites are the second kind.

There is a very well-defined minimum velocity in figure 6.1, which is particularly noteworthy in that it is far less than the velocity for either constituent. An extremum in velocity can be obtained from the Reuss formalism when the volume fraction is

$$vf_2 = \frac{1}{2} \left\{ \frac{1}{1 - K_1/K_2} - \frac{1}{\rho_2/\rho_1 - 1} \right\} \tag{6.1}$$

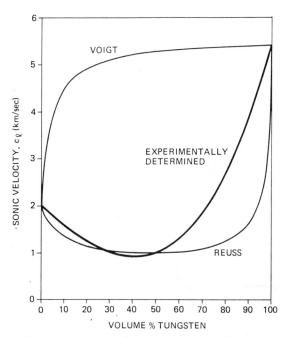

Figure 6.1 Voigt–Reuss bounds for a vinyl–tungsten composite system compared with the experimentally determined curve. (From Lees and Davidson, 1977b.)

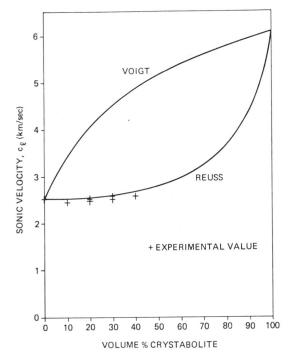

Figure 6.2 Voigt–Reuss bounds for a polymethacrylate–crystabolite composite system. Experimental values fall on the Reuss bound. (From Lees and Davidson, 1977b.)

The extremum velocity is given by

$$\frac{c_m}{c_1} = 2\sqrt{\frac{(1 - K_1/K_2)(\rho_2/\rho_1 - 1)}{(\rho_2/\rho_1 - K_1/K_2)^2}} \qquad (6.2)$$

where c_1 = sonic velocity of component 1; c_m = extremum velocity; K = longitudinal modulus; ρ = density (Lees and Davidson, 1977b).

The predicted minimum velocity ratio is 0.49 for a volume fraction of 0.47, where the measured minimum is 0.41 for a volume fraction of 0.4. The uncertainty and limitations of the experimental methodology may account for the discrepancy.

A more bonelike composite system was evaluated using fluorapatite (FAP)-filled epoxy (Lees and Davidson, 1977a). The results plotted in figure 6.4 show a surprising difference from the previous figures. The measured sonic velocities are all *greater* than the Reuss curve calculated with the normal epoxy K modulus, suggesting the introduction of an additional factor. It is known that the elastic moduli of highly cross-linked polymers are greater than for less densely cross-linked polymers (Burhans *et al.*, 1965). It was concluded in the study that a surface-active material

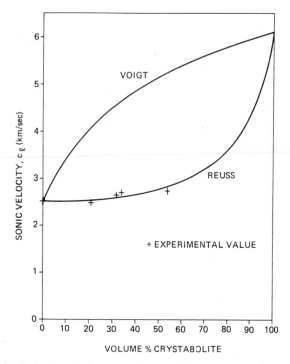

Figure 6.3   Voigt–Reuss bounds for an epoxy–crystabolite composite system. Experimental points fall on the Reuss bound. (From Lees and Davidson, 1977b.)

like apatitic mineral can affect the cross-linking density, as well as the length of the cross-links of epoxy during the hardening process of polymerisation, and the effect is influenced by the volume fraction of the apatitic component. It was estimated that the maximum longitudinal modulus for epoxy is 15.2×10^9 N/m^2, compared with 8×10^9 N/m^2 for unfilled epoxy, a factor of almost 2. The upper curve in figure 6.4, based on the maximum value for K, shows that all the measured values for the sonic velocity fall between the two Reuss curves.

The group sonic velocity at 10 MHz has been determined for a wide range of compact mineralised tissues, together with the density of the wet tissue and its composition. A representative sampling is plotted in figure 6.5, where the volume fraction of the contained mineral was calculated from the tissue composition and density. A Reuss curve was calculated for a minimum longitudinal modulus for collagen, and a similar curve was found for a maximum longitudinal modulus using values for the appropriate parameters given in the paragraphs below. All the measured data fall between the two Reuss curves, which suggests that the elastic properties of the organic component are changed by the mineralisation process, perhaps

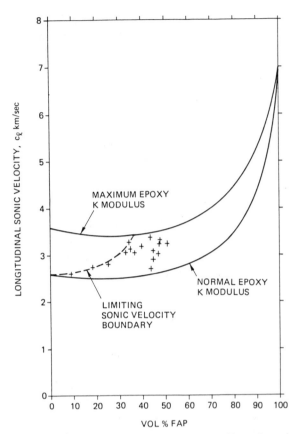

Figure 6.4 Epoxy-fluorapatite composite system. The lower Reuss bound was calculated using the longitudinal modulus of pure epoxy. The upper Reuss bound was obtained by using the maximum possible value for this modulus associated with the shortest cross-link. (From Lees and Davidson, 1977a.)

by increasing cross-linking density or by changing the properties of molecular collagen. Unlike mineralised epoxy, the tissues calcify by a complex process after the organic solid is formed. The structural changes in the tissues must be induced by specific cell-controlled and cell-mediated reactions.

It is difficult to assign a value to the longitudinal modulus of the organic matrix, and equally difficult for the apatitic mineral component. The matrix includes about 10 per cent non-collageneous matter, which may not have a significant role in the elastic properties of the composite. It is known that collagen is stiffer and tougher than most organic matter, and it is likely that only the collagen contributes to the tissue stiffness. Collagen is a complex anisotropic material. The sonic velocity for the bulk matrix is much less than for molecular collagen, indicating a difference between the elastic characteristics of the macroscopic structure and those of the fibrillar bundles of collagen molecules (Lees *et al.*, 1983b). The extremely small dimensions of the apatitic crystallites, of the order of 10 to 100 nm, indicate that the mineral interacts directly with the 300 nm long collagen molecules, or with the collagen molecules bundled into fibrils, and that the elastic properties of molecular collagen are the appropriate parameters.

The sonic phase velocity at 10 GHz in rat tail tendon fibre collagen was determined optically using Brillouin scattering by Cusack and Miller (1979). The sonic wavelength at this frequency is comparable to the length of a single collagen molecule. The axial velocity for the wet tissue is 2.64 km/sec while the radial value is 1.89 km/sec. In contrast, the axial sonic group velocity at 10 Mhz in bovine demineralised bone matrix is 1.82 km/sec and in the radial direction it is 1.69 km/sec (Lees *et al.*, 1983b). The density of wet molecular collagen is 1.33 g/cc, where the density of wet bovine bone matrix is 1.18 g/cc (Lees and Heeley, 1981). The lower bound in figure 6.5 was calculated on the basis of the minimum longitudinal modulus ($K = 4.75 \times 10^9$ N/m^2), using the Cusack–Miller radial sonic velocity and the molecular density of collagen. The corresponding Cusack–Miller axial K is 9.27×10^9 N/m^2.

Gilmore and Katz (1968) measured the sonic velocity in HAP to be 6.85 km/sec, from which the longitudinal modulus can be found when the density of the material is known by the expression given in table 6.2. The density of pure HAP is 3.17 g/cc, but the value for bone mineral is less definite. A reasonable value appears to be 3.0 g/cc (Lees, 1987a), for which the longitudinal modulus is 140.8×10^9 N/m^2.

The longitudinal modulus for the collagen in the upper curve in the figure was calculated by inverting the Reuss formalism. An estimated upper limit for the collagen axial modulus in bone of 22.4×10^9 N/m^2 was derived for a cow tibia specimen, where the density is 2.07 g/cc, the axial sonic velocity is 4.26 km/sec and the mineral volume fraction is 0.481. The ratio of the maximum axial longitudinal modulus for mineralised collagen to the axial modulus for unmineralised collagen is 2.41 according to these estimates. Similarly, an estimate for the maximum collagen radial modulus in bone of 13.6×10^9 N/m^2 was found for a cow tibia specimen, density 2.08 g/cc, radial sonic velocity 3.32 km/sec and mineral volume fraction of 0.449. This value is 2.87 times Cusack's value for rat tail tendon collagen, which is reasonably close to the ratio of the axial moduli. It shows that the collagen in fully mineralised bone is stiffer in all directions than in the unmineralised collagen.

ANISOTROPY IN BONE

The structure of compact bone in long bones is visibly anisotropic,

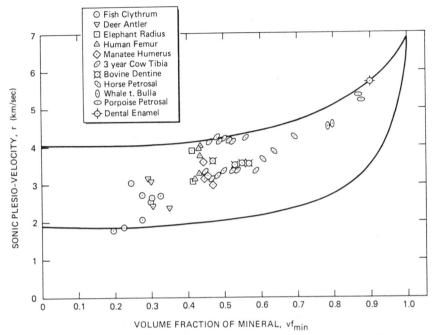

Figure 6.5   Sonic plesio-velocity for various mineralised tissues as a function of the volume fraction of the contained mineral. Orientation of the specimen was ignored.

particularly in the midsection of the bone. The anisotropy is even more obvious microscopically by observing the order of the bone fibres, the orientation of osteons, and the orientation of collagen fibrils in demineralised tissues. The fibrous structure may appear twisted, but a major component of the orientation is parallel to the bone axis. Moreover, bone composition varies locally (from point to adjacent point), as well as more systematically around the cross-section. The bone structure is penetrated by blood vessels, nerve passageways and tendon attachment sites. Cortical bone is clearly inhomogeneous anatomically, as well as anisotropic, which is reflected in its mechanical properties. It is to be expected that the elastic properties and the sonic velocity must vary with orientation, as well as with the location of the sample around the bone axis. The scattering of the plotted points in figure 6.5 is in part a reflection of the inhomogeneity and anisotropy.

Some tissues are much less anisotropic than others. These include the otic bones and dentine. The distinction between the two classes of bone can be demonstrated by ultrasound, as shown below in a subsequent section.

It is difficult to measure the sonic velocity of inhomogeneous anisotropic media. The sonic beam can be deflected and split by the birefringence of homogeneous anisotropic crystalline media (Musgrave, 1970; Fedorov, 1968). If the medium is also inhomogeneous, the problems are even more difficult. The unknown sonic path must be longer than the thickness of the specimen, and the transit time correspondingly greater than indicated by the thickness. If the specimen is made very thin, the difference between the sonic path and the thickness should be small and the measured transit time almost that corresponding to the measured specimen thickness. The observed value should be closer to the true sonic velocity. The term 'plesio-velocity' has been adopted to distinguish the measured from the true value (Lees *et al.*, 1979a).

Specimens used in these experiments were about 2 mm thick or less, and at least 1 cm by 1 cm in area. The sonic beam diameter used in the pulse echo mode was no more than 4 mm, smaller than the area of the specimens. The specimens were cut from the bone sample on a slow-speed diamond abrasive saw cooled by water. The individual specimens were ground on a surface grinder with water cooling to provide two flat, parallel sides. The final specimens were uniformly thick within 2 μm. Details of the protocol are given in the references (Lees *et al.*, 1979a, b).

Figure 6.6 displays the anisotropic velocity distribution associated with the propagation of longitudinal sonic waves in the cortical part of an adult midshaft bovine tibia (Lees *et al.*, 1979b). The specimens were prepared in pairs to assure the reliability and reproducibility of the measurements. The upper part of the figure depicts the sites of radial and tangential specimens, while the lower part shows the location of the axial specimens. The orientation refers to the nominal direction of sonic propagation. The pulse echo method using a pulse of 100 ns duration was employed to determine the transit time, which requires the sonic pulse to traverse the sound path twice. The ratio of the specimen thickness divided by half the transit time is defined as the sonic plesio-velocity.

Three numbers are shown with each specimen. The first is the value of the sonic plesio-velocity for the normal fully mineralised wet specimen, the second that for the completely dried specimen and the third that for the wet demineralised bone matrix in the demineralising solution. The axial velocity is always greater. The individual values for all the specimens are shown in figure 6.6, but mean values for each orientation and condition are given in this text. The mean axial value for this bone is 3.89 ± 0.04 km/sec, compared with a mean radial value of 3.21 ± 0.04 km/sec. The standard deviation probably reflects the variability of this property in the tissue, rather than the uncertainty of the measurement process.

The plesio-velocity for the dried bone is greater in every direction than for the corresponding wet-state value, but more so in the axial direction, where the mean value increases 9 per cent from 3.89 to 4.24 km/sec. The mean radial value increases 6 per cent from 3.21 to 3.40 km/sec, which shows an increase in the anisotropy when bone is dried. The water comes

TANGENTIAL (T) AND "RADIAL" (R) SPECIMENS

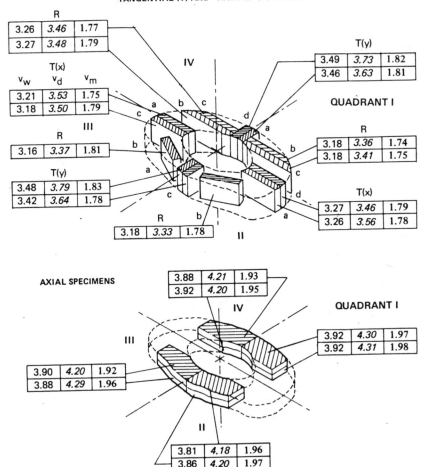

Figure 6.6 Distribution of the sonic plesio-velocity in a sample of cow tibia with orientation. v_w = wet bone, v_d = dried bone, v_m = demineralised bone matrix. (From Lees *et al.*, 1979b.)

mostly out of the organic matter (Lees and Escoubes, 1987). There is no evidence that the mineral properties differ whether wet or dry, but the properties of collagen undergo a large change when collagen is dried. Cusack and Miller (1979) found the longitudinal sonic velocity at 10 GHz for wet rat tail tendon collagen to be 2.64 km/sec axially and 1.89 km/sec radially, while the corresponding values for dry material are 3.64 and 2.94. The axial velocity increases 38 per cent and the radial velocity 56 per cent when rat tail tendon collagen is dried. The sonic velocity of mineralised collagen may not experience as great a change when dried, but the change

in the properties of its collagen is surely the source of the velocity increase
in bone.

The sonic plesio-velocity is much lower in the demineralised state, but
the anisotropy persists. The mean velocity axially for bone matrix in
demineralising solution is 1.96 ± 0.02 km/sec and radially it is 1.77 ± 0.02
km/sec. When the demineralising solution (0.5 M EDTA, pH 7.5) is
replaced by 0.15 M saline, the mean plesio-velocity decreases to 1.82 km/
sec axially and 1.69 km/sec radially (Lees *et al.*, 1981).

The higher sonic velocity in wet rat tail tendon fibre collagen, both
axially and radially at 10 GHz, compared with the bone matrix values at
10 MHz, must reflect the influence of the liquid contained in the bone
matrix. At 10 GHz, the sonic wavelength is comparable to the length of a
single collagen molecule, but the sonic wavelength is 1000 times larger at
the lower frequency. The least volume of bone matrix excited by the
10 MHz radiation must contain tens of thousands of collagen molecules,
together with the water between molecules, and the tissue must be
considered as a water–collagen composite. The volume fraction of collagen
in the demineralised bone matrix was estimated to be 0.564 and the rest of
the volume to be 0.15 M saline with a density of 1 g/cc (Lees and Heeley,
1981). The sonic speed in the saline is taken as 1.5 km/sec and the density
of the wet collagen molecule as 1.33 g/cc. Application of the Reuss
formalism to a collagen–water composite using the values given in table 6.3
yields 1.82 km/sec for the axial and 1.64 km/sec for the radial velocities,
quite close to the measured quantities.

It is seen in table 6.3 that anisotropy is greatest in collagen fibrils and
least for the water–collagen composite and wet demineralised bone matrix.
The intermediate anisotropy of wet bone shows the influence of both water
and mineral on the elastic properties of hard tissues.

Table 6.3   Anisotropy in sonic plesio-velocity

Tissue	Axial	Radial	Ratio	Frequency
	mean (km/sec)			
Cow bone wet	3.89	3.21	0.83	10 MHz
dry	4.24	3.40	0.80	
Cow matrix wet	1.82	1.69	0.93	
Rat tail tendon wet	2.64	1.89	0.72	10 GHz
dry	3.64	2.94	0.81	
Reuss composite	1.82	1.64	0.90	
(0.436 water, 0.564 collagen)				

BONE SHRINKAGE

Variation of the specimen thickness with water content was observed
during the procedure for determining composition. Three kinds of frac-

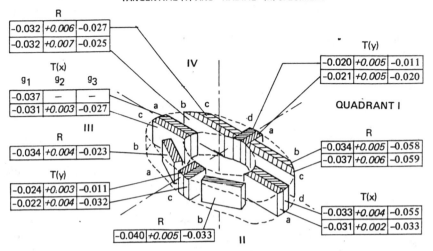

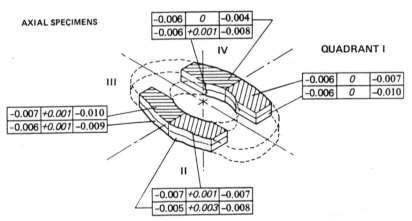

Figure 6.7 Distribution of fractional dimensional changes in a sample of cow bone with orientation. t_w = wet thickness, t_d = dry thickness, t_r = rehydrated thickness, t_m = demineralised bone matrix thickness;

$$g_1 = \frac{t_d - t_w}{t_w} = \text{shrinkage};$$

$$g_2 = \frac{t_r - t_w}{t_w} = \text{rehydrated bone dimensional change};$$

$$g_3 = \frac{t_m - t_w}{t_w} = \text{dimensional change after demineralisation.}$$

tional change are defined in the legend to figure 6.7. The first number shows the *shrinkage* when the bone specimen is dried, the second the variation from the original thickness when the bone specimen is rewetted, and the third shows a loss in thickness when the bone is demineralised. The average axial shrinkage of 0.006 is an order of magnitude less than the average radial shrinkage of 0.035. It was concluded that it is the *organic* phase which is responsible for such large dimensional changes. The X-ray diffraction spacing of soft-tissue collagen decreases both axially and radially when the tissue is dried and the shrinkage is much less axially than radially (Brodsky, 1982), just like in long bone. The anisotropic shrinkage of bone is additional evidence that the mineral must be dispersed through the organic phase and cannot be present as a monolithic solid.

The second set of numbers in figure 6.7 shows that a structural change is induced by dehydration, since the rewetted thickness is slightly greater than the original value. Again the effect is anisotropic, being least axially and largest radially. It is also to be noted from the third set of numbers that the demineralised matrix shrinks anisotropically and that the magnitude of the changes is very much like the shrinkage in the first set of values for the dehydrated, fully mineralised tissue. The reason for these dimensional changes has not been investigated, but they indicate that the organic phase suffers macroscopic dimensional modification with mineral as well as water content, matching the dependence of the sonic velocity on these parameters noted in the previous section.

SOME PARAMETERS INFLUENCING THE SONIC PLESIO-VELOCITY

The data plotted in figure 6.5 display the plesio-velocity only as a function of mineral content for wet tissues. Figures 6.6 and 6.7 disclose the existence and influence of other factors in a single type of compact bone. The contribution of these factors can be studied more carefully by extending the types of hard tissues over the maximum range of density. Figure 6.8(a–c) shows the effect of orientation and type of wet compact tissue on the longitudinal plesio-velocity (Lees *et al.*, 1983a). Values for long bone are plotted in figure 6.8(a, b) for the axial and radial directions. Figure 6.8(c) shows the variation of the quantity for hyperdense tissues, including bovine dentine and bovine enamel. The points refer to average values of many specimens in each instance. Figure 6.9(a–c) shows the dried tissue values. A least-squares line was fitted to the data in each case and listed in table 6.4. At least four parameters have been identified that affect the sonic velocity and the elastic properties of hard tissues: density, orientation in the tissue, water content and order in the matrix fibres.

The linear dependence on density is related to the factors that control density, namely the mineral content, organic matter and water content. This relationship is described in more detail below. Porosity is a possible fifth parameter, but its effect has not been determined.

The orientation dependence of physical properties, including elastic

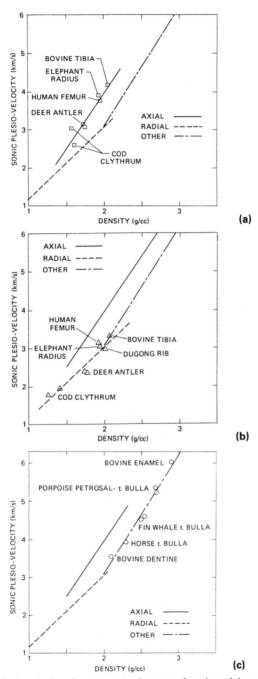

Figure 6.8 Sonic plesio-velocity of wet compact tissue as a function of the wet tissue density: (a) parallel to bone axis, (b) perpendicular to the bone axis in the radial direction, (c) hyperdense tissues. (From Lees *et al.*, 1983a.)

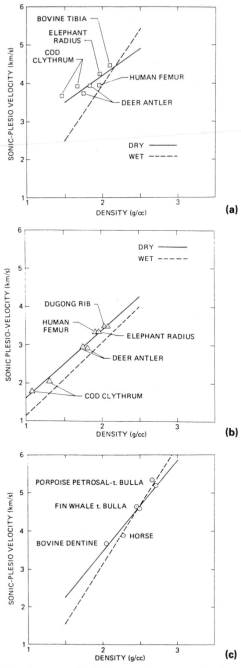

Figure 6.9 Sonic plesio-velocity of dried compact tissue as a function of the wet tissue density: (a) axial direction, (b) radial direction, (c) hyperdense tissues. (From Lees *et al.*, 1983a.)

Table 6.4   Least-squares fitted lines for sonic plesio-velocity as a function of density and water content

1.	Axial wet	$v = 2.891\rho_b - 1.821 \pm 0.16$ km/sec
2.	Axial dry	$v = 1.140\rho_b + 1.907 \pm 0.13$ km/sec
3.	Radial wet	$v = 1.882\rho_b - 0.700 \pm 0.15$ km/sec
4.	Radial dry	$v = 1.818\rho_b - 0.277 \pm 0.08$ km/sec
5.	Hyperdense wet	$v = 3.141\rho_b - 3.193 \pm 0.14$ km/sec
6.	Hyperdense dry	$v = 2.593\rho_b - 1.785 \pm 0.16$ km/sec

The standard deviation was calculated from the deviation of the observed sound velocity from the line for a given density

wave propagation, appears to be correlated with the orientation of the bone matrix fibres. The lack of anisotropy in the otic bones is presumed to be associated with a corresponding lack of anisotropy in the matrix. Hyperdense bone has much less organic matter than do long bones, little or no blood supply (like dentine and enamel) and apparently is not subject to remodelling or mineral turnover. The embryological development is different, and, once formed, the internal structures of hyperdense bone, like the internal structures of the enamel and dentine of teeth, do not change. Dimensional changes between wet and dried states appear to be essentially independent of orientation (Lees and Escoubes, 1987).

Dental enamel, unlike the otic bones, does have orientation-dependent properties. Enamel contains practically no organic matter and that small amount of organic matter is a different protein from collagen. It is an almost purely apatitic substance, in which an organic network is thinly dispersed, barely separating the crystallites, which may be the reason it fits with the other hyperdense tissues. The cited value is for propagation normal to the surface. The physical properties of the hyperdense tissues other than enamel are probably due to the matrix fibres being different from and less well ordered than in long bone. For the highest-density tissues, the mineral properties contribute much more to the properties of the composite than where the mineral concentration is lower.

EQUATORIAL DIFFRACTION SPACING OF THE COLLAGEN IN HARD TISSUES

The dimensional changes when bone is dried were attributed to the organic matrix, especially the fibrous collagen structure, but direct evidence would be more convincing. Until recently (White *et al.*, 1977), the molecular structure of collagenous tissue was studied primarily by X-ray and electron diffraction (Brodsky and Eikenberry, 1982; Rougvie and Bear, 1953; Katz, 1973). It was assumed that the equatorial diffraction spacing in the mineralised tissue is the same as in the demineralised state, despite the reports by Eanes *et al.* (1970, 1976), who found the spacing to be 1.33 nm for fresh wet mineralised turkey leg tendon and 1.13 nm for dried,

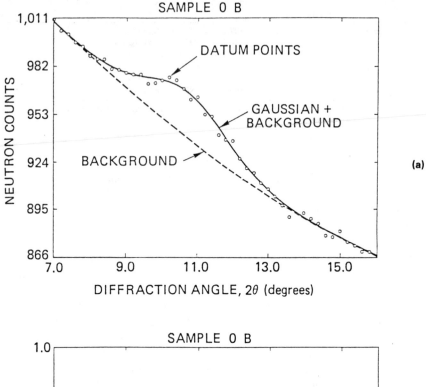

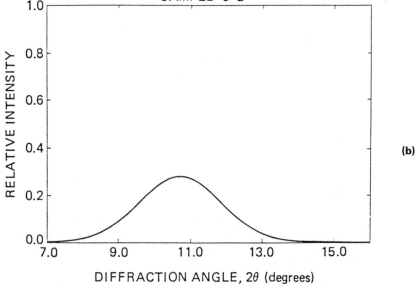

Figure 6.10   Typical example of neutron diffraction pattern from bone. (a) The curve is the sum of a Gaussian and a second-order polynomial representing the contribution of the background fitted to the data by least squares. (b) The Gaussian extracted from the previous curve. The peak of the Gaussian is taken as the equatorial spacing. (From Lees *et al.*, 1987b.)

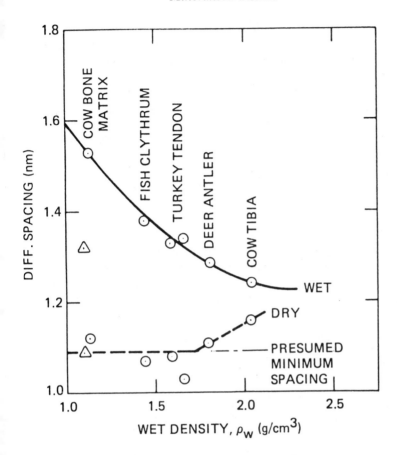

△ = RAT TAIL TENDON (X-RAY DIFFRACTION, Katz and Li)

Figure 6.11 Equatorial diffraction spacing of representative hard tissues as a function of wet tissue density. The solid-line curve is given by equation 6.3. The broken-line curve represents an approximation of the dry state spacing. The values for rat tail tendon collagen were added for comparison. (From Lees *et al.*, 1984b.)

compared with 1.44 nm for fresh wet unmineralised turkey leg tendon and 1.12 nm for dried. White *et al.* (1977) examined the axial diffraction pattern of wet mineralised turkey leg tendon using neutrons, and concluded that the axial long spacing, D, was the same as for wet unmineralised collagen, 67 nm. Since neutrons are affected by the nucleus and not by the electron density, neutron diffraction can sense the collagen structure in fully mineralised tissues, where X-rays and electrons are much more strongly influenced by the electron-dense mineral content.

Lees *et al.* (1984b) used neutron diffraction to determine the equatorial diffraction spacing of fully mineralised tissues as a function of the wet density. The tissues were examined in the normal wet state and then after being fully dehydrated. The typical diffraction pattern, seen in figure 6.10, was considered to be the sum of two curves, a background represented by a second-order polynomial and a Gaussian. The data are fitted by the computer in the least-squares sense to the complex curve. The equatorial spacing is calculated from the locus of the Gaussian peak. Figure 6.11 displays the results, showing that collagen spacing in the wet tissue decreases as the density increases and that the dried tissue spacing is essentially the same (1.1 nm) for all mineralised tissues as for unmineralised tissue. The relationship between the equatorial spacing, d_w, and wet tissue density, ρ_w, has been found empirically to be (Lees, 1987a)

$$d_w = C_0 + C_1/\rho_w \tag{6.3}$$

($C_0 = 0.8876$, $C_1 = 0.7213$).

The decreased spacing for dried tissues confirms the previous inference that it is the contained structural organic matter that induces the shrinkage of bone when dried. There are, however, two additional important conclusions from these data. Since the equatorial diffraction spacing for

Table 6.5   Equatorial diffraction spacing for various tissues

		Wet density, ρ_w (g/ml)	Diffraction spacing	
			Wet d_w (nm)	Dry d_d (nm)
Tissue				
Cow tibia matrix		1.13	1.53 ± 0.006	1.12 ± 0.006
Codfish clythrum		1.44	1.38 ± 0.02	1.07 ± 0.02
Mineralised turkey tendon	1	1.66	1.34 ± 0.03	1.03 ± 0.03
	2	1.58	1.33 ± 0.06	1.08 ± 0.01
Deer antler		1.80	1.29 ± 0.02	1.11 ± 0.06
Cow tibia		2.04	1.24 ± 0.002	1.16 ± 0.006

Table 6.6   Equatorial diffraction spacing for dried non-mineralised collagen tissues

Tissue	Equatorial diffraction spacing (nm)
Kangaroo tail tendon	1.07[a]
Rat tail tendon	1.10
Uncalcified turkey tendon	1.12
	1.08
Demineralised rat bone	1.09
Demineralised normal chick bone	1.09
Demineralised lathyritic chick bone	1.09
Mineralised turkey tendon	1.13
	1.08
Mean	1.09 ± 0.02

[a] Extrapolated from published data.

dried tissue is about 1.1 nm, essentially the same whether the tissue is mineralised or not, as seen from Tables 6.5 and 6.6, *there cannot be any mineral within the collagen fibril* except possibly in the hole zone region of colinear collagen molecules. If there were mineral between the collagen molecules the collagen spacing would not decrease as observed. Second, since the spacing of the demineralised bone matrix is 1.53 nm, *the collagen fibrils must become compacted during the mineralisation process* and the compaction appears to be greater as the mineral content increases.

The observed variation of the equatorial spacing in mineralised type I collagen tissues extends the range of this property that has been observed before. The spacing for tail tendon fibre collagen is usually given as 1.33 nm, compared with 1.53 for bone matrix (Brodsky and Eikenberry, 1982). A possible packing model for all these examples of type I collagen was advanced by Lees *et al.* (1984a).

A GENERALISED PACKING MODEL

Most models for a three-dimensional collagen structure have been proposed for tail tendon collagen (Chapman, 1984; Hulmes and Miller, 1979; White *et al.*, 1977). The well-known Hodge–Petruska *D*-stagger overlap is a condition that must be satisfied by any model, but is incomplete in itself. The Hulmes and Miller (1979) 'quasi-hexagonal' packing model was proposed to conform with the X-ray diffraction patterns of stretched rat tail tendon collagen, where the equatorial pattern indicates a degree of crystallinity not observed with other collagenous tissues. Woodhead-Galloway (1984) devised the 'liquid crystal' model to explain the diffuse equatorial diffraction pattern, like figure 6.10, observed with most type I collagen tissues, together with the well-structured axial diffraction pattern, which he described as a one-dimensional crystal. The generalised packing model was devised to account for the observed variation of the equatorial diffraction spacing associated with diffuse diffraction patterns and is not a completed three-dimensional model.

The equatorial packing of the Hulmes–Miller packing model is given schematically by figure 6.12. The six apices and the centre are occupied by seven collagen molecules, with axes perpendicular to the page. The Hulmes–Miller spacings are identified with the altitudes of the triangle and are the interplanar distances between rows of molecules. The sides of the triangle are the intermolecular distances, and the point of interest is that these are comparable to the spacing (1.53 nm) given by the peak of the diffuse equatorial diffraction pattern for demineralised bone matrix. Lees (1981) proposed a quadrilateral packing model for demineralised bone collagen, as distinct from the Hulmes–Miller quasi-hexagonal model for tail tendon collagen. Since all these tissues are made of type I collagen, a scheme is required that can accommodate the wide range of the observed

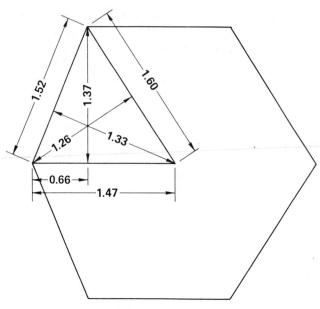

Figure 6.12   A representation of the Hulmes–Miller 'quasi-hexagonal' packing model. Each vertex and the mid-point correspond to collagen molecules. (From Lees *et al.*, 1984a.)

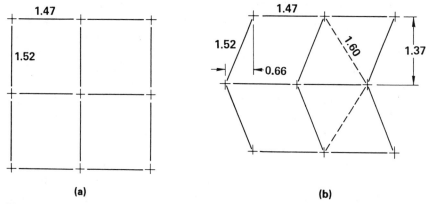

Figure 6.13   The scheme of the generalised packing model. The rectangles are transformed into hexagons by displacing one plane of molecules with respect to its neighbours. (From Lees *et al.*, 1984a.)

spacings. Figure 6.13 demonstrates how a rectangular quadrilateral pattern can be transformed into the quasi-hexagonal one by sliding the middle plane 0.66 nm to the left with respect to the two adjacent planes. The intermolecular distances are invariant, but the interplanar distances are changed as the rectangles become rhomboidal.

A more complete exposition is given by figure 6.14, where examples show how a continuous range of packing can be generated for various collagen tissues as the midplane is displaced. The sides of the rhomboid connecting four collagen molecules are intended to be symbols for projections of intermolecular cross-links at the ends of molecules. While the intermolecular cross-links may not be identical for all tissues, and there may be small deviations from the rat tail collagen values, the validity of the hypothesis is unaffected. The altitude on the left is identical to the diffuse equatorial diffraction spacing of each tissue. Only the internal angles of the rhomboid vary from one packing model to the next. It is to be observed that when the equatorial spacing is reduced to 1.09 nm, the collagen molecules are in contact. This explains why all the dried tissues have the same equatorial diffraction spacing. The molecules cannot pack more tightly.

According to the Hodge–Petruska *D*-stagger scheme, no more than one-fifth of the collagen molecules in a fibril can have their ends in the same plane. The intermolecular cross-links appear to be in the end region of the collagen molecules, between the telepeptides (Eyre *et al.*, 1984). Cross-links impose stereospecific constraints between the molecules defining the geometry between the molecules at the interconnecting region. Collagen molecules may be regarded as long, slender rods with a diameter of 1.23 nm and a length of about 295 nm (Lees, 1986). For most of the length of the molecule, there are no intermolecular cross-links, and there should be no restraints from this source on the relative displacements of adjoining molecules between their ends. The order imposed by the cross-links can be invoked only for the 20 per cent of the molecular ends in any plane, unless another influence exists. The structure of the collagen fibril is a network of long, slender molecules tied together at their ends by a meshwork of cross-links. The locus of maximum intensity in the equatorial diffraction pattern is taken to imply that the most probable location for the collagen molecule is the nominal molecular axis connecting the two cross-linked ends of the molecule. There is also the possibility that the molecule is twisted along its length, as well as being tilted with respect to the fibril axis (Chapman, 1984). A schematic drawing of a collagen fibril equatorial cross-section is given in figure 6.15. A few sets of four collagen molecule ends linked together are given by the clear circles. The shaded circles represent the mid-region of other collagen molecules and are displaced in a seemingly random pattern. The Woodhead-Galloway (1984) model should be applicable, provided the packing factor is defined by the order fixed by the cross-links at the ends of the molecules. The reproducible equatorial diffraction spacing observed for a specific tissue, according to this interpretation, reflects the stereospecific relationships of the reference framework.

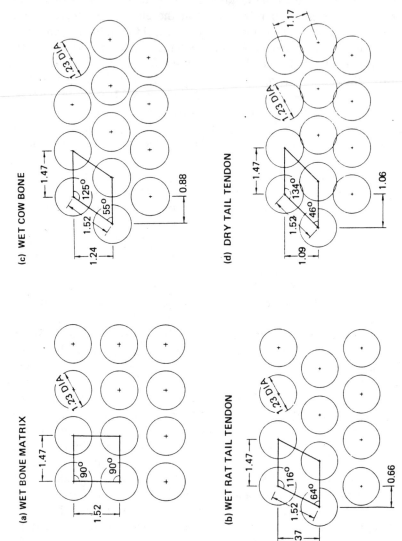

Figure 6.14   Examples of the generalised packing model for several collagen tissues. (From Lees, 1986.)

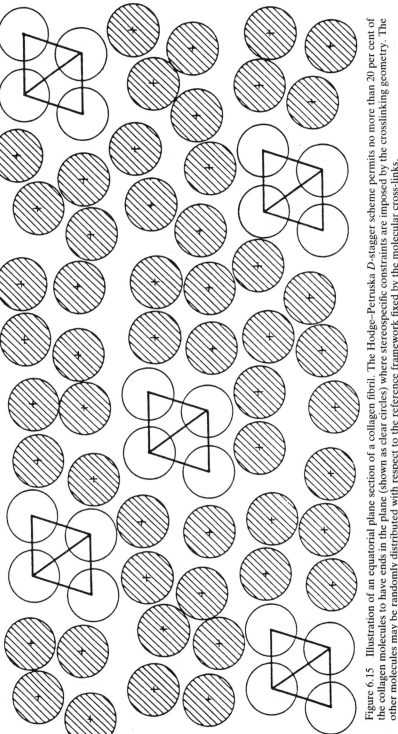

Figure 6.15   Illustration of an equatorial plane section of a collagen fibril. The Hodge–Petruska *D*-stagger scheme permits no more than 20 per cent of the collagen molecules to have ends in the plane (shown as clear circles) where stereospecific constraints are imposed by the crosslinking geometry. The other molecules may be randomly distributed with respect to the reference framework fixed by the molecular cross-links.

THE COMPOSITION OF HARD TISSUES

The organic, mineral and water content of a hard tissue may be regarded as the major components of calcified tissues. While the organic phase consists of many compounds that are of considerable importance, these details are outside the range of interest. Three measurements suffice to make the determinations: the weight of the tissue when water saturated, its dried mineralised weight and the weight of the dried demineralised tissue. The density of the fully mineralised wet tissue is used as the independent variable. The weight difference between the wet and dried mineralised tissue is assumed to be the water contained in the specimen. The dried demineralised tissue weight is taken as the organic content. The weight difference between the dried mineralised and dried demineralised tissue is presumed to be the mineral weight. Each specimen is processed intact as a block and is not pulverised. A study of the demineralisation process showed that all of the organic matter is retained in the specimen, within the

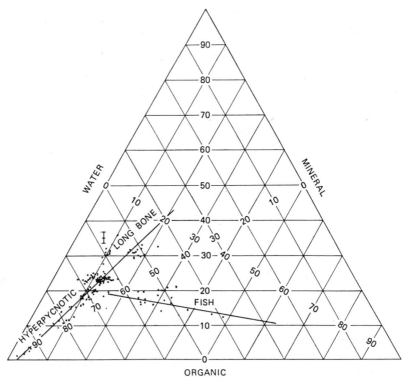

Figure 6.16 Weight fractions of the three major components for hard tissues of varying densities. Two groups are apparent, one for mammalian calcified tissues and another for fish clythrum.

limits of experimental limits (1 per cent uncertainty). The processing was done at 23 °C.

Figure 6.16 summarises the available data. Each side in the triangular plot represents one of the three components as the weight fraction of the entire wet specimen. Each point represents three weight fractions with the sum of one. The data break into two groups, one for fish clythrum and the other for mammalian bone for the entire density range from deer antler (1.7 g/cc) to porpoise petrosal (2.7 g/cc). The fish clythrum is acellular and very porous (Lees *et al.*, 1983a). The water content can vary widely with porosity, even if the solid content remains the same. The line indicates that the organic content is almost constant, whereas the mineral and water components vary widely. In contrast, the water weight fraction of mammalian bone varies much less than the organic content. This implies a consistent structural pattern for all mammalian hard tissues that is different from fish clythrum. The extremely small amount of organic matter in some hyperdense bone (as little as 2 per cent in some cases) is of particular interest. Since bone becomes mineralised after the organic structure is laid down, there must be a loss of organic matter during the mineralisation process, which can be substantial for high-density bone. It was noted above that there is compaction of the collagen fibrils in bone, which appears to be accompanied by a loss of the organic matter.

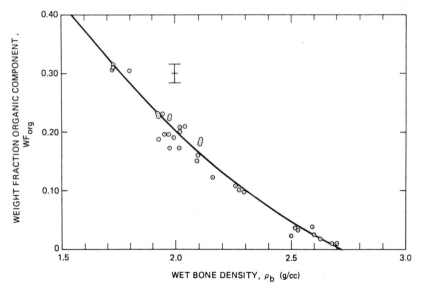

Figure 6.17 The organic weight fraction of mammalian hard tissues as a function of wet-tissue density. The curve is given by the polynomial

$$WF_{org} = 1.472 - 0.894\rho_b + 0.129\rho_b^2 \pm 0.016$$

(From Lees, 1987a.)

This observation is more obvious in figure 6.17, where the organic weight fraction is plotted against the wet-tissue density. The lightest tissue was deer antler, the densest from porpoise petrosal. The matching curve in figure 6.18 shows the mineral content increases monotonically with the wet density. The scatter of the plotted data probably reflects the effect of the variability in the bone structure with tissue type.

At first sight, the curvature of the plots in these two figures may be puzzling, since the density should be linearly dependent on its composition:

$$\rho_w = vf_{min}\rho_{min} + vf_{org}\rho_{org} + vf_{H_2O}\,\rho_{H_2O}$$

$$vf_{min} + vf_{org} + vf_{H_2O} = 1 \qquad (6.4)$$

(vf = volume fraction.)

The expression assumes that the density of each component is constant,

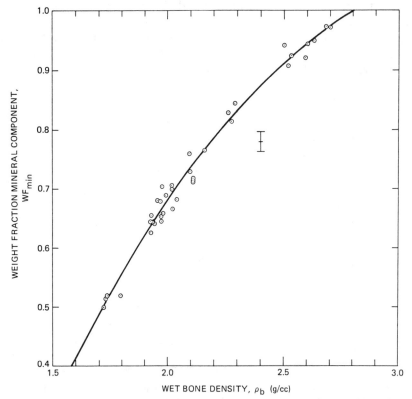

Figure 6.18 The mineral weight fraction of mammalian hard tissues as a function of wet-tissue density. The curve is given by the polynomial

$$WF_{min} = 1.322 + 1.429\rho_b - 0.215\rho_b^2 \pm 0.017$$

but the density of the organic component must increase as the collagen becomes more compact with mineral content. A more careful analysis (Lees *et al.*, 1987a) shows three factors influence the weight fraction of the organic component. The first is the actual loss of organic matter. Second, an increase of mineral concentration will decrease the *relative* amount of organic matter even though the weight is constant. The third effect is the increased density of the collagén fibrils. The interactions of these three effects results in the curve seen in figure 6.17.

Figure 6.9 indicates a linear relationship between sonic plesio-velocity and wet-tissue density, at least within the accuracy of the data. If density is replaced by either organic or mineral content weight fraction, the dependence becomes non-linear. The ultimate source of the non-linearity should be traceable to the modification of the bone collagen by the mineralisation process, but the work is incomplete.

CONCLUSIONS

Ultrasonics has been successfully employed to study the ultrastructure of hard tissues when used with information from other modalities. Only the longitudinal sonic velocity was used in these experiments, but other ultrasonic modes and properties can provide useful information and have been employed (Adler and Cook, 1975; Garcia *et al.*, 1978; Lakes *et al.*, 1986; Lang, 1970, van Buskirk and Ashman, 1981). The amplitude of low-energy ultrasonic waves is small, of the order of a fraction of a nanometer. Conventional tests relating strain to stress require macroscopic displacements that invoke the viscoelastic aspects of biological matter. The rate of application of stress in such tests, as well as the previous history and the duration of the test, influence the results, whereas ultrasonic tests can be applied repeatedly with reproducible results. Care must be used in trying to relate more conventional test results with ultrasonic data. Stress–strain tests are essentially isothermal, where ultrasound wave propagation is essentially adiabatic (although there is heat loss through thermal conduction). Both will shows comparable changes, since higher sonic velocity relates to higher elastic moduli, but it is more difficult to make the relation a quantitative one.

It is of particular interest and good fortune that the longitudinal sonic velocity appears to correlate with molecular level properties. Shear waves and attenuation are sensitive to structure at the microscopic level, owing to interfaces in the tissue that may make interpretation difficult in complex material like bone. The data assembled here show the anisotropic longitudinal sonic velocity in bone to be closely correlated with the anisotropic properties of the organic matrix. Further, the anisotropy is correlated with the structure of the collagen fibrils. The sonic velocity is highest along the bone axis and along the fibril axis, which is roughly parallel to the bone axis. The dimensional changes of long bone when it is dried are equally anisotropic and congruent with the anistropic dimensional changes experienced by the collagen in bone, as revealed by neutron diffraction.

According to the Lees–Davidson hypothesis (Lees and Davidson, 1977a), compact bone is a Reuss solid, in which the collagen is modified by the mineralisation process to increase its elastic moduli. It also appears that the amount of modification of the collagen depends on the wet density of the tissue and the weight fraction of the mineral component. Figure 6.5 shows that the longitudinal sonic plesio-velocity is greater than can be accounted for using the longitudinal modulus of unmineralised collagen, but less than if the maximum possible longitudinal modulus is employed. Neutron diffraction showed the equatorial diffraction spacing in compact long bone to vary inversely with tissue density, indicating that the collagen in bone is modified and different from the same collagen when demineralised. Comparison of the equatorial diffraction spacing of dried bone with the same wet bone showed most of the mineral must be between the collagen fibrils. Other properties of calcified tissues are being investigated to learn more about this modification. Some of the characteristics of mineralised collagen are described in more detail in the next chapter.

REFERENCES

Adler, A. and Cook, K. V. (1975). Ultrasonic parameters of freshly frozen dog tibia. *J. Acous. Soc. Am.*, **58**, 1107–8

Anderson, O. L. (1965). Determination and some uses of isotropic elastic constants of polycrystalline aggregates using single crystal data. In *Physical Acoustics* (ed. W. P. Mason), Vol. **III**, part B, Academic Press, New York, pp. 43–95

Bonar, L. C., Lees, S. and Mook, H. A. (1985). Neutron diffraction studies of collagen in fully mineralized bone. *J. Molec. Biol.*, **181**, 265–70

Brodsky, B. and Eikenberry, E. F. (1982). Characterization of fibrous forms of collagen. *Methods of Enzymology*, **82**, 107–17

Burhans, A. S., Pitt. C., Sellers, R. F. and Smith, S. G. (1965). High performance epoxy resin systems for fiber reinforced composites. *21st Annual Meeting of the Reinforced Plastics Division, Society of the Plastics Industry*, personal communication

Chapman, J. A. (1984). Molecular organization in the collagen fibril. In *Connective Tissue Matrix* (ed. D. W. L. Hukins), Macmillan, London and Basingstoke

Currey, J. D. (1964). Three analogies to explain the mechanical properties of bone. *Biorheol.*, **2**, 1–10

Currey, J. D. (1969a). The mechanical consequences of variation in the mineral content of bone. *J. Biomech.*, **2**, 1–11

Currey, J. D. (1969b). The relationship between the stiffness and the mineral content of bone. *J. Biomech.*, **2**, 477–80

Cusack, S. and Miller, A. (1979). Determination of the elastic constants of collagen by Brillouin light scattering. *J. Molec. Biol.*, **135**, 285–7

Eanes, E. D., Lundy, D. R. and Martin, G. N. (1970). X-ray diffraction study of the mineralization of turkey leg tendon. *Calcif. Tiss. Res.*, **6**, 239–48

Eanes, E. D., Martin, G. N. and Lundy, D. P. (1976). The distribution of water in calcified turkey leg tendon. *Calcif. Tiss. Res.*, **20**, 313–16

Eyre, D. R., Paz, M. A. and Gallop, P. M. (1984). Cross-linking in collagen and elastin. *Ann. Rev. Biochem.*, **53**, 717–48

Fedorov, F. I. (1968). *Theory of Elastic Waves in Crystals.* Plenum Press, New York

Garcia, B. J., McNeill, K. G. and Cobbold, R. S. C. (1978). Propagation of ultrasound in bone: longitudinal and shear wave reflection and transmission coefficients. *Third International Symposium on Ultrasonic Imaging and Tissue Characterization*, National Bureau of Standards, Gaithersburg

Gilmore, R. S. and Katz, J. L. (1968). Elastic properties of apatites. In *Proceedings of an International Symposium on Structural Properties of Hydroxyapatite and Related Compounds*, National Bureau of Standards, Washington, DC

Hill, R. (1952). The elastic behavior of crystalline aggregates. *Proc. Phys. Soc. Lond. A*, **65**, 349–54

Hulmes, D. J. S. and Miller, A. (1979). Quasi-hexagonal packing in collagen fibrils. *Nature*, **282**, 878–80

Katz, J. L. (1971). Hard tissue as a composite material. I. Bounds on the elastic behavior. *J. Biomech.*, **4**, 455–73

Katz, E. P. and Li, S. T. (1973). Structure and function of bone collagen fibrils. *J. Molec. Biol.*, **80**, 1–15

Lakes, R., Yoon, H. S. and Katz, J. L. (1986). Ultrasonic wave propagation and attenuation in wet bone. *J. Biomed. Eng.*, **8**, 143–8

Lang, S. B. (1970). Ultrasonic method for measuring elastic coefficients of bone and results on fresh and dried bovine bones. *IEEE Trans. Biomed. Eng.*, **17**, 101–5

Lees, S. (1981). A mixed packing model for bone collagen. *Calcif. Tiss. Int.*, **33**, 591–602

Lees, S. (1986). Water content in type I collagen tissues calculated from the generalized packing model. *Int. J. Biol. Macromol.*, **8**, 66–72

Lees, S. (1987a). Considerations regarding the structure of the mammalian mineralized osteoid from viewpoint of the generalized packing model. *Conn. Tiss. Res.*, **16**, 281–303

Lees, S. (1987b). Possible effect between the molecular packing of collagen and the composition of bony tissues. *Int. J. Biol. Macromol.*, **9**, 321–6

Lees, S. and Davidson, C. L. (1977a). The role of collagen in the elastic properties of calcified tissues. *J. Biomech.*, **10**, 473–486

Lees, S. and Davidson, C. L. (1977b). Ultrasonic measurements of some mineral filled plastics. *IEEE Trans. Sonics Ultrason.*, **SU24**, 222–5

Lees, S. and Escoubes, M. (1987). Vapor pressure isotherms, composition and density of hyperdense bones of horse, whale and porpoise. *Conn. Tiss. Res.*, **16**, 305–322

Lees, S. and Heeley, J. D. (1981). Density of a sample bovine cortical bone matrix and its solid constituents in various media. *Calcif. Tiss. Int.*, **33**, 499–504

Lees, S., Gilmore, R. S. and Kranz, P. R. (1973). Acoustic properties of tungsten-vinyl composites. *IEEE Trans. Sonics Ultrason.*, **SU20**, 1–2

Lees, S., Cleary, P. F., Heeley, J. D. and Gariepy, E. L. (1979a). Distribution of sonic plesio-velocity in a compact bone sample. *J. Acoust. Soc. Am.*, **66**, 641–6

Lees, S., Heeley, J. D. and Cleary, P. F. (1979b). A study of some properties of a sample of bovine cortical bone using ultrasound. *Calcif. Tiss. Int.*, **29**, 107–17

Lees, S., Heeley, J. D. and Cleary, P. F. (1981). Some properties of the organic matrix of a bovine cortical bone sample in various media. *Calcif. Tiss. Int.*, **33**, 83–6

Lees, S., Ahern, J. M. and Leonard, M. (1983a). Parameters influencing the sonic velocity in compact calcified tissues of various species. *J. Acoust. Soc. Am.*, **74**, 28–33

Lees, S., Heeley, J. D., Ahern, J. M. and Oravecz, M. G. (1983b). Axial phase velocity in rat tail tendon fibers at 100 MHz. *IEEE Trans. Sonics Ultrason.*, **SU30**, 85–90

Lees, S., Pineri, M. and Escoubes, M. (1984a). A generalized packing model for type I collagens. *Int. J. Biol. Macromol.*, **6**, 133–6

Lees, S., Bonar, L. C. and Mook, H. A. (1984b). A study of dense mineralized tissue by neutron diffraction. *Int. J. Biol. Macromol.*, **6**, 321–6

Lees, S., Barnard, S. M. and Churchill, D. (1987a). The variation of sonic plesio-velocity in dose dependent lathyritic rabbit femurs. *Ultrasound Med. Biol.*, **13**, 19–24

Lees, S., Barnard, S. M. and Mook, H. A. (1987b). Neutron studies of collagen in lathyritic bone. *Int. J. Biol. Macromol.*, **9**, 32–8

Musgrave, M. J. P. (1970). *Crystal Acoustics*, Holden-Day, San Francisco

Rougvie, M. A. and Bear, R. S. (1953). An X-ray diffraction investigation of swelling by collagen. *J. Am. Leather Chem. Assn*, **48**, 735–51

Selvig, K. A. (1970). Periodic lattice images of hydroxyapatite crystals in human bone and dental hard tissues. *Calcif. Tiss. Res.*, **6**, 227–38

Termine, J. D., Eanes, E. D., Greenfield, D. J., Nylen, M. U. and Harper, R. A. (1973). Hydrazine-deproteinated bone mineral. *Calcif. Tiss. Res.*, **12**, 73–90

van Buskirk, W. C. and Ashman, R. B. (1981). The elastic moduli of bone. In *Mechanical Properties of Bone* (ed. S. C. Cowin), American Society of Mechanical Engineers, New York, 131–43

Voegel, J. C. and Frank, R. M. (1977). Ultrastructural study of apatite crystal dissolution in human dentine and bone. *J. Biol. Buccale*, **5**, 181–94

Weiner, S. and Price, P. A. (1986a). Disaggregation of bone into crystals. *Calcif. Tiss. Int.*, **39**, 365–75

Weiner, S. and Traub, W. (1986b). Organization of hydroxyapatite crystals within collagen fibrils. *FEBS Lett.*, **206**, 262–6

White, S. W., Hulmes, D. J. S., Miller, A. and Timmins, P. A. (1977). Collagen-mineral axial relationship in calcified turkey leg tendon by X-ray and neutron diffraction. *Nature*, **266**, 421–5

Woodhead-Galloway, J. (1984). Two theories of the structure of the collagen fibril. In *Connective Tissue Matrix* (ed. D. W. L. Hukins), Macmillan, London and Basingstoke, 133–60

7
Some characteristics of mineralised collagen

Sidney Lees

INTRODUCTION

According to Albert Szent-Gyorgyi, 'Discovery consists of looking at the same thing as everyone else and thinking something different.' The ideas and suggestions presented in this chapter do not quite satisfy Szent-Gyorgyi's paradigm, since some new facts were added to the older data. However, the previously available information should have sufficed for an acute observer. It is well known that the type I collagen in bone differs from that in soft tissue. For example, the collagen in bone cannot be split by collagenase until the tissue is demineralised. Also, the collagen in bone requires a much higher temperature to gelatinise.

In these two examples, it is only by the loss of the mineral that collagenase becomes effective and the melting-point temperature is drastically reduced. There may be a loss of some non-collagenous factors along with the loss of mineral, and these components may modify the collagen properties, but there is no direct evidence. The question is whether it is the apatitic crystallites that act directly on the collagen or if there are other factors that may depend on the presence of the crystallites. There is reason to believe that the calcium ions interact with the collagen in other ways than as calcium phosphate crystallites.

In the previous chapter, a comparison of the ultrasonic properties of mineralised and demineralised tissues led to the conclusion that the longitudinal modulus of collagen must be greater in the mineralised state, and that one source of the stiffening may be higher cross-linking density of the collagen or some similar process. Most of the data in that chapter referred to macroscopic quantities, except for the neutron diffraction studies. The latter showed that the equatorial diffraction spacing decreases with wet tissue density, implying that the collagen fibrils are more tightly compacted in the more mineralised tissue. Preliminary results found by small-angle neutron diffraction indicate that the axial D-spacing is 63 nm for cow tibia and deer antler. For mineralised turkey leg tendon it is 67 nm, just as for wet demineralised bone matrix and tail tendon collagen. While Rougvie and Bear (1953) showed the axial D-spacing to decrease from about 67 nm for wet tissue to 63 nm after drying, only two values have been observed for wet mineralised tissue, either 63 or 67 nm. The resolution of this situation remains to be undertaken. At this point, it has been demonstrated that at least four properties of mineralised collagen distinguish it from the demineralised substance: the resistance to collagenase, the high gelatinising temperature, the higher elastic moduli and the decreased equatorial diffraction spacing. It will now be shown that there are other differences in properties between mineralised and unmineralised collagen.

OSTEOLATHYRISM AND CROSS-LINKING DENSITY

The stiffness of collagen is attributable to the intermolecular cross-linking, whether mineralised or not. These linkages form a three-dimensional meshwork, giving stiffness and toughness to tendons and ligaments, as well as high values for the elastic moduli (Piez, 1984; Veis, 1984). The cross-linking pattern seems to be specific to each type of tissue. Each cross-linking process involves a complex series of reactions. One series, based on the oxidation of lysine and hydroxylysine mediated by an enzyme, lysyl oxidase, has been extensively explored. Detailed information of the cross-linking pattern, as well as the control of the cross-linking pattern, is difficult to obtain because of the relatively small number of cross-links, often fewer than one per thousand amino acid residues (Reiser and Last, 1986).

Miller (1984) noted that lysyl-derived cross-links are the major ones in fibrillar collagens, including the bone matrix, but that the literature suggests many others not involving lysine. A situation where the cross-linking can be decreased should be associated with a decrease in the stiffness of the tissue, which for mineralised tissues can be detected by a decrease in the sonic velocity. Osteolathyrism is just such a condition, where lysyl oxidase is irreversibly inhibited by the drug beta-amino-propionitrile (BAPN). The reduced cross-linking density is evidenced by reduced mechanical strength and loss of tissue stability (Spengler *et al.*, 1977; Broek *et al.*, 1981; Glimcher *et al.*, 1966). It has been shown *in vitro* that the inhibition is concentration dependent (Tang *et al.*, 1983), suggesting that the effect on bone stiffness should be dose dependent. Other observations indicate that it may not be proportional to the dose level, and in fact there may be a minimum dose required to elicit the lathyritic condition. It is known, for example, that BAPN is converted to cyanoacetic acid (CAA), which is non-lathrogenic, in the liver and possibly elsewhere in the body (Fleisher *et al.*, 1979), and that sequestering and other similar effects exist. Moreover, the administration of the drug is episodic, so that the body concentration varies during the day.

Despite these reservations, dose dependence of many physical and chemical characteristics has been demonstrated in rabbits intoxicated with BAPN from eight weeks of age to early maturity when twenty-two weeks old. In these experiments sections of the cortical bone from femoral diaphyses were compared as a function of the drug dosage. The results show a decrease in lysyl oxidase mediated cross-linking density, an increase in equatorial diffraction spacing, a decrease in the mean radial sonic plesio-velocity, a decrease in the mean wet-bone density, and modification of the gross morphology and histology (Lees *et al.*, 1987a, b; 1988). The density of the lysyl oxidase mediated cross-links was measured in terms of the hydroxypyridinium concentration in the demineralised matrix (Eyre *et al.*, 1984). A comparable measure is given by the fraction of the bone matrix that is insoluble in 0.5 M acetic acid, since the cross-linked collagen is presumably not acid soluble. Figure 7.1 shows that the acid insoluble fraction (AIF) decreases as the BAPN dosage increases, as expected. The curve is derived from experimental values, using the average value for each dosage level. The curve is interpreted to demonstrate that intermolecular collagen cross-linking decreases as the systemic level of BAPN increases, since according to the literature only lysyl oxidase is inhibited by this drug.

It is seen that the insoluble fraction responds to the least amount of BAPN and that the response is most prominent at low dosages. In fact, most of the effect takes place for dosage less than 0.2 g/kg/day, which is interesting because overt symptoms of osteolathyrism become manifest only when the dosage exceeds this value. The observation suggests that a

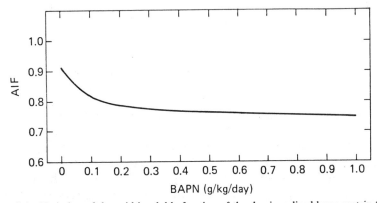

Figure 7.1 Variation of the acid-insoluble fraction of the demineralised bone matrix (AIF) with BAPN dosage. A smooth curve was drawn through the average value for 0, 0.05, 0.1, 0.2, 0.4, 0.6 and 1.0 g BAPN/kg bodyweight/day.

compensatory mechanism may be at work that offsets the loss of cross-linking density until the capacity of the mechanism is saturated. Alternatively, it may indicate a redundancy in cross-linking density in normal bone. Also, it should be noted that the minimum value of AIF is 0.75, showing that a significant fraction of the matrix collagen is cross-linked despite the effects of BAPN. More extensive inhibition was reported by Glimcher *et al.* (1966) where the drug was applied to fetal chick eggs, before much mineralisation or significant collagen turnover took place.

The next set of figures represent the variation of properties of osteolathyritic bone with BAPN dose. In almost all instances, smoothed curves were derived from averaged values. Several samples were prepared from each femur, up to a maximum of six. Bone density varies within a single bone as well as from one femur to the next. The maximum density appears to be 2.1 g/cc for all dosages, as shown in figure 7.2. In these experiments the minimum density decreased from about 2.0 g/cc to 1.75 g/cc, almost linearly with dosage. Clearly, there is a dispersion of bone properties, which increases with BAPN dose, showing that the drug effect is not equal everywhere in the body. This corresponds to clinical observations for neurolathyrism, in which some parts of the body are more paralysed than others.

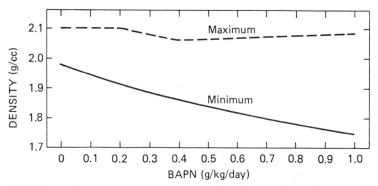

Figure 7.2   The minimum and maximum compact-bone density observed in osteolathyritic rabbit femur as a function of BAPN dosage. The drug does not act equally upon all parts of the bone.

The equatorial diffraction spacing of the collagen in fully mineralised bone (measured by neutron diffraction) *increases* with dosage, as shown in figure 7.3. The rate of increase is somewhat higher at low dosage, but the spacing increases monotonically. The increase corresponds to the decreasing minimum density and to the average density shown in figure 7.4(a). This is a relationship in accord with figure 6.11, where it was shown that the spacing varies inversely with the wet density for normal bone.

The mean density of all the bone samples, as well as the dispersion of

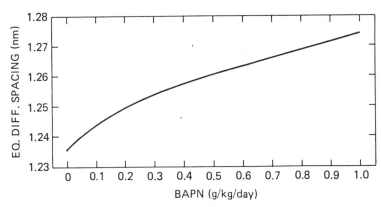

Figure 7.3 Equatorial diffraction spacing of collagen in fully mineralised compact femur bone with BAPN dosage. Comparison with figure 7.1 shows the spacing to decrease with cross-linking density. The relationship is more effective at higher BAPN dose levels where the cross-linking density is least.

this parameter as given by the standard deviation, is displayed in figure 7.4(a). As in figure 7.2, the mean bone density decreases with BAPN dose, while the variability increases. The variation is monotonic and almost linear in both parameters, although the rate at which the mean bone density decreases is steeper for low dosage. Likewise, the mean sonic plesiovelocity decreases with dosage, as seen in figure 7.4(b), while again the dispersion of this parameter increases. The effect on the sonic velocity is more intense at low dosages; i.e., the slope is steeper much like the curve in figure 7.1. This is interesting, because the osteolathyritic symptoms are absent at the low dosages.

The longitudinal elastic modulus is defined as

$$K = \rho c^2$$

where ρ is the density and c the longitudinal sonic velocity. The quantity in figure 7.4(b) is not the true longitudinal velocity because of inhomogeneity and anisotropy of bone. It is defined as the *plesiovelocity*, to indicate that it is almost the true value because the specimen is so thin that its thickness is almost the true sonic path. The quantity plotted in figure 7.5 employs the mean bone density and the mean sonic plesiovelocity of figure 7.4, and not the properties of a single bone specimen. The reference, $\bar{k}_0$, is calculated from the zero BAPN dose specimen. It can be seen in the figure that the longitudinal modulus decreases to slightly less than 80 per cent of the control.

Figure 7.6 shows the dependence of the longitudinal modulus on the cross-linking density, expressed as AIF. The early impact of low BAPN dosage is clearly seen, with the greatest changes occurring at the lowest

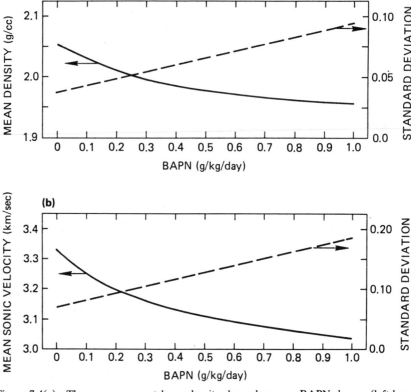

Figure 7.4(a) The mean compact bone density dependence on BAPN dosage (left-hand scale). The dispersion of this quantity expressed as the standard deviation is given by the dashed line (right-hand scale). (b) The mean sonic plesiovelocity compared with its dispersion (standard deviation) as a function of BAPN dosage.

dosage. It is equally clear that while there is a large effect on the cross-linking density for the least BAPN dose level as expressed by AIF, the impact on the elastic moduli is greater at the higher dosages, where overt symptoms of the pathology can be observed. It is further evidence for the existence of a compensatory process for small weaknesses of the mineralised tissue, remarked on previously.

While it is evident that lysyl-oxidase-mediated cross-linking has a marked effect on bone properties and on mineralisation, it must be noted that the sample undergoing the most extreme change still has the properties of bone comparable to deer antler. It is most likely that additional factors participate in controlling the formation of bone.

It is observed that investigations of cross-linking in collagen have been directed to the discovery of covalent organic groups, either in soft connective tissue collagen like rat tail tendon or in the demineralised

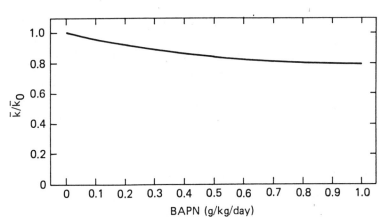

Figure 7.5   The decrease of the longitudinal modulus with BAPN dosage.

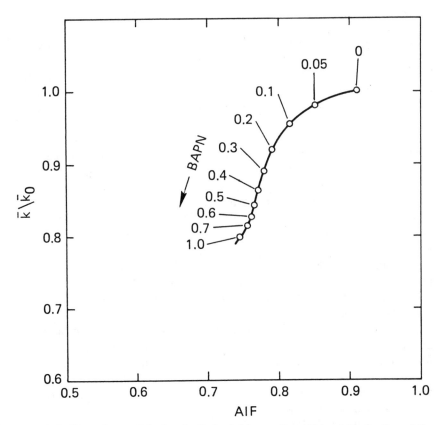

Figure 7.6   Dependence of the longitudinal modulus on the acid-insoluble fraction of the demineralised bone matrix. The BAPN dosage is indicated on the curve.

matrix of hard tissues. In no instance has there been an attempt to distinguish the cross-links in fully mineralised hard tissue from those in the demineralised tissue. It has always been assumed that *all* intermolecular connections are carbon based. Yet it was seen in figure 6.11 that the spacing is 1.24 nm in fully mineralised cow bone, compared with 1.53 nm in the demineralised matrix. The demineralisation process destroys the intermolecular factors that compact the collagen fibrils, which may or may not be carbon based.

THERMODYNAMIC CONSIDERATIONS

It has long been noted that heat affects the collagen in mineralised tissues differently from the way that non-mineralised collagen reacts. It is well known that soft-tissue collagen denatures and forms gelatine above its 'melting point' of 60 °C, where the ordered pattern of interconnected molecules is broken down. A much higher temperature is required to extract gelatine from bone. Two kinds of temperature-dependent effects are presented here.

Bonar and Glimcher (1970) investigated the consequences of heating collagen on its X-ray diffraction pattern. Three types of tissues were examined: tendons, demineralised bone matrix and fully mineralised bone, obtained from chicken, rat, cow and guinea-pig. Wide-angle and low-angle X-ray diffraction patterns of the soft tissue disappear after the tissue is heated above the melting point.

In this investigation, one set of tissue samples was heated to 65 °C, one set to 82.5 °C and a third set to 100 °C, each for 30 minutes. After heating, the bone specimens were demineralised in 0.5 M EDTA solution at alkaline pH. Both types of X-ray diffraction patterns were prepared for all specimens and compared with the controls.

The diffraction patterns were destroyed for tendons and demineralised bone matrix, although under certain circumstances the bone matrix wide-angle diffraction pattern could be recovered. Bones heated to 100 °C for 30 minutes and then demineralised yielded diffraction patterns identical both axially and equatorially to those of the controls. Heating at a temperature that denatures soft-tissue collagen has no effect on the fully mineralised collagen.

The investigators concluded that the stabilising effect may be a purely mechanical phenomenon, with the mineral by its mere presence within the fibrils physically restraining the collagen. Alternatively, they said that chemical interactions between calcium and phosphate ions with the amino-acid residue side chains, as well as with the collagen molecule backbone, may play a role.

A second thermal effect has been observed when differential scanning calorimetry (DSC) is employed. This instrument enables various thermodynamic parameters to be measured as the temperature is increased at a uniform rate. Protein denaturation is manifest by a peak of input energy at a critical temperature (Privalov and Tiktopulo, 1970), which for collagen has been found to depend on the specific composition of the collagen, the conditions of the test and the structure of the collagenous tissue. Privalov (1982), for example, reported the peak temperature for solutions of collagen to vary from 6 °C, for Antarctic ice fish, to 41 °C, for chick skin collagen, and 52 °C, for *Ascaris* cuticle collagen. Intact rat skin collagen has a peak at 59 °C (Flandin *et al.*, 1984). The peak for normal human demineralised bone matrix is 60 °C (Herbage *et al.*, 1982). We have made DSC measurements on wet-bone matrix, dry-bone matrix and fully mineralised dry bone. The temperatures of the input energy peak for our preliminary results were 58 °C for wet cow-bone matrix, 94 °C for dry cow-bone matrix and 173 °C for fully mineralised dry cow-bone.

Privalov's data show the temperature at which the collagen molecules suffer denaturation, where the others refer to the denaturation temperature of collagen structures interconnected by cross-links. It is presumed that the lowest temperatures correspond to the unravelling of the triple-helical chains, where the higher temperatures relate to the disruption of the intermolecular cross-links, as well as to the denaturation of the collagen molecules. This interpretation is supported by Flandin *et al.* (1984), where it can be seen that a 50–55 °C peak predominates in lathyritic rat skin collagen, owing to the decreased intermolecular cross-link density. The different denaturation temperatures between wet cow-bone matrix and dry cow-bone matrix collagen shows the powerful effect of water on the structural characteristics of collagen. The much higher peak temperature for denaturation of the collagen in intact bone demonstrates that mineralised collagen differs significantly from the same collagen in the demineralised state. Again, as for the X-ray diffraction studies, the mineralised condition strongly modifies the characteristics of collagen.

The thermal studies show positively and clearly that the difference between mineralised and non-mineralised collagen must reside in the chemical state of the collagen and not simply in a mechanical property of the embedded crystallites. Again, since the loss of calcium induces such great changes, it seems likely that calcium interacting with the collagen molecules is the source of the modification of properties.

WATER CONTENT OF MINERALISED TISSUE

Pineri *et al.* (1978) identified five regimes (or hydration shells) for the water in rat tail tendon. The first two regimes refer to water within the collagen molecule needed to tie the three α-chains into a single molecular structure by means of water bridges, as described by Ramachandran (1976). Regime I water (0.01 g/g dry collagen) can only be removed at high temperatures, destroying the triple helix. Regime II water (0.100 g/g) is removable at 20 °C by evaporation. The same amount of Regime II water was found in bovine bone matrix (Lees, 1981). However, Regime II water cannot be detected from vapour pressure isotherm studies of intact bone or mineralised turkey leg tendon (Lees and Escoubes, 1987).

The inability to detect Regime II water may not correspond to its *absence* in bone. It only demonstrates that Regime II water cannot be extracted by evaporation at room temperature. It has been shown that there is water within the fibrils but outside the molecules (Lees, 1986) and that the intrafibrilar water can be extracted at room temperature (Lees *et al.*, 1984). The individual collagen molecules are surrounded by water, and, since these are all type I collagens with the same chemical composition, except for inorganic matter like calcium ions, the water content of mineralised collagen should be the same as for soft tissue collagen. Some factor associated with the mineralised state prevents the removal of Regime II water.

The heat of hydration for the calcium ion is 589.3 kJ/mol (Monk, 1961), showing very tight binding to water. As discussed below, because of the presence of apatitic crystallites, the effective calcium ion concentration in the mineralised collagen fibrils must be higher than in soft tissue. As the tissue dries, the amount of free water decreases and the concentration of calcium ions within the fibril increases. Hydrated calcium ions can exchange with water molecules in the fibril structure. It may be that during the process of drying the Regime II water in bone collagen becomes bound to calcium ions, and consequently water is more difficult to extract from bone.

MOBILITY OF THE COLLAGEN MOLECULE WITHIN THE FIBRIL

Torchia and his associates have detected angular motion of the individual collagen molecules within the three-dimensional mesh of the collagen fibril (Batchelder *et al.*, 1982; Jelinski *et al.*, 1980; Sarker *et al.*, 1983, 1985). In these experiments, specific amino acids were replaced with isotope-labelled equivalents. For example, glycine was replaced by [1-^{13}C]glycine in one experimental series and by [2-^{13}C]glycine in a second series. Leucine and alanine were labelled with deuterium in previous earlier experiments. Such labelling made it possible to detect the isotope by the chemical shift in the solid-state NMR spectrum. Their analysis led to the conclusion that the collagen molecule rotates about the molecular backbone; that is, about the long axis of the molecule. It has also been concluded that segments of the whole molecule can and do rotate about the long axis as well, and that even individual amino acid side chains can rotate about the same axis. The collagen molecule was shown to have two stable azimuthal orientations. The angular motion corresponds to a jump by the molecule from one

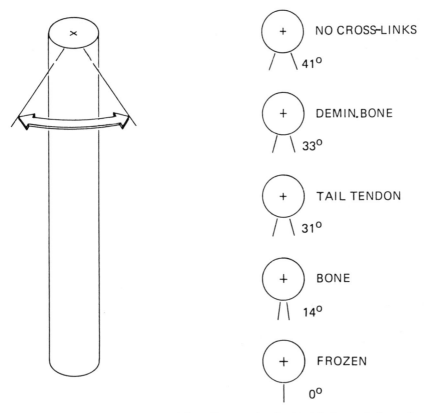

Figure 7.7   Angular displacement of the collagen molecule about its long axis for various situations.

orientation to the other. The process for the whole molecule takes place on a time scale of 10^{-4} seconds, whereas for segmental jumps the time scale is of the order of nanoseconds. These two orientations correspond to energy wells and the molecule is thermally activated to hop from one well to the other.

Four kinds of tissue were examined in their studies of soft and hard collagen tissues. The first was reconstituted collagen fibrils, where there are no cross-links between collagen molecules. The second tissue was rat tail tendon fibres, in which the molecules are highly ordered and cross-linked. The third was demineralised rat calvaria and rat tibia, while the fourth was the same fully mineralised bone. In the first instance, the work was done at 22 °C, which was repeated at −35 °C where the bulk water is frozen. The results are summarised in figure 7.7, which shows the angular displacement to be ±41 ° for reconstituted collagen fibrils, decreasing to ±14 ° for bone and to 0 ° for all frozen tissues.

It should be noted especially that only motion about the long axis is reported in these studies. Brillouin scattering studies show the existence of translational modes, both along the long axis and in the perpendicular direction (Cusack and Miller, 1979). Apparently these motions do not induce a detectable signal in NMR.

The magnitude of the angular displacement, even for fully mineralised bone, indicates that the molecules do not interconnect along their length between their teleopeptide ends. The intermolecular connections can only be at the ends of the molecules. The ability of collagen molecules to organise into stable fibrils without intermolecular cross-links, as demonstrated by reconstituted collagen, shows that the order in this instance arises from the field interaction between adjacent molecules that is due to the molecular structure. The existence of two energy wells implies that adjacent molecules interact to create the energy wells, even in the absence of cross-links. The presence of cross-links reduces the angular displacement, apparently in response to the elastic restraint, which modifies the locus of the energy wells. The difference between the angular displacement of demineralised bone and tail tendon collagens suggests a difference in the cross-linking structure. These measurements may be related to the difference in the equatorial diffraction spacing of these two tissues, 1.33 nm for tail tendon collagen and 1.53 nm for demineralised bone matrix collagen.

The azimuthal displacements for mineralised tissues demonstrate again that there is no mineral between adjacent molecules. The absence of angular displacement in frozen tissue where the extramolecular water is frozen proves the point. This is further confirmation of the previous conclusion that mineral is unlikely to exist between adjacent molecules. The significant decrease in angular displacement between demineralised and mineralised tissue might be attributed to mechanical constraints imposed by hole-filling crystallites. Alternatively, it may indicate a greatly augmented elastic restraint, due either to a non-crystalline mineralisation of the cross-link between molecules, or to the presence of additional mineral-organic cross-links augmenting the purely organic cross-linking density.

PHOSPHORYLATED COLLAGEN IN THE BONE MATRIX

Phosphorylated organic components have been detected in mineralised tissues for many years (Glimcher, 1984; Veis, 1984), but mostly as non-collagenous compounds like phosphoserine and phosphothreonine. However, it has been demonstrated that there are phosphate groups bound to bone collagen and not to soft tissue collagen (Cohen-Solal et al., 1979a, b; 1981). Initially, γ-glutamyl phosphate was identified in the α-2 chains of chicken bone collagen (Cohen-Solel et al., 1979b). This study showed there to be approximately four atoms of organic phosphorus per collagen

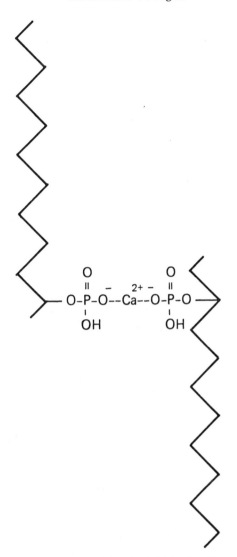

Figure 7.8 Intermolecular linkage by calcium ion bridging in collagen.

molecule. It was demonstrated that no organic phosphorus is present in other collagens. Subsequently, γ-glutamyl phosphate was identified in collagen from turkey bone, calf bone, monkey bone, rat bone, turkey calcified tendon and calf calcified cartilage.

Veis (1984) has investigated phosphophoryn, found in abundance in dentine and much less so in bone. He pointed out that a linear chain polyion of high charge like a phosphophoryn has high binding affinity for small counterions, particularly calcium ions. He showed that a calcium ion can bind two organic phosphate groups, thereby coupling two adjacent molecules. It is seen in figure 7.8 how two collagen molecules can be linked by the glutamyl phosphate groups in the α-chains. The multiple phosphorylation provides sites for complex meshing of the collagenous structure in addition to the organic cross-links like the lysyl-oxidase-mediated processes. These additional intermolecular linkages, present only in the fully mineralised tissue, may be representative of the hypothesised increased cross-linking density in bone, which vanishes during demineralisation. There may be other unknown intermolecular linkages.

INFLUENCE OF THE CALCIUM-RICH ENVIRONMENT

The local environment of collagen molecules within a mineral-embedded fibril must be different from the environment of soft-tissue collagen. The presence of a calcium phosphate mineral surrounding and in intimate contact with the fibrils suggests that the fluid bathing the collagen is saturated in calcium and phosphate ions. The fluid around a soft-tissue collagen fibril may be supersaturated with respect to calcium phosphates also, but the presence of inhibiting agents, which prevent crystallisation or deposition of calcium phosphate, results in a very low *effective* calcium ion concentration. On the other hand, the effective calcium ion concentration in the presence of apatitic crystallites must be presumed to be much higher to prevent dissolution of the crystallites. There is a limitation to this assumption, in that the crystallites have been shown to be embedded in organic matter (Lees and Escoubes, 1987). It is also believed that organic matter, like the GLA protein, regulates the size of the crystallites (Glimcher, 1984). There are probably additional active agents that make the bony tissue environment different from that of soft tissue, but it is suspected that calcium plays a dominant role, since demineralisation drastically changes the properties of hard tissue. The interaction by other active agents may enhance the influence of calcium.

The electrical field around the collagen molecule is created by the collagen molecule itself, as well as by the nearby neighbours and the fluid filling the intervening space. The resultant local field within the molecule, which is due to all the intramolecular interactions as well as to the interacting fields from the closest neighbours, is the source of the observed stability and structural characteristics for the individual molecules and the comparable properties of the collagenous fibrous structure. If the local environment is changed, the conformation of individual collagen molecules, as well as the complex meshwork of molecules, may be altered. The higher effective calcium ion concentration in the presence of calcium phosphate crystals represents a likely alteration of the local environment.

It can be demonstrated readily that the local environment affects the collagen molecular configuration. The *D*-spacing, as well as the equatorial diffraction spacing of tail tendon collagen, decreases as the water content of the tissue is reduced (Rougvie and Bear, 1953). The *D*-value goes from 67 to 63 nm, while the equatorial spacing decreases from 1.33 to 1.09 nm.

A second example was reported by Nemetschek *et al.* (1983b), where water in rat tail tendon collagen was replaced by various linear chain alcohols of a homologous series. Three types of experiment were undertaken. In the first, alcohol–water solutions of varying concentration were used. The second was a sequence of 100 per cent 1-alcanols with the number of carbons increasing from 1 to 12. In the third, the sequence consisted of 2-alcanols. The *D*-spacing for collagen in ethanol–water solutions decreased from 67.0 to 66.4 nm as the ethanol concentration increased to 100 per cent. The *D*-spacing decreased monotonically to 64.8 nm as the number of carbons increased to 12 for the 100 per cent 1-alcanol sequence. For the 2-alcanol sequence, the least *D*-spacing was 63.3 nm, just as for dried collagen fibres. However, unlike dried collagen, the equatorial diffraction spacing increased, as if the molecules became shorter and squatter (Nemetschek *et al.*, 1983a; Folkhard *et al.*, 1984).

Conformational polymorphism has been observed in polyions (Manning, 1979), particularly for DNA molecules, where at least four conformations are known (Soumpasis, 1986, Brady *et al.*, 1986). The B-form is a right-handed double helix, while the Z-form is left-handed (see figure 7.9). The transition from B to Z (Soumpasis, 1984, 1987) can be induced by increasing the salt concentration, e.g. NaCl. The pitch angle has been

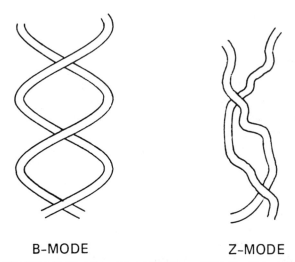

B–MODE   Z–MODE

Figure 7.9 The DNA B–Z conformational transformations. The B-form is a right-handed helix, while the Z-form is left-handed.

reported to change with sodium ion concentration, from 50° when $[Na^+] = 0.02$ M to 15° at 1.0 M, along with other parameters of the helix (Brady *et al.*, 1986). Similar changes were observed as a function of the temperature.

Soumpasis (1986) identified two situations. In the first the small ions bind to specific sites of the molecule and induce B–Z transformations at millimolar concentrations of appropriate salts. These low concentrations can change the charge distribution of the polyion. In the second instance, the small ions collect in a diffuse cloud around the polyion, statistically screening the electrical field. Soumpasis (1986) observed that the diffuse cloud requires high ion concentration for DNA in solution, where specific site ion binding is effective at low ion concentration in solid DNA. It cannot be predicted, on the basis of present information, what may be true for collagen. The tenor of the literature, as exemplified by Glimcher (1984) and Veis (1984), favours specific site ion binding. It is already noted that certain sites in bone collagen favour calcium bridging (Cohen-Solal *et al.*, 1981), but the presence of a relatively high calcium ion concentration, together with other active agents in the fluid, filling the relatively wide intermolecular volume, may induce conformational transformations by either mechanism.

The apparent absence of Regime II water was interpreted to be a consequence of a high calcium ion concentration. The *D*-spacing for collagen in fully mineralised cow bone was found to be 63 nm, whether the bone is wet or dry, whereas in the wet demineralised bone collagen it is 67 nm and 63 nm for dried collagen. These measurements suggest that mineralised collagen undergoes a conformational transformation in the presence of high calcium ion concentration, but it is unclear whether this is due to specific site binding or to a diffuse ion cloud.

PHYSICOCHEMICAL CONSIDERATIONS

It was pointed out in the beginning of this chapter that collagenase cannot attack mineralised collagen. There are many agents that react with non-mineralised collagen to which the mineralised tissue is resistant. Osteoclasts demineralise bone in their immediate environment before the collagen fibrils can be lysed (Heersche, 1978). Tissues are stained with histochemical reagents to distinguish microscopic structures. The Van Gieson stain is specific for collagen, which appears bright red in the microscope (Cowdry, 1952). Van Gieson will not stain mineralised collagen, and it is necessary to demineralise before staining.

When bone is dried it undergoes shrinkage (Lees *et al.*, 1979), which is reversed when the bone is rewetted. Attempts to wet the dried bone with various alcohols were unsuccessful. A small increase in weight was detected after a long exposure to ethanol, but this was probably due to penetration of some pores in the bone. Non-mineralised collagen reacts obviously to alcohol and becomes quite rigid in 100 per cent ethanol (Lees *et al.*, 1981a; Nemetschek *et al.*, 1983a, b).

These instances demonstrate that mineralised collagen reacts differently from non-mineralised or demineralised tissues. Two possible reasons are proposed. Either the specific reaction sites on the collagen molecule are blocked in the mineralised state, or the mineralised structure between collagen fibrils limits accessibility to the collagen. Wooley (1984) pointed out that collagenase activity is reduced by a factor of 20 for fibrils compared with collagen in solution. It is inferred that it is necessary for the disrupted collagen molecules to be removed so as to expose new layers of molecules to the enzyme. Further, the reference suggests that cross-linking acts to retain the disrupted fragments in place in the fibril. Mineralised collagen presents an even more difficult situation, where the extrafibrillar mineral-filled volume presents a mechanical cage-like restraint to trap the collagen molecular fragments. Only when the tissue is demineralised can the collagen fragments be cleared from the site.

It is more likely that the large size of the collagenase molecule keeps it outside the mineral crystallites, tightly clustered around the collagen fibril. It is also important to note that the individual crystallites are embedded in a non-collagenous organic coating, which reduces the intercrystalline spacing (Lees and Escoubes, 1987). Water can probably penetrate the coating by its solubility properties. The limited effectiveness of Van Gieson staining, as well as the alcohols, suggest that it is difficult for particles larger than a water molecule to be transported through the mineralised extrafibrillar space.

RECAPITULATION

In Chapter 6 it was shown that the composition of bone varies widely with its wet density. The increase in the mineral weight fraction is associated with a larger decrease in the organic content and with a lesser decrease in the water content, as illustrated in figures 6.16, 6.17 and 6.18. Evidence has been given in Chapters 6 and 7 that most of the mineral must lie *between* collagen fibrils and that only the hole region between collinear collagen molecules can possibly provide space for mineral crystallites within the fibrils. Other important characteristics of mineralised tissue are summarised here.

(1)	Chemical resistance	Cleavage by collagenase is resisted. Histochemical agents are ineffective. Alcohols are not absorbed.
(2)	Thermodynamic stability	Much higher temperatures are required to denature mineralised collagen.

(3) Cross-linking density

Mineral content appears to depend on intermolecular cross-linking density of collagen. Lysyl-oxidase-mediated cross-linking is a factor, but other types of cross-linking may also be important.

(4) Phosphorylation

Bone collagen has at least four phosphate groups per collagen molecule. Soft-tissue collagen has none. Calcium ions may bridge adjoining collagen molecules

(5) Collagen molecule mobility

Solid-state NMR shows mineralised collagen molecules rotate about the long axis between two stable azimuthal positions. Angular displacement is less than half that for demineralised collagen.

(6) Elastic moduli

Elastic moduli appear to depend on collagen stiffened by increased cross-linking density and other types of intermolecular linkages

(7) Intermolecular structure

Equatorial diffraction spacing of bone collagen is inverse to the wet-bone density. Dried-bone spacing is reduced to the same value as dried soft-tissue collagen

(8) Conformational transformation

Axial D-spacing of mineralised turkey leg tendon is 67 nm. For deer antler and for cow bone, it appears to be 63 nm, whether the bone is wet or dry. This may depend on the effective calcium ion concentration.

(9) Absence of Regime II water

Higher effective calcium ion concentration may bind the residual water during drying.

This list shows that mineralised collagen is different from the same collagen after demineralisation, as well as from soft tissue collagen. The mineralisation process is accompanied by modification of the collagen in the matrix by two possible sources. Some modifications are associated with the mineralisation process, like the replacement of soft matter with mineral crystallites, or phosphorylation of collagen. Other modifications may come about because of the calcium-rich environment in the presence of calcium phosphate crystallites, such as conformational transformation or calcium bridging between the ends of collagen molecules. The drastic changes observed when calcium is removed implicate calcium as a potent agent in modifying collagen properties.

The different thermodynamic properties, as well as the marked structural modifications revealed by neutron diffraction, imply that mineralised collagen is chemically different from soft tissue and from demineralised collagens. It is necessary to study the mineralised state of collagen, as well as after demineralisation, because the latter is incomplete.

It is inferred that mineralised collagen is stiffened as a consequence of calcium bridging, as well as by other intermolecular linking processes. Moreover, the individual collagen molecule may be stiffened by the conformational transformation in the presence of high calcium ion concentration, as indicated by the shorter *D*-spacing. Dried collagen, which also has a *D*-spacing of 63 nm, is stiffer than the wet tissue. The closer intermolecular packing, revealed by the inverse dependence of the equatorial diffraction spacing with wet tissue density, should make the fibril stiffer. Crystallites in the hole zones would stiffen the intermolecular cross-links and transmit forces between molecules without buckling. The extrafibrillar crystallites confine the collagen fibril (not the individual molecules) within channels, thereby preventing columnar buckling. These several effects combine to stiffen the structure and to enable it to support compressive loads.

REFERENCES

Batchelder, L. S., Sullivan, C. E., Jelinski, L. W. and Torchia, D. A. (1982). Characterization of leucine side-chain reorientation in collagen fibrils by solid-state ^{2}H NMR. *Proc. Natl Acad. Sci. USA*, **79**, 386–9

Bonar, L. C. and Glimcher, M. J. (1970). Thermal denaturation of mineralized and demineralized bone collagens. *J. Ultrastruct. Res.*, **32**, 545–51

Bonar, L. C., Lees, S. and Mook, H. A. (1985). Neutron diffraction studies of collagen in fully mineralized bone. *J. Molec. Biol.*, **181**, 265–70

Brady, G. W., Satkowski, M., Foos, D. and Benheim, C. J. (1986). Environmental influences on DNA superhelicity. Ionic strength and temperature effects on superhelix conformation in solution. In *Biomolecular Stereodynamics*, Vol. IV (eds R. H. Sarma and M. H. Sarma), Adenine Press, Guilderland

Broek, D. L., Eikenberry, E. F., Rietzek, P. P. and Brodsky, B. (1981). Collagen structure in tendon and bone. In *The Chemistry and Biology of Mineralized Connective Tissue* (ed. A. Veis), Elsevier, New York, pp. 79–84

Cohen-Solal, L., Lian, J. B., Kossiva, D. and Glimcher, M. J. (1979a). Identification of organic phosphorus and O-phosphothreonine in non-collageneous proteins and their absence from phosphorylated collagen. *Biochem. J.*, **177**, 81–98

Cohen-Solal, L., Cohen-Solal, M. and Glimcher, M. J. (1979b). Identification of gamma-glutamyl phosphate in the alpha2 chains of chicken bone collagen. *Proc. Natl Acad. Sci. USA*, **76**, 4327–30

Cohen-Solal, L., Maroteaux, P. and Glimcher, M. J. (1981). Presence of gamma-glutamyl phosphate in the collagens of bone and other calcified tissues and its absence in the collagens of unmineralized tissues. In *The Chemistry and Biology of Mineralized Connective Tissues* (ed. A. Veis), Elsevier North Holland, New York, pp. 7–11

Cowdry, E. V. (1952). *Laboratory Technique in Biology and Medicine*, Williams and Wilkins, Baltimore

Cusack, S. and Miller, A. (1979). Determination of the elastic constants of collagen by Brillouin light scattering. *J. Molec. Biol.*, **135**, 39–51

Eyre, D. R., Paz, M. A. and Gallop, P. A. (1984). Cross linking in collagen and elastin. *Ann. Rev. Biochem.*, **53**, 717–48

Flandin, F., Buffevant, C. and Herbage, D. (1984). A differential scanning calorimetry analysis of the age related changes in the thermal stability of rat skin collagen. *Biochim. Biophys. Acta*, **791**, 205–11

Fleisher, J. H., Spear, D., Brendel, K. and Chvapil, M. (1979). Effect of pargyline on the metabolism of BAPN by rabbits. *Toxicol. Appl. Pharmacol.*, **47**, 61–9

Folkhard, W., Knorzer, E., Mosler, E. and Nemetschek, T. (1984). Packing of collagen molecules modified with 2-propanol. *J. Molec. Biol.*, **177**, 841–4

Glimcher, M. J. (1984). Recent studies of the mineral phase in bone and its possible linkage to the organic matrix by protein-bound phosphate bonds. *Phil. Trans. R. Soc. Lond. B*, **304**, 479–508

Glimcher, M. J., Friberg, U. A., Orloff, S. and Gross, J. (1966). The role of the inorganic crystals in the stability characteristics of collagen in lathyritic bone. *J. Ultrastruct. Res.*, **15**, 74–86

Heersche, J. N. M. (1978). Mechanisms of osteoclastic bone resorption: a new hypothesis. *Calcif. Tissue Res.*, **26**, 81–4

Herbage, D., Borsali, F., Buffevant, Ch., Flandin, F. and Aguercif, M. (1982). Composition, cross-linking and thermal stability of bone and skin collagens in patients with osteogenesis imperfecta. *Metab. Bone Dis. Rel. Res.*, **4**, 95–101

Jelinski, L. W., Sullivan, C. E. and Torchia, D. A. (1980). ^{2}H NMR study of molecular motion in collagen fibrils. *Nature*, **284**, 531–4

Lees, S. (1981). A mixed packing model for bone collagen. *Calcif. Tiss. Int.*, **33**, 591–602

Lees, S. (1986). Water content in Type I collagen tissues calculated from the generalized packing model. *Int. J. Biol. Macromol.*, **8**, 66–72

Lees, S. and Escoubes, M. (1987). Vapor pressure isotherms, composition and density of hyperdense bones of horse, whale and porpoise. *Conn. Tiss. Res.*, **16**, 281–303

Lees, S., Heeley, J. D. and Cleary, P. F. (1979). A study of some properties of a sample of bovine cortical bone using ultrasound. *Calcif. Tiss. Int.*, **29**, 107–17

Lees, S., Heeley, J. D. and Cleary, P. F. (1981). Some properties of the organic matrix of a bovine cortical bone sample in various media. *Calcif. Tiss. Int.*, **83**, 83–6

Lees, S., Bonar, L. C. and Mook, H. A. (1984). A study of dense mineralized tissue by neutron diffraction. *Int. J. Biol. Macromol.*, **6**, 321–6

Lees, S., Barnard, S. M. and Churchill, D. (1987a). The variation of sonic plesiovelocity in dose-dependent lathyritic rabbit femurs. *Ultrasound Med. Biol.*, **13**, 19–24

Lees, S., Barnard, S. M. and Mook, H. A. (1987b). Neutron studies of collagen in lathyritic bone. *Int. J. Biol. Macromol.*, **9**, 32–8

Lees, S., Eyre, D. R. and Barnard, S. M. (1989). BAPN dose dependence of mature crosslinks in bone matrix collagen of rabbit compact bone: corresponding variation of several physical properties. To be published

Manning, G. S. (1979). Counterion binding in polyelectrolyte theory. *Acc. Chem. Res.*, **12**, 443–9

Miller, E. J. (1984). Chemistry of the Collagens. In *Extracellular Matrix Biochemistry* (eds K. A. Piez and A. H. Reddi), Elsevier, New York, p. 57

Monk, C. B. (1961). *Electrolytic Dissociation*. Academic Press, London, p. 261

Nemetschek, T., Jelenik, K., Knorzer, E., Mosler, E., Nemetschek-Gansler, H., Riedl, H. and Schilling, V. (1983a). Transformation of the structure of collagen. *J. Molec. Biol.*, **167**, 461–79

Nemetschek, T., Knorzer, E., Folkhard, W., Gerken, W., Jelenik, K., Kuhleman, C., Mosler, E. and Nemetschek-Gansler, H. (1983b). Hydratwasseraustausch und alkanol-induzierte molekulare unordnungen an kollagen. *Z. Naturforsch.*, **38c**, 815–28

Piez, K. A. (1984). Molecular and aggregate structures of the collagens. In *Extracellular Matrix Biochemistry* (eds K. A. Piez and A. H. Reddi), Elsevier, New York

Pineri, M. H., Escoubes, M. and Roche, G. (1978). Water–collagen interactions: calorimetric and mechanical experiments. *Biopolymers*, **17**, 2799–815

Privalov, P. L. (1982). Stability of proteins: proteins which do not present a single cooperative system. In *Advances in Protein Chemistry* (eds C. B. Anfinsen, J. T. Edsall and F. M. Richards), Academic Press, New York, pp. 1–104

Privalov, P. L. and Tiktopulo, E. I. (1970). Thermal conformational transformation of tropocollagen. I. Calorometric study. *Biopolymers*, **9**, 127–39

Ramachandran, G. N. and Ramakrishnan, C. (1976). Molecular structure. In *Biochemistry of Collagen* (eds G. N. Ramachandran and A. H. Reddi), Plenum Press, New York, pp. 45–84

Rougvie, M. A. and Bear, R. S. (1953). An X-ray diffraction investigation of swelling by collagen. *J. Am. Leather Chem. Assoc.*, **48**, 735–51

Reiser, K. M. and Last, J. A. (1986). Biosynthesis of collagen crosslinks: *in vivo* labelling of neonatal skin, tendon and bone in rats. *Conn. Tiss. Res.*, **14**, 293–306

Sarker, S. K., Sullivan, E. S. and Torchia, D. A. (1983). Solid state ^{13}C NMR study of collagen molecular dynamics in hard and soft tissues. *J. Biol. Chem.*, **258**, 9762–7

Sarker, S. K., Sullivan, E. S. and Torchia, D. A. (1985). Nanosecond fluctuations of the molecular backbone of collagen in hard and soft tissues: a carbon-13 NMR relaxation study. *Biochem.*, **24**, 2348–54

Soumpasis, D. M. (1984). Statistical mechanics of the B–Z transition of DNA: contribution of diffuse ion interactions. *Proc. Natl Acad. Sci. USA*, **81**, 5116–20

Soumpasis, D. M. (1986). Ionic stabilization and modulation of nucleic acid conformations in solution. In *Biomolecular Stereodynamics*, Vol. **IV** (eds R. H. Sarma and M. H. Sarma), Adenine Press, Guilderland

Soumpasis, D. M., Robert-Nicoud, M. and Jovin, T. M. (1987). B–Z DNA conformational transition in 1:1 electrolytes: dependence upon counterion size. *FEBS Lett.*, **213**, 341–4

Spengler, D. M., Baylink, D. J. and Rosenquist, J. B. (1977). Whole bone mechanical properties: evidence for an effect of bone matrix. *J. Bone Joint Surg.*, **59A**, 670

Tang, S. S., Trackman, P. C. and Kagan, H. M. (1983). Reaction of aortic lysyl oxidase with beta-aminopropionitrile. *J. Biol. Chem.*, **258**, 4331–38

Veis, A. (1984). Bones and teeth. In *Extracellular Matrix Biochemistry* (eds K. A. Piez and A. H. Reddi), Elsevier, New York, pp. 352

Wooley, D. E. (1984). Mammalian collagenases. In *Extracellular Matrix Biochemistry* (eds K. A. Piez and A. H. Reddi), Elsevier, New York

8
The interaction of phosphoproteins with calcium phosphate

C. Holt and M. J. J. M. van Kemenade

INTRODUCTION

This review is concerned with some of the well-characterised phosphoproteins that interact with calcium phosphate as part of their biological function, and phosphoproteins that have been used frequently in laboratory studies of phosphoprotein–calcium phosphate interactions. This heterogeneous group comprises the phosphophoryns from teeth, the bone phosphoproteins, the caseins from milk, the statherins and acidic proline-rich proteins of saliva, osteonectin and the egg phosvitins. The prominence given here to the caseins is largely a reflection of our own research interests, but it can be justified as bringing this well-studied group of phosphoproteins more to the attention of researchers in the field of tissue mineralisation.

Before examining each of these groups of proteins, it is necessary to set out in general terms what is meant by saying that phosphoproteins interact with calcium phosphate. Phosphoproteins can influence the mechanisms of formation of calcium phosphate phases; they can inhibit or promote nucleation of a particular phase and its subsequent growth, inhibit or promote the transformation of a precursor phase into a thermodynamically more stable phase or influence which of several more stable phases actually forms. They can influence the rate of dissolution of individual phases in complex deposits, affect crystal size and morphology, the aggregation of crystals into clusters and much else besides. At a fundamental level, therefore, we wish to know about the stereochemistry, kinetics and thermodynamics of adsorption of the phosphoprotein at the surface of a calcium phosphate phase or cluster of ions. The systems we are dealing with, however, present some particularly severe problems in attempting to acquire fundamental information of general validity: the phosphoproteins, as a group, are difficult to isolate in pure form and tend to have flexible conformations in solution; they are difficult to crystallise, so there is a dearth of structural information on them. On the other hand, calcium phosphates are notoriously variable in chemical composition, impurity content and degree of crystallinity: hydroxyapatite (HAP, $Ca_5OH(PO_4)_3$) is difficult to prepare as large crystals under laboratory conditions, octacalcium phosphate (OCP, $Ca_4H(PO_4)_3$) is commonly found in an expitaxial relationship with HAP, and β-tricalcium phosphate (β-TCP, $Ca_3(PO_4)_2$) in biology is invariably formed with Mg^{2+} replacing a significant fraction of the Ca^{2+}. Brushite (dicalcium phosphate dihydrate DCPD, $CaHPO_4.2H_2O$), however, can be obtained as large, well-formed, crystals of perfect stoichiometry, and therefore is the preferred phase for work in well-defined systems, even though it is thermodynamically unstable with respect to the more basic phases under physiological conditions.

In this review, each phosphoprotein is first considered separately in terms of its biosynthesis, primary structure, structure in solution, calcium binding behaviour and interaction with calcium phosphate. In the concluding section, an attempt is made to bring together aspects that are common to several members of the group, and we speculate indulgently on the fundamentals (stereochemistry, kinetics and thermodynamics) of the binding of phosphoproteins to calcium phosphate in relation to the structure of the proteins and their biological functions.

THE CASEINS

General properties

Bovine caseins, and possibly all caseins, are of four types: α_{s1}-, α_{s2}-, β- and κ-casein. Of these, κ-casein is distinctly different in primary structure, post-translational processing and sensitivity to precipitation by calcium. Consequently, the four caseins have been divided into the Ca^{2+}-sensitive (α_{s1}-, α_{s2}- and β-) and the Ca^{2+}-insensitive (κ-) caseins. In cow's milk, all four caseins, together with about 7 per cent (by weight) calcium phosphate, are found in colloidal, spherical, particles known as casein micelles. The historical division of caseins according to precipitation by Ca^{2+} is still of use, since it reflects also the strength of interaction of the individual caseins with calcium phosphate. In the casein micelle, the caseins are linked through their phosphoseryl (SerP) residues to the calcium phosphate which is present as finely dispersed ion clusters throughout the protein matrix. Because κ-casein interacts only weakly with calcium phosphate, its function is different: some of the κ-casein lies on the surface of the micelle with the C-terminal macropeptide projecting into the surrounding serum to form a protective 'hairy' layer which gives the casein micelle great thermal stability. On the other hand, the hairs are easily 'clipped' by the enzyme chymosin to cause aggregation of micelles. This is the first stage of the cheese-making process.

Each of the caseins has a distinct character, dependent only in part on the differences in degree of phosphorylation. For example, β-casein has a hydrophilic head and hydrophobic tail, giving it a polar character, much like a surfactant. Four of the five SerP residues are in an acidic N-terminal peptide, in the sequence

$$\overset{15}{\text{-SerP}}\text{-Leu-SerP-SerP-SerP-}\overset{21}{\text{Glu}}\text{-Glu-}$$

with the fifth SerP at position 35. Similar clusters of SerP residues are found in α_{s1}- and α_{s2}-caseins which contain 8–9 and 10–13 phosphorylated residues, respectively. The most hydrophilic casein is α_{s2}-casein, which has an unusual distribution of charges such that, at about neutral pH, the N-terminal 68 residues have a net charge of -27 compared with a net charge of about $+13$ in the C-terminal 60 residues. Fully phosphorylated α_{s2}-casein has its phosphoamino acids concentrated largely in three clusters along the polypetide chain. The guinea pig α_{s1}-casein also contains three clusters of phosphorylated residues, but in the bovine homologue the most N-terminal of these is deleted. In contrast to α_{s2}-casein, the C- and N-terminal peptides of α_{s1}-casein are hydrophobic.

The κ-caseins are, like β-caseins, polar molecules but with a hydrophilic peptide in the C-terminal, rather than the N-terminal, half of the molecule. The phosphorylation of κ-casein is of marginal importance to its biological function since in some non-ruminant species the homologous protein is unphosphorylated. Although a small proportion of bovine κ-casein has two or more phosphorylated residues, the sites of phosphorylation are not clustered together, as in the Ca^{2+}-sensitive. Possibly, phosphorylation acts *in vivo* to increase the hydrophilic nature of the C-terminal macropeptide, rather than to enhance the interaction of this casein with calcium phosphate. Primary and predicted secondary structures for the four bovine caseins are shown in figures 8.1 to 8.4.

The caseins were, at one time, regarded as archetypal 'random coil' proteins, but this now seems to have been an exaggeration. No studies of secondary structure in the native casein micelle have been reported, and, since the individual caseins are almost invariably isolated in a denatured state, and contain many Pro residues, the relevance of the structural results obtained to the native structure must be open to doubt. In one study, however, a comparison of results on the circular dichroism (CD) spectrum of β-casein, isolated with and without the use of a denaturing agent (Graham *et al.*, 1984) indicated that the proportions of regular secondary structure were about the same, irrespective of the method of isolation.

```
1                   10                      20                      30
R  P  K  H  P  I  K  H  Q  G  L  P  Q  E  V  L  N  E  N  L  L  R  F  F  V  A  P  F  P  E
   t                    t                 α  α  α  α  α  α  α  α  α  α           t  α  α

                                   P                  P     P
31                  40                      50                      60
V  F  G  K  E  K  V  N  E  L  S  K  D  I  G  S  E  S  T  E  D  Q  A  M  E  D  I  K  Q  M
α  α  α  α  α  α  α  α  α  α  α  α  α  t  t  t  t        α  α  α  α  α  α  α  α  α  α  α  α

               P        P  P  P                    P
61                  70                      80                      90
E  A  E  S  I  S  S  S  E  E  I  V  P  N  S  V  E  Q  K  H  I  Q  K  E  D  V  P  S  E  R
α  α  α  α        t  t           t  t  t  α  α  α  α  α  α  α  α  α  α        t  t  t

                                                            P
91                  100                     110                     120
Y  L  G  Y  L  E  Q  L  L  R  L  K  K  Y  K  V  P  Q  L  E  I  V  P  N  S  A  E  E  R  L
   t              α  α  α  α  α  α  α  α  α  α                 t     α  α  α  α  α  α

121                 130                     140                     150
H  S  M  K  E  G  I  H  A  Q  Q  K  E  P  M  I  G  V  N  Q  E  L  A  Y  F  Y  P  E  L  F
α  α  α  α  α  α  α  α  α  α  α  α  α     t     t  t  α  α  α  α  α           α  α  α  α  α

151                 160                     170                     180
R  Q  F  Y  Q  L  D  A  Y  P  S  G  A  W  Y  Y  V  P  L  G  T  Q  Y  T  D  A  P  S  F  S
α  α  α  α  α  α     t  t  t  t  t  t  β  β  β  β  β  β  β  β  β  β        t  t  t  t  t  t

181                 190
D  I  P  N  P  I  G  S  E  N  S  E  K  T  T  M  P  L  W
t  t  t  t  t  t  t  t  t     t
```

Figure 8.1   Primary structure of bovine α_{s1}-casein B (Grosclaude *et al.*, 1973; Mercier *et al.*, 1971) and predicted secondary structure (Holt and Sawyer, 1988) of the unphosphorylated molecule by the methods of Eliopoulos *et al.* (1982), as modified (Sawyer *et al.*, 1986). α = α-helix, β = extended β-structure, t = β-turn. The nine sites of phosphorylation are shown by a P, but Ser-41 is phosphorylated in only a small proportion of the molecules.

```
                 P  P  P                 P
1                10                      20                      30
K  N  T  M  E  H  V  S  S  S  E  E  S  I  I  S  Q  E  T  Y  K  Q  E  K  N  M  A  I  N  P
α  α  α  α  α                             α  α  α  α  α  α  α        t  t

P                                                          P  P  P
                 40                      50                      60
S  K  E  N  L  C  S  T  F  C  K  E  V  V  R  N  A  N  E  E  E  Y  S  I  G  S  S  S  E  E
   β  β  β  β  α  α  α  α  α  α  α  α  α  α  α  α        t  t  t  t  t  t

P
                 70                      80                      90
S  A  E  V  A  T  E  E  V  K  I  T  V  D  D  K  H  Y  Q  K  A  L  N  E  I  N  Q  F  Y  Q
α  α  α  α  α  α  α  α  α  α  α  α  α     α  α  α  α  α  α  α  α  α  α  α  α  α  α  α  α
                 β  β  β  β  β  t

91               100                     110                     120
K  F  P  Q  Y  L  Q  Y  L  Y  Q  G  P  I  V  L  N  P  W  D  Q  V  K  R  N  A  V  P  I  T
   β  β  β  β  t  t  t  β  β  β  β     t           t

                    P     P                          P
121                 130                     140                     150
P  T  L  N  R  E  Q  L  S  T  S  E  E  N  S  K  K  T  V  D  M  E  S  T  E  V  F  T  K  K
                     t              α  α  α  α  α  α  α  α  α  α  α  α  α  α  α

151                 160                     170                     180
T  K  L  T  E  E  E  K  N  R  L  N  F  L  K  K  I  S  Q  R  Y  Q  K  F  A  L  P  Q  Y  L
α  α  α  α  α  α  α  α  α  α  α  α  α  α  α  α  α                                      β

181                 190                     200
K  T  V  Y  Q  H  Q  K  A  M  K  P  W  I  Q  P  K  T  K  V  I  P  Y  V  R  Y  L
β  β  β  β  α  α  α  α  α  α  α                 β  β  β  β  β  β  β  β  β  β
```

Figure 8.2   Primary structure of bovine α_{s2}-casein A (Brignon *et al.*, 1976; 1977) and predicted secondary structure of the unphosphorylated molecule (see figure 8.1). The sites of phosphorylation for the 11-P microvariant are shown, but there are at least two further sites.

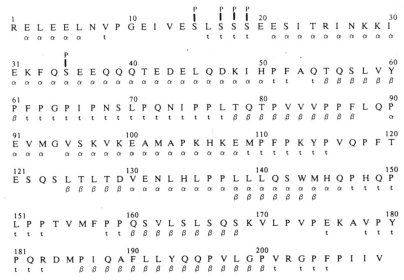

Figure 8.3 Primary structure of bovine β-casein A² (Ribadeau Dumas *et al.*, 1972; Grosclaude *et al.*, 1973) and predicted secondary structure of the unphosphorylated molecule (figure 8.1). Sites of phosphorylation are shown by a P.

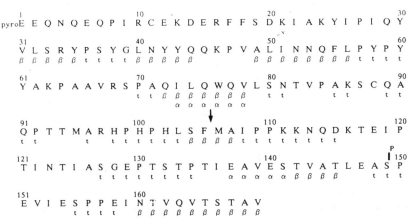

Figure 8.4 Primary structure of bovine κ-casein B (Mercier *et al.*, 1973) and predicted secondary structure of the unphosphorylated molecule (see figure 8.1). The single site of phosphorylation (P) and site of cleavage by the enzyme chymosin (↓) are shown.

The results of optical rotatory dispersion (ORD), CD, hydrodynamic and nuclear magnetic resonance (NMR) measurements indicate that the caseins have a rather open structure in solution with many of the amino acid sidechains exposed to solvent and relatively flexible (Andrews *et al.*, 1979; Sleigh *et al.*, 1983; Humphrey and Jolley, 1982; Graham *et al.*, 1984; Raap *et al.*, 1983; Rollema *et al.*, 1984; Griffin *et al.*, 1986; Payens and

Vreeman, 1982). In solution, ^{31}P-NMR relaxation measurements (T_1 and T_2) indicate that the SerP residues are mobile in β-casein, but their chemical shifts and some other aspects of their behaviour are still uncertain. Humphrey and Jolley (1982) found the same chemical shifts for the four SerP residues in the N-terminal cluster in the isolated phosphopeptide as in the whole molecule, whereas, in virtually the same experiment, Sleigh *et al.* (1983) reported that these resonances were shifted upfield by about one p.p.m. in the whole molecule, perhaps as a result of interaction with hydrophobic or acidic amino acids in the rest of the protein to increase the effective pK of the SerP residues. Neither Sleigh *et al.* (1983) nor Humphrey and Jolley (1982) measured the pH dependence of chemical shifts at high enough pH to determine whether there were interactions with basic moieties in the proteins, as has been seen in osteonectin, phosvitin and phosphophoryn.

Although the caseins behave in solution as open and flexible molecules, with more β-strand and β-turn than α-helical structure, secondary structure predictions for the unphosphorylated chains (figures 8.1 to 8.4) indicate that the α-helical segments are predominantly close to sites of phosphorylation (Holt and Sawyer, 1988). Indeed, the predicted structure around many of the clustered potential sites of phosphorylation forms an α-helix–loop–α-helix motif or a variation thereof, in which one or other of the predicted α-helices is occasionally replaced by unordered structure or a β-strand. The loop contains the sites of phosphorylation, often predicted to be in β-turn or non-regular conformations (Holt and Sawyer, 1988). In the native β-casein molecule, the α-helix content was increased by partial dephosphorylation, and, compared with the phosphopeptide alone, further α-helical structure was induced at a lower concentration of TFE (Chaplin *et al.* 1988). These results illustrate that the β-casein molecule near the sites of phosphorylation is not in a stable conformation in aqueous solution, but it can easily assume a stable conformation in the presence of a structure-forming solvent. The conditions that apply in the native casein micelle, where the phosphorylated residues are immobilised by binding to the calcium phosphate and the polypeptide chains are closely apposed, could be ones that allow the predicted secondary structural motif around the sites of phosphorylation to be stable.

Binding Ca^{2+} to $α_{s1}$- or β-caseins induces little change in their CD spectra, in spite of site binding by many ions, with association constants in the mM range. The moderate binding constant, conformational flexibility and multiplicity of binding sites argue against there being helix–loop–helix (EF hand) high-affinity binding sites in the caseins. Instead, there is much evidence that the binding sites involve the phosphoamino acids, particularly at lower levels of binding, and, because a significant fraction of these are protonated at milk pH (6.7), H^+ ions are displaced. Binding is an antico-operative process, involving a large number of similar sites: Parker and Dalgleish (1981) adopted an approach that has much to recommend it for these kinds of proteins over the more usual models of binding used in biochemistry. They assumed a linear free-energy relationship between the free-energy change for successively bound ions and hence described the binding isotherms in terms of a base binding constant, K_0, for the first ion bound, and a parameter, N_s $(0 \leqslant N_s \leqslant 1)$, measuring the degree of anti-cooperativity. The total number of binding sites is infinite in this model, but in practice the antico-operative nature of the binding provides an upper limit to the number of ions bound at any given free Ca^{2+} ion concentration. Both K_0 and N_s were found to increase with pH and temperature, with a positive enthalpy of reaction indicating that the process is driven entropically. When the average binding constant for binding the first five Ca^{2+} to β-casein is compared to that for the first eight Ca^{2+} to α_{s1}-casein, very similar values result, emphasising the similarity of the two caseins in this regard, when scaled according to their SerP content. As we shall see, the strength of interaction with Ca^{2+} closely parallels the strength of binding to calcium phosphate.

The native casein micelle

Casein micelles are formed in vesicles derived from the Golgi apparatus of the mammary secretory cell. Vesicles, containing casein and the other milk proteins, bleb off the distal face of the Golgi stack and migrate to the apical membrane, where exocytosis occurs. During migration, the vesicles swell, Ca^{2+} and phosphate accumulate in the vesicle, casein micelles are formed and lactose is synthesised (figure 8.5). Holt (1983) has proposed how these various processes are interrelated. Briefly, vesicles swell osmotically because of the synthesis of lactose coupled to net anion transport across the vesicle membrane, which results in a progressive dilution of the casein. A membrane-bound Ca^{2+}-ATPase actively transports Ca^{2+} from the μM concentration in the cytoplasm of the secretory cell to the mM free ion concentration within the vesicle (West and Clegg, 1981; Neville and Staiert, 1983). Phosphate accumulation is intimately linked to lactose synthesis, since the uridine diphosphate (UDP) produced in the reaction is further degraded to uridine monophosphate (UMP) and inorganic phosphate (P_i) before the nucleotide can return to the cytoplasm (Kuhn and White, 1977). At some stage, presumably, the solubility product for calcium phosphate is exceeded and nucleation occurs either on the Ca^{2+}-sensitive caseins or in free solution, but, if the latter, the ion cluster is very soon coated with casein, since only small clusters of ions are found in the micelle. Aggregation of the caseins proceeds with the formation of more calcium phosphate, until the micelles stop growing due to the accumulation of κ-casein in their surface (Schmidt, 1982; Slattery and Evard, 1973).

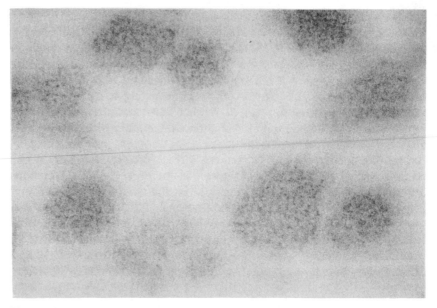

Figure 8.5 Electron micrograph of a thin section of unstained casein micelles showing the more electron dense regions of calcium phosphate embedded in the matrix of phosphoproteins. (Reproduced from plate 2 of Knoop *et al.*, 1979.)

The conditions under which casein micelle formation occurs are known only in outline. The casein concentration is probably higher than in milk, possibly as high as about 100 g/l (Jenness and Holt, 1987), the free Ca^{2+} concentration is probably in the low mM range, the ionic strength probably higher than in milk (0.08 M) and the pH possibly lower (Orci *et al.*, 1987). Under these conditions, and in the presence of Mg^{2+} and citrate, an acidic amorphous calcium phosphate may be expected.

Casein micelles can be digested with a non-specific protease, under conditions that prevent the calcium phosphate dissolving. The resulting calcium phosphate-rich material, designated micellar calcium phosphate (MCP), is amorphous, as judged by X-ray and electron diffraction, contains the phosphopeptides of the three Ca^{2+}-sensitive caseins and has a high proportion of protonated phosphate groups (Lyster *et al.*, 1984; Holt *et al.*, 1986; Holt *et al.*, 1988a). Its infrared spectrum and X-ray absorption spectrum near the K-edge of Ca^{2+} are consistent with an acidic amorphous calcium phosphate (Holt *et al.*, 1988b). Likewise, the form of the solubility product observed in milk serum is consistent with an acidic calcium phosphate (Holt, 1982).

The α_{s1}- and α_{s2}-caseins have several clusters of SerP residues along their sequences, so the possibility exists that one of their SerP clusters can be bound to calcium phosphate at one site, while another SerP cluster can be bound to a different calcium phosphate nucleus to give a cross-linked network. Casein micelles dissociate when calcium phosphate is removed, even when the free Ca^{2+} is two to three times larger than in milk, demonstrating that it is the calcium phosphate and not Ca^{2+} that is the cross-linking agent. Nevertheless, the binding of the casein to the calcium phosphate is dependent on the free calcium ion concentration, and is sufficiently weak at less than 1 mM Ca^{2+} to allow some micellar dissociation even without the colloidal calcium phosphate dissolving (Holt *et al.*, 1986). If dissociation is brought about by reducing the colloidal calcium

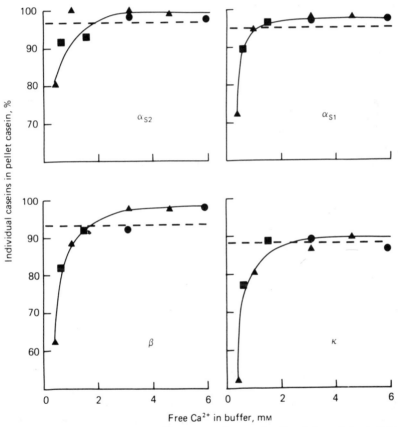

Figure 8.6   Effect of serum free Ca^{2+} concentration on the dissociation of the individual caseins from bovine casein micelles. The dashed line represents the percentage of each casein in the casein micelle prior to dialysis against buffers of different free Ca^{2+} concentration but each saturated with respect to calcium phosphate. The experiment demonstrates that solution composition affects the strength of binding of phosphoproteins to the calcium phosphate. At a given free Ca^{2+} concentration, the strength of binding was in the order of the SerP content of the individual caseins: α_{s2}->α_{s1}->β->κ-casein. (Reproduced from figure 3 of Holt *et al.*, 1986.)

phosphate content at constant free Ca^{2+} concentration or by reducing free Ca^{2+} concentration at constant colloidal phosphate content, the ease with which the Ca^{2+}-sensitive caseins dissociate is, in both cases, closely related to their SerP content: β- > α_{s1}- > α_{s2}-casein, as shown in figure 8.6.

Inhibitory effect of caseins on the spontaneous precipitation of calcium phosphate

At the pH of milk, 37 °C, and with free Ca^{2+} and phosphate concentrations similar to those in milk, but without Mg^{2+}, a fast precipitation of HAP occurs (van Kemenade and de Bruyn, 1987; 1988). According to the Ostwald rule of stages, both OCP and brushite should form as precursor phases, but these are sufficiently unstable under the given conditions that neither was detected. Addition of very low concentrations of casein (greater than 10^{-8} M) leads to a dramatic increase in the time which elapses before precipitation accelerates rapidly, although the rate of growth thereafter is hardly affected. At casein concentrations above 5×10^{-8} M, OCP is formed and it does not transform into the more stable HAP (van Kemenade and de Bruyn, 1988).

The inhibitory effect of casein on precipitation kinetics can be expressed by means of the relaxation time, t_R, defined as the time between the attainment of the target pH and the time at which maximum growth occurs. The growth rate is usually measured by the amount of base required to keep pH constant. With casein, the relaxation time was a linear increasing function of casein concentration which can be understood in terms of adsorption of casein on the active growth sites of the crystal surface. In the Langmuir adsorption model, the fraction of occupied sites, Θ, at concentration C is

$$\Theta = C/(C + K) \tag{8.1}$$

where K is the concentration at which $\Theta = 0.5$, and, by considering the growth rate at sites that are occupied and unoccupied, we obtain:

$$t_R(0)/t_R(C) = \Theta b + (1 - \Theta) \tag{8.2}$$

where $t_R(0)$ and $t_R(C)$ are the relaxation times at casein concentrations zero and C respectively, and b $(0 \leqslant b \leqslant 1)$ is a measure of the reduction in the incorporation of crystal monomers at an occupied growth site. For whole casein, $K = 3.6 \times 10^{-9}$ M, indicating a very high adsorption affinity and $b = 7 \times 10^{-3}$, indicating the virtually complete blockage of every occupied site, leading to the observed linear relationship between t_R and C. Moreover, for the individual caseins (α_{s1}-, β- and κ-), K decreased with increase in SerP content, such that all relaxation time measurements fell on the same straight line when plotted as a function of SerP concentration (figure 8.7). Confirmation that the SerP content was the single most

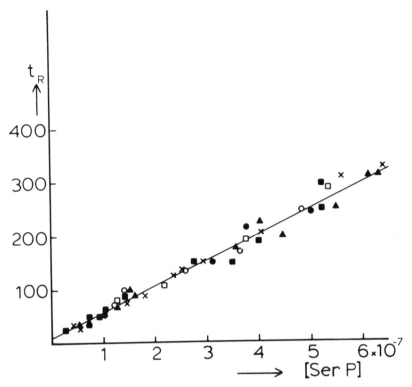

Figure 8.7   Variation in relaxation time with the concentration of SerP residues for: ●, whole casein; ▲, α_{s1}-casein; ■, β-casein; ×, κ-casein; ○, 20% dephosphorylated whole casein; □, a 40% dephosphorylated whole casein. The solution conditions prior to spontaneous precipitation were pH 6.7, $T = 37\,°C$, $KNO_3 = 0.15$ M, total Ca = 4.5 mM and total $P = 3.9$ mM.

important factor in growth rate inhibition was obtained by partial dephosphorylation of β-casein, where it was found that the loss of inhibitory activity was proportional to the decrease in SerP content. When casein concentrations are re-expressed as SerP concentrations, the Langmuir adsorption model gives $K = 2.3 \times 10^{-8}$ M SerP for all the caseins studied and $b \simeq 0$ (van Kemenade and de Bruyn, 1988). This low value of K can be explained by a mononuclear growth mechanism which generally applies for precipitations at relatively low supersaturation (Hartman, 1982). As expected for this mechanism, the growth rate was proportional to the square of the available surface area. In the mononuclear growth model, the rate at which a new layer is built up on a crystal surface is limited by the rate of formation of nuclei on the smooth surfaces. A high proportion of the crystals therefore have flat faces, with, typically, 10^7 growth sites/m² and only a small proportion of kinked surfaces with $\approx 10^{12}$ growth sites/m².

Effective inhibition of growth can therefore occur when only 10^8–10^{10} growth sites/m^2 are occupied by casein, which, in the conditions used, would not have depleted the free casein concentrations appreciably.

Effect of casein on nucleation

At very low casein concentrations there was a reduction in relaxation time, pointing to a stimulation of nucleation, possibly by the caseins acting as nucleation centres. Addition of SerP markedly reduced the relaxation time, and, since this amino acid has been shown to inhibit HAP growth by adsorption at growth sites, the implication is that it stimulates nucleation (van Kemenade and de Bruyn, 1988).

This observation has implications for the formation of casein micelles in the Golgi vesicles. The calcium phosphate could precipitate directly on the protein in a way which is easily controlled by the secretory cell, so that a highly dispersed, high-surface-area, high-energy, amorphous calcium phosphate is produced.

Selective inhibition of calcium phosphate phases

Stabilisation of precursor phases is often seen in biological mineralisation processes, and is believed to be the result of preferential adsorption of ions or macromolecules on the growth sites of the more stable phases. For example, Mg^{2+} inhibits the growth of different phases in the order of effectiveness DCPD $\ll$ OCP $<$ HAP. Effectively, under conditions where all three phases might be expected, DCPD is actually produced. Another example is provided by polyphosphonates which allow di- and tri-hydrates of calcium oxalate to form by inhibiting the more stable monohydrate phase (Liu *et al.*, 1982). Since many crystallisations, and especially calcium phosphate precipitations, proceed through the initial formation of precursor phases, selective inhibition is a potentially important means by which biological mineralisation processes can be controlled.

The effect of the individual α_{s1}-, β- and κ-caseins on the seeded growth of HAP, OCP and DCPD has been studied. In seeded growth experiments, carefully controlled solution conditions and pure seed crystals allow the growth of a single phase to be studied, without the marked induction times found in spontaneous precipitation experiments. In figure 8.8, the reductions in growth rates are seen to be in the order HAP $<$ OCP $<$ DCPD for all caseins at pH values of 7.4, 6.4 and 5.5 respectively. The growth of the thermodynamically most stable phase is, surprisingly, the least affected (van Kemenade and de Bruyn, 1988). There is an extremely strong inhibition of DCPD growth, with complete inhibition observed at a casein concentration of 5×10^{-8} M α_{s1}-casein. For all phases, the order of inhibition was the order of increasing SerP content:

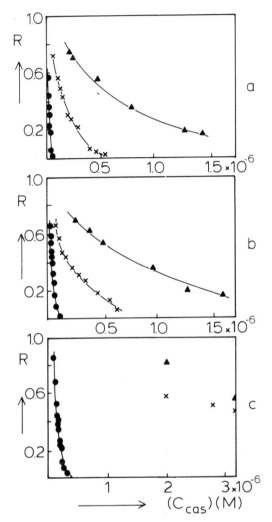

Figure 8.8   Growth rate retardation in the seeded growth of hydroxyapatite (▲), octacalcium phosphate (×) and dicalcium phosphate dihydrate (●) as a function of increasing concentrations of (a) α_{s1}-casein, (b) β-casein and (c) κ-casein. The retardation R is defined as the ratio of growth rate at casein concentration C to that in the absence of casein.

κ-<β-<α_{s1}-casein. Values of K and b for each casein and calcium phosphate phase are given in Table 8.1 (van Kemenade and de Bruyn, 1988) and the significance of the negative b-values is that the caseins can completely suppress growth at less than monolayer coverage. This is never seen in spontaneous precipitations, where a larger number of growth sites are distributed over different and smaller particles.

In view of the increasing growth inhibition, HAP<OCP<DCPD, one

Table 8.1 Values for K and b for the inhibition of the seeded growth of HAP at pH 7.4, OCP at pH 6.4 and DCPD at pH 5.5 by individual caseins (van Kemenade, 1988)

Hydroxyapatite	K ($M \times 10^{-7}$)	$-b$
α_{s1}-casein	8.2 ± 0.8	0.27 ± 0.08
β-casein	10 ± 2	0.4 ± 0.1
κ-casein	30 ± 20	—

Octacalcium phosphate	K ($M \times 10^{-7}$)	$-b$
α_{s1}-casein	1.23 ± 0.08	0.05 ± 0.03
β-casein	1.4 ± 0.1	0.23 ± 0.05
κ-casein	30 ± 10	—

Dicalcium phosphate dihydrate	K ($M \times 10^{-9}$)	$-b$
α_{s1}-casein	5.2 ± 1.0	0.21 ± 0.11
β-casein	21 ± 5	0.6 ± 0.2
κ-casein	65 ± 7	0.31 ± 0.07

might expect HAP to be the preferred phase in spontaneous precipitations in the presence of caseins. However, if HAP is formed heterogeneously on small clusters of a precursor phase (van Kemenade and de Bruyn, 1987; Meyer and Eanes, 1978; Madsen and Thorvardarson, 1984), the formation of HAP may be inhibited by retarding the formation of these precursor phases or their subsequent transformation into HAP. At pH 6.7 and 37 °C, slow growth of OCP is observed, stabilised against HAP growth. At pH 6.0 and 37 °C, DCPD is stabilised at the expense of OCP and HAP. At pH 7.4, an ACP precursor phase is formed and casein strongly inhibits its transformation into crystalline phases. Therefore, if an amorphous phase forms inside the Golgi vesicle during the secretion process, the casein can be expected to stabilise this phase.

Another factor that may contribute to the stabilisation of precursor phases is the aggregation of crystallites. Aggregation reduces the surface area available for heterogeneous nucleation of the more stable phases. Whereas large aggregates of OCP at pH 6.7 and DCPD at pH 6.0 form in the presence of Ca^{2+}-sensitive α_{s1}- and β-caseins, no aggregation was seen with κ-casein (van Kemenade, 1988). Concomitantly, α_{s1}- and β-caseins stabilised the precursor phases whereas κ-casein did not.

Effect of caseins on the morphology of brushite crystals

The habit of a crystal results from the different rates of growth of the various faces. According to the Curie–Wulff rule, the habit is dominated by those faces showing the lowest rates of advancement (Chernov, 1984).

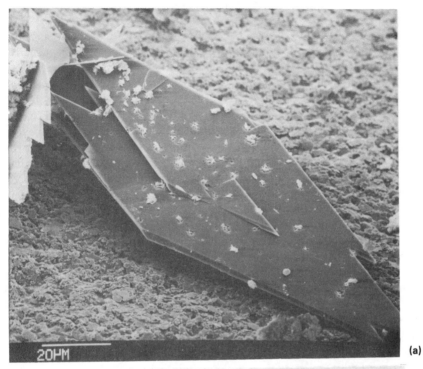

(a)

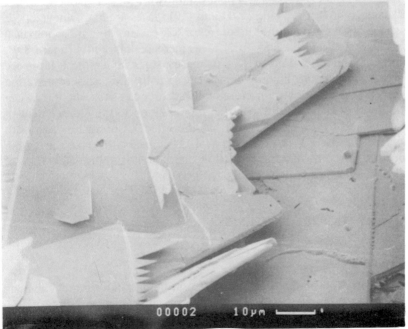

(b)

Figure 8.9 Scanning electron micrographs of dicalcium phosphate dihydrate crystals grown in the absence (a) and the presence (b) of 5×10^{-8} M casein. The greater morphological importance of the {101} faces can be seen in (b).

Selective adsorption at different surfaces can therefore alter crystal habit. A number of factors have been shown to be important in selective adsorption, such as the charge density and atomic spacings on the various faces. A biological example is provided by the experiments of Addadi and co-workers on the stereochemistry of adsorption of acidic Asp-rich proteins from a mollusc on the surfaces of crystals of calcium dicarboxylic acids (Addadi and Weiner, 1985; Addadi et al., 1985). The rigid calcium-loaded acidic proteins adopt a β-sheet conformation which can bind to the {10Ī} and {101} faces of calcium malonate, where Ca–Ca and carboxylate–carboxylate repeating distances of 0.681 nm match the distance between alternate side chains along the protein polypeptide chain of a β-strand (0.67–0.70 nm). In contrast, the {100} face has the highest calcium density but does not preferentially interact with the protein.

Numerous studies have shown preferential adsorption onto fast-growing faces. These faces contain a large number of high-energy growth sites, where an adsorbing molecule can form a larger number of bonds to the surface than if the adsorption were on a perfectly flat plane. According to the Bravais–Friedel rule (Hartman, 1973), the fast-growing surfaces are often the high-index faces, the rationale being that the attachment energy will be inversely related to the interplanar spacing, d_{hkl}, and will therefore increase with increasing indices.

Typical DCPD crystals have a platey habit with well developed smooth {010} faces. The fast-growing {101} and {10Ī} faces are hardly developed. However, when grown in the presence of casein, the morphological importance of the {101} and {10Ī} faces increases markedly (figure 8.9), pointing to preferential adsorption at these planes. Since these faces are expected to have the highest density of growth sites, this observation suggests that the caseins are preferentially adsorbed at sites where they can make the most bonds with the surface. In addition to the enlargement of the {101} and {10Ī} faces, casein has the effect of producing sawtooth structures on the edges of the crystal. It appears that, at the casein adsorption sites, growth does not follow the crystallographic orientation of the former interface (van Kemenade, 1988).

SALIVARY PHOSPHOPROTEINS

General properties

Approximately 30 per cent of the protein in human parotid and submandibular saliva comprises a closely related group of acidic Pro-rich proteins. Four members of this group (PRP1–4) have been studied in detail and found to be phosphoproteins. The amino acid sequence of PRP1 is shown in figure 8.10; PRP2 differs from PRP1 in the substitution Asn-4→Asp-4,

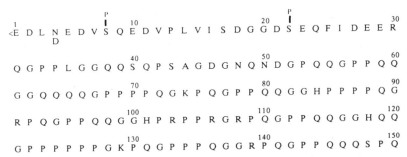

Figure 8.10   Primary structure of the acidic Pro- rich proteins (PRPs) from human saliva (Wong *et al.*, 1979; Wong and Bennick, 1980). The sequence shown is PRP1, whereas the substitution Asn-4→Asp-4 generates the sequence of PRP2 and termination of the sequence at residue 106 generates PRP3. PRP4 is the same as residues 1–106 of PRP2. The TX peptides are residues 1–30.

PRP3 comprises the first 106 residues of PRP1 and PRP4 is the same as the first 106 residues of PRP2. The PRP3 and PRP4 components could arise by proteolytic cleavage from the larger proteins as a result of the action of the salivary proteinase kalikrein (Wong and Bennick, 1981), but Schlesinger and Hay (1986) have argued that partial gene duplication, rather than post-translational modification, is responsible, and this is supported by a study of genetic polymorphism in a large human population (Azen, 1978).

The PRPs contain two SerP residues at positions 8 and 22, and the first 30 amino acids, comprising the TX peptide, form a highly acidic N-terminal domain. In contrast, the remainder of the protein is hydrophobic giving the molecule a polar character, like β-casein. The Pro residues tend to occur in runs, one of which in PRP1 and PRP2 is as long as 6 residues; since homopeptides of five or more Pro groups can form the poly-Pro secondary structure, it is possible that this element of conformation can exist in PRP1 and PRP2 (Deber *et al.*, 1970), but no evidence of such a structure has been found experimentally. The CD spectrum of PRP3 (Bennick, 1975) suggests little regular secondary structure, and, since the NMR longitudinal relaxation rates of selected and non-selected protons are well fitted to single exponential curves (Braunlin *et al.*, 1986), there is evidence of significant mobility of amino acid residues throughout the protein. Further evidence of mobility is that the linewidth of bound $^{43}Ca^{2+}$ is the same whether bound to the TX peptide or to the whole PRP3 molecule (Braunlin *et al.*, 1986), despite the large difference of molecular weight. Nevertheless, the SerP residues are able to interact with basic residues since the chemical shift of bound $^{43}Ca^{2+}$ and the ^{31}P nucleus of the SerP residues show changes at high pH, well above the pK of the phosphate group (Braunlin *et al.*, 1986; Bennick *et al.*, 1981). This behaviour is reminiscent of that observed in phosvitin and phosphophoryn, but may not be due to an interaction of groups well separated in the primary structure; a similar pH-dependent transition is seen in the TX peptide, where the SerP groups may be interacting with Arg-30.

Binding sites for Ca^{2+} involve SerP and Asp residues, mainly, if not exclusively, on the N-terminal part of the proteins (Bennick *et al.*, 1981; Braunlin *et al.*, 1986). The association constant ($\approx 2 \times 10^3$ M^{-1}; Braunlin *et al.*, 1986) indicates fairly strong binding at pH 7.2. Bennick *et al.* (1981) found two classes of binding sites, one of high affinity ($K_a = 2.5 \times 10^5$ M^{-1}) and a larger number of weaker binding sites. The total binding capacity for Ca^{2+} was less in PRP3 than in the TX peptide and still less in the longer PRP1 protein under comparable conditions of measurement (Bennick *et al.*, 1981) which could be due to an interaction between the N-terminal region and the remainder of the molecule.

Statherin (Greek *statheropio*, I stabilise) is unusual among well-characterised phosphoproteins in being rich in Tyr residues. The primary structure (figure 8.11) shows two adjacent SerP residues, together with two adjacent Arg and two adjacent Glu residues in a highly polar N-terminal region, but the remaining two-thirds of the molecule is highly hydrophobic. The sequence appears to be unrelated to those of the acidic, Pro-rich phosphopeptides. The sequence -SerP-SerP-Glu-Glu- is also found in all the Ca^{2+}-sensitive caseins that have been sequenced, where it is believed to comprise the primary recognition site for the phosphokinase(s) (Mercier and Gaye, 1983), and in avian riboflavin-binding protein (Fenselau *et al.*, 1985).

```
     P  P
  1  |  |              10                    20                    30
  D  S  S  E  E  K  F  L  R  R  I  G  R  F  G  Y  G  Y  G  P  Y  Q  P  V  P  E  Q  P  L  Y

                          40
  P  Q  P  Y  Q  P  Q  Y  Q  Q  Y  T  F
```

Figure 8.11   Primary structure of statherin from human saliva. (Schlesinger and Hay, 1977.)

Using ^{1}H- and ^{31}P-NMR spectroscopy, Elgavish *et al.* (1984) showed that statherin has a uniquely stable and well-defined structure, which contrasts with many of the other phosphoproteins considered here. In the ^{1}H spectrum, distinct differences were found between the observed resonances and a calculated spectrum for a random-coil polypeptide of the same amino acid composition. Moreover, a remarkable degree of structural stability was generated, with many features independent of pH in the range 1.9–9.4 and of temperature from 22 to 87 °C where denaturation occurred. Even in 6-mM-guanidine hydrochloride, statherin demonstrated features of a folded polypeptide. Another unusual finding was the broad ^{31}P resonance, of line-width 300 Hz, whether or not the protein solution had been treated with chelex resin to remove Ca^{2+} and paramagnetic species (Humphrey and Jolley, 1982). A typical ^{31}P linewidth for a freely rotating phosphate moiety would be only 5–10 Hz, as exemplified by the PRPs.

Interaction of the salivary phosphoproteins with calcium phosphate

The PRPs and statherin are preferentially absorbed from saliva onto the tooth enamel to form the precursor molecules of the acquired enamel pellicle (Kousvelari *et al.*, 1980). Because of their ability to bind Ca^{2+}, they are a possible reservoir, buffering the free-calcium-ion activity in saliva and hence help to maintain it in a state of supersaturation with respect to calcium phosphates and carbonates (Bennick *et al.*, 1981; Saitoh *et al.*, 1985).

Macaque PRPs and statherin inhibit precipitation in solutions that are supersaturated with respect to basic calcium phosphates (Grøn and Hay, 1976; Hay *et al.*, 1979; Oppenheim *et al.*, 1982), whereas the human PRPs are inactive at physiological concentrations (Oppenheim *et al.*, 1982). Both PRPs and statherin were found to be powerful inhibitors of the seeded growth of calcium phosphate phases (Hay *et al.*, 1979; Oppenheim *et al.*, 1982), and although assay conditions have differed slightly between investigations, the statherins, with their stable conformation, appear to be more effective. Both the PRPs and the statherins have two SerP residues per mole, and, for both proteins, the amino terminal peptides are of prime importance in controlling the slowly forming crystal nuclei. However, with statherin the Pro- and Tyr-rich hydrophobic region is also thought to be involved (Hay *et al.*, 1979). When the TX peptide of PRP3 was cleaved by thermolysin to give two monophosphorylated peptides, the inhibitory activity of each was much less than the original molecule, showing the importance of both phosphorylated residues when acting together (Hay *et al.*, 1987).

The inhibition of crystal growth by the acidic PRPs can be related to their strength of binding to the crystal surface (Moreno *et al.*, 1979), which is primarily a function of the N-terminal region and the binding capacity for Ca^{2+} (Bennick *et al.*, 1981). Thus, the inhibition of crystal growth is modulated by the interaction of the N-terminal region with the rest of the molecule.

Moreno *et al.* (1982) made a particularly detailed study of the adsorption thermodynamics on apatites of acidic PRPs and the TX peptide from PRP1. From the adsorption isotherms measured at 4 and 37 °C, the adsorption free energy (per unit area of surface, ΔG), the adsorption enthalpy (ΔH) and entropy (ΔS) were calculated. Langmuir adsorption isotherms were obtained; i.e., they had the form

$$Q = K_a N_m C/(1 + K_a C) \qquad (8.3)$$

where Q is the amount absorbed per m^2 of surface, N_m is the maximum number of adsorption sites per m^2 of surface, K_a is the affinity constant and C the protein concentration (mM). Moreno *et al.* (1982) then decomposed ΔG into partial free-energy changes for the apatite and polypeptide (subscripts 1 and 2 respectively):

$$\Delta G = \Delta \bar{G}_1 + Q \Delta \bar{G}_2 \qquad (8.4)$$

with

$$\Delta \bar{G}_2 = RT \log_e[Q/\{K_a(N_m - Q)\}] \qquad (8.5)$$

Equation (8.4) is homogeneous because $\Delta \bar{G}_1$ is in units of energy per m^2 rather than the more usual units of energy per mol. Standard methods were then used to derive $\Delta \bar{H}_1$, $\Delta \bar{H}_2$, $\Delta \bar{S}_1$ and $\Delta \bar{S}_2$.

The adsorption affinity constant K_a is determined by the N-terminal region alone (Table 8.2), since the values for the TX peptide, PRP1 and PRP3, are the same in spite of the large differences of size. Likewise, K_a values for PRP2 and PRP4 are not significantly different from each other, but are reduced by the effect of substituting Asp for Asn at position 4. The value of N_m is greatest, as expected, for the smallest (TX) polypeptide, but the maximum binding capacity for the PRP1 and PRP2 proteins is greater than that for the smaller PRP3 and PRP4 chains, presumably reflecting some difference of conformation or orientation at the surface.

Table 8.2   Adsorption parameters for PRPs on hydroxyapatite at 37 °C (Moreno *et al.*, 1982)

Polypeptide	$K_a \times 10^{-6}$ (M^{-1})	N_m (μmol/m^2)
TX (PRP1)	25.3	0.28
PRP1	26.7	0.20
PRP3	26.0	0.16
PRP2	18.1	0.20
PRP4	21.0	0.18

The enthalpy of adsorption was positive, and increased monotonically with the amount absorbed, so adsorption must be driven by increases in entropy. The net positive enthalpy change was the result of a positive $\Delta \bar{H}_2$, which always outweighed a negative contribution from the apatite. The net positive change in entropy was similarly dominated by the contribution from the protein, since $\Delta \bar{S}_1$ was always small by comparison. The positive $\Delta \bar{S}_2$ could arise from the disruption of ion pairs, such as the putative SerP–Arg interactions (Braunlin *et al.*, 1986), breaking of hydrogen-bonds and removal of the hydration shells of adsorbing groups.

Further studies on the thermodynamics of adsorption of phosphoproteins to calcium phosphates are desirable to see if the process is, in general, entropically driven. The possible significance of this is discussed in relation to biological function in the final section.

DENTINE PHOSPHOPHORYNS

General properties

Phosphoproteins constitute the major fraction of non-collagenous proteins extracted from all mammalian sources of dentine so far examined (Linde, 1985). Most studies have concentrated on the more abundant, highly phosphorylated phosphoprotein (HPP) sometimes called the phosphophoryns (Veis, 1985), but other fractions of medium (MPP) and low (LPP) degrees of phosphorylation can be isolated from rat dentine. Dephosphorylation of the HPP fraction allows two components of different composition to be separated. The HPPs are not found in predentine layers, but are synthesised by the odontoblast and rapidly transported to the site of mineralisation (Jontell and Linde, 1983; MacDougal *et al.*, 1985) where they appear to be essential to the process of calcification.

The most intact and purified bovine phosphophoryn isolated by Stetler-Stevenson and Veis (1983) had $M_r \approx 155\,000$ and of the 1130 amino acid residues, 970 were found to be either Asp or Ser(P). Nearly 90 per cent of the Ser residues were phosphorylated, making this one of the most acidic proteins known. The amino acid sequence is unknown, but evidence of $-(\text{Asp–SerP})_n-$ as well as poly–Asp and poly–SerP blocks has been obtained (see Linde, 1985).

Bovine dentine phosphophoryn behaves in solution somewhat like an anionic random coil polyelectrolyte (Lee *et al.*, 1977). Solutions of the protein show non-ideal behaviour at low concentration, even with 0.5 M background electrolyte (Stetler-Stevenson and Veis, 1987). For example, the binding capacity for Ca^{2+} increases with protein concentration, and can, apparently, even exceed the total anion charge on the polyelectrolyte (Stetler-Stevenson and Veis, 1987). As Ca^{2+} is bound, the viscosity of phosphophoryn solutions decreases, possibly owing to intramolecular cross-linking, but some reduction of the intrinsic viscosity would be expected to occur, even if the cations bind to a single site because of the reduced mutual repulsion of charges along the polypeptide chain. Binding of Ca^{2+} also induces a conformational change in phosphophoryn, as measured by CD spectroscopy, with an increase in extended β-structure. Electron micrographs of rotary shadowed molecules show that a thickening of the chain occurs at intervals along its length. These thickened regions are described as having a disk-like morphology (Cocking-Johnson *et al.*, 1983) but it is not possible to relate them to any particular part of the primary structure.

The flexible nature of phosphophoryn is demonstrated by ^{1}H-NMR spectroscopy, which shows relatively narrow linewidths characteristic of a considerable degree of segmental mobility (Cookson *et al.*, 1980). The terminal functional groups of neighbouring Asp and SerP side chains may, however, be able to form hydrogen-bonded structures that give the protein an open or extended conformation in the absence of bound ions. Cookson *et al.* (1980) studied the effect of binding Mn^{2+} as a model for the interaction with Ca^{2+}. The binding affinity was high for the first ten or so Mn^{2+} ions bound ($10^6 M^{-1}$), with the $\beta(CH_2O$ resonance of SerP residues most affected and the $\beta(CH_2)$ resonance of Asp less so, but conditions of fast exchange were observed in spite of the strong binding constant. Cookson *et al.* (1980) resolved the apparent paradox by their ion shuttle hypothesis. An ion landing at a particular site is able to move reasonably freely between adjacent sites, creating the conditions of fast exchange, but nevertheless remains bound to the protein. Other phosphoproteins, such as phosvitin and the Ca^{2+}-sensitive caseins, also have clusters of SerP and Glu or Asp acid residues, so similar ion shuttles might be present in these macromolecules.

Interaction of dentine phosphophoryns with calcium phosphate

The ion shuttle hypothesis describes how the protein can bind Ca^{2+} in a dynamic but strong complex. Other work, by ^{31}P-NMR spectroscopy, has shown that ternary complexes of Ca^{2+}, phosphate and protein can form spontaneously from metastable solution (Lee *et al.*, 1983). The ^{31}P peaks of SerP and P_i groups were broadened by adding Ca^{2+} to phosphate-buffered phosphophoryn solutions under conditions were precipitation of calcium phosphate was not expected. Since the narrow linewidth of orthophosphate was not seen in the ternary system, either the orthophosphate was completely bound to the protein or conditions of fast exchange between free and bound P_i prevailed. These results are significant in demonstrating that a flexible phosphoprotein has properties that appear suited to a role as a nucleator of calcium phosphate precipitation, or as a stabiliser of metastable calcium phosphate solutions (see the final section).

The adsorption of bovine dentine phosphophoryn to HAP has been studied (Fujisawa *et al.*, 1986) and shown to follow a Langmuir binding isotherm with an adsorption constant of 54 ± 16 ml/mg and total binding capacity of 0.25 ± 0.02 mg/m^2 surface. Both dephosphorylation and blocking the carboxyl groups reduced the adsorption affinity, demonstrating the importance of these functional groups for binding, as with the PRPs, but the total binding, capacity was, for both chemical modifications, increased.

A number of investigations have been made of the effect of phosphophoryn preparations on the spontaneous precipitation of calcium phosphate from solution with results that are, at first sight, conflicting. Termine and Conn (1976) used a buffered solution at pH 7.4 with Ca^{2+} and HPO_4^{2-} concentrations of 4.4 and 3.0 mM respectively, prior to precipitation. In the absence of stabiliser, precipitation occurred within 10–15 min of mixing to give an amorphous product. At a phosphophoryn concentration of 200 mg/l, an ACP was again found which converted to HAP in 18–24 h, compared with 8–10 h in the absence of protein. At the higher phosphophoryn concentration of 500 mg/l, the ACP was indefinitely stable, but later work under similar conditions (Termine *et al.*, 1980) showed that Ca^{2+}-loaded phosphophoryn was much less effective as a stabiliser. This result could indicate that the protein significantly perturbed the free ion concentrations in the precipitation medium, particularly at the higher concentrations used. Nawrot *et al.* (1976) also studied spontaneous precipitation from a supersaturated solution (Boskey and Posner, 1973), but at a free Ca^{2+} concentration that was considerably higher: about 20 mM. In such a buffer, the phosphophoryn should be in a more ordered conformation than at low free Ca^{2+}. At very low phosphophoryn concentrations, an ACP was produced, but at above 10 mg/l the product isolated was a poorly crystalline apatite. Therefore Nawrot *et al.* (1976) concluded that the phosphophoryn was able to nucleate HAP from solution. If this is so, then the findings of Termine and co-workers (Termine and Conn, 1976; Termine *et al.*, 1980) suggest that the more flexible Ca^{2+}-free conformation is not so effective at nucleating HAP, but may be able to nucleate an ACP, as well as stabilise it, once formed. Udich *et al.* (1986) observed that Ca^{2+}-loaded phosphophoryn had a different effect on the rate of precipitation of ACP, and on its subsequent crystallisation in agar gels compared to phosphophoryn that was initially free of Ca^{2+}. In their one-dimensional diffusion experiments, the phosphophoryn was without effect on the time required for crystal formation from the initial phase, but the Ca^{2+}-loaded protein actually decreased the stability of the first-formed material.

These somewhat confusing results illustrate the difficulties inherent in studies of spontaneous precipitation where a multitude of factors, including solution composition, amount of precipitate formed, particle size, stability of intermediate phases and mechanisms of reaction, can all influence the time taken for crystals to form.

Termine *et al.* (1980) examined the effect of phosphophoryn on the seeded growth of calcium phosphate at pH 7.4 and found that the protein introduced a lag phase before growth of OCP on the HAP seed crystals occurred. When Ca^{2+}-loaded phosphophoryn (or phosvitin) was used, the inhibitory action towards apatite formation was reduced.

PHOSVITINS

General properties

The phosvitins are derived by proteolytic cleavage from vitellogenins and occur, concentrated, in lipid-rich cyclosomes in the yolk of vertebrate eggs. Their biological function is unkown, though they constitute by far the

```
1                      10                        20                        30
A E F G T E P D A K T S S S S S S A S S T A T S S S S S S A
                       40                        50                        60
S S P N R K K P M D E E E N D Q V K Q A R N K D A S S S S R
                       70                        80                        90
S S K S S N S S K R S S S K S S N S S K R S S S S S S S S
                      100                       110                       120
S S S R S S S S S S S S S S N S K S S S S S S K S S S S S
                      130                       140                       150
R S R S S S K S S S S S S S S S S S S S K S S S S R S S S
                      160                       170                       180
S S S K S S S H H S H S H H S G H L N G S S S S S S S R S
                      190                       200                       210
V S H H S H E H H S G H L E D D S S S S S S S V L S K I W

    G R H E I Y Q
```

Figure 8.12   Primary structure of phosvitin deduced from the nucleotide sequence of part of the chicken vitellogenin gene. (Byrne *et al.*, 1984.)

largest single fraction of phosphorus in the egg. Phosvitins are not known to be involved in calcification, but, as highly phosphorylated proteins, they have been used in some experimental studies of *in vitro* calcification. Also, as flexible macromolecules, which can, under a variety of conditions, assume a more regular conformation, they are exemplars of the class of highly phosphorylated flexible proteins that are largely the subject of this review.

The complete amino acid sequence of a phosvitin (figure 8.12) has been deduced from the structure of a chicken vitellogenin gene (Byrne *et al.*, 1984). Of the 217 amino acid residues, 123 are Ser, 93–95 per cent of which are phosphorylated (Rosenstein and Taborsky, 1970). In the middle of the sequence, runs of up to 14 contiguous Ser residues occur, alternating with the basic residues Arg and Lys, and occasionally Asn. The remaining 27 ser residues are in the C-terminal portion, which is also particularly rich in His residues.

At pH 7, phosvitin has a relatively open and flexible structure but at pH 2 it undergoes a transition to a form with a much higher proportion of regular secondary structures, primarily β-sheet (Perlmann, 1973; Braunlin *et al.*, 1984; Vogel, 1983; Renugopalakrishnan *et al.*, 1985; Prescott *et al.*, 1986). All eleven His residues, however, are only partly exposed to solvent and titrate with an unusually high $pK = 7.45$. Vogel (1983) suggested that the His residues are protonated and interact, electrostatically and via hydrogen bonds, with SerP residues. The more ordered structure may be stabilised by interaction with positively charged species and occurs at a higher pH. For example, phosvitin forms a complex rich in β-sheet with the basic macromolecules polylysine and protamine at pH 3–5 (Perlmann and Grizzuti, 1971). Addition of certain non-solvents also promoted the formation of β-sheet (Perlmann and Grizzuti, 1971), as did freezing and thawing cycles (Taborski, 1970). It appears, therefore, that while phosvitins are relatively flexible molecules at neutral pH, they are close to being able to form more ordered structures once the high charge on the backbone is partly neutralised. Whether this occurs when phosvitin binds to calcium phosphate has not been established. Films of the protein alone, prepared from solution at pH 3.3, gave X-ray diffraction rings characteristic of β-strands and sheets, but no ordered conformations were detected in films made from phosvitin solution at pH 7.3 (Traub and Perlmann, 1972).

The SerP residues at physiological pH are partly protonated, as measured by the pH dependence of the chemical shifts of ^{31}P nuclei in the SerP (and possibly one ThrP) residues. Approximately 80 per cent of the residues titrated with pK = 5.79 (Vogel, 1983), a value appreciably lower than observed in the caseins (Humphrey and Jolley, 1982; Sleigh *et al.*, 1983), and indicating a considerable degree of interaction between SerP residues. The ^{31}P nuclei also are perturbed at pH ≈ 10, indicating some interaction with the basic residues of the protein. In the primary sequence, virtually all the basic residues are found to be adjacent to Ser residues, but the ^{31}P-NMR results indicate that all SerP groups are able to sense the basic ones. In phosphophoryn, an extensive hydrogen-bonded network for the ionic side chains was proposed (Cookson *et al.*, 1980) on the basis of similar titration results.

From the positions and intensities of the Raman amide I and III bands of phosvitin in neutral solution, Prescott *et al.* (1986) concluded that some secondary structure other than the well known α-helix, β-strand or β-turn was dominant. This structure, which is a feature of highly phosphorylated proteins, has previously been assigned to a 'random coil' or unordered structure in earlier structural studies, but Prescott *et al.* (1986) considered it to be a novel conformational state. Such a view is not inconsistent with what else is known about phosvitin: the flexible nature seen by intrinsic viscosity and ^{1}H-NMR measurements can result from the motion of segments of the polypeptide chain (up to 50 residues) about hinge regions distributed through the sequence (Bhandari *et al.*, 1986). The hydrogen-bonded network can exist within segments, and interactions between segments can strongly influence the overall, average, conformation of the protein.

Another interesting point to emerge from the Raman studies of Prescott *et al.* (1986) is that lyophilization from neutral as well as acidic solutions produced a β-sheet structure as indicated by the amide I and III resonances. These findings, together with the absence of diffraction rings in the measurements of Traub and Perlmann (1972), suggest that there is short-range but not long-range ordering of β-strands in the films prepared from neutral pH solutions.

Phosvitin binds Ca^{2+} with a moderately strong binding constant

(≈ 400 M^{-1} at pH 6.8, $I = 0.02$) and a binding capacity approximately equal to the total negative charge, assuming dianionic SerP residues (Grizzuti and Perlmann, 1973). Like the Ca^{2+}-sensitive caseins, phosvitin is precipitated at high levels of binding and at about neutral pH there is no large-scale conformational rearrangement (Grizzuti and Perlmann, 1973; Renugopalakrishnan, 1985).

Interaction of phosvitin with calcium phosphate

The interaction of phosvitin with calcium phosphates has been studied in precipitating systems, where it appears to stabilise ACP or OCP (Termine and Posner, 1970; Termine *et al.*, 1980). Phosvitin appears to be about as effective as dentine phosphophoryn in increasing the relative lifetime of metastable phases, but in the precipitating system of Boskey and Posner (1973), phosvitin still produced an ACP, whereas the phosphophoryn induced the formation of poorly crystalline HAP (Nawrot *et al.*, 1976). The role of phosvitin as an agent that can possibly mediate in the nucleation of calcium phosphate from solution is suggested by the experiments of Banks *et al.* (1977). They found that calf skin collagen did not nucleate calcium phosphate when incubated in synthetic solutions, but when phosvitin was cross-linked to the collagen, mineralisation did occur. Moreover, the apatite crystals formed on the collagen fibrils with their c-axes aligned with the fibre axis, as in a normal hard tissue.

BONE PHOSPHOPROTEINS

Compared with the dentine system, the bone phosphoprotein fraction comprises a lesser proportion of the total non-collagenous proteins. Moreover, the proteins are less highly phosphorylated and have roughly equal numbers of Asx and Glx residues (Table 8.3). In further contrast to the HPPs of dentine, a smaller proportion of the Ser residues are phosphorylated, but ThrP is also found (Uchiyama *et al.*, 1985). Bone phosphoproteins are most actively synthesised by osteoblasts, and then, like the HPPs of dentine, are passed to the mineralisation front (Landis *et al.*, 1984), but their precise role in the calcification process is unclear.

The CD spectra of two chicken bone matrix phosphoprotein fractions indicate a preponderance of extended β-structure, with little or no α-helix between pH 4 and pH 7.4 (Renugopalakrishnan, 1986). Analysis of the infrared amide I band after resolution enhancement by Fourier self-deconvolution largely confirmed the results from the CD measurements.

Table 8.3   Amino acid and sugar content of an $M_r = 44\,000$ phosphoprotein from rat bone[a]

	Residues (mol)
Amino acid	
Glu	58
Asp	57
Ser	30
SerP	12
Thr	12
ThrP	1 (1.3)
Ala	21
Leu	18
Pro	18
Lys	16
His	14
Val	14
Gly	13
Arg	10
Phe	9
Tyr	6
Ile	6
Met	3
Cys	1 (0.3)
Monosaccharide	
Galactose	11.6
N-Acetylneuraminic acid	10.4
N-Acetylgalactosamine	4.7
N-Acetylglucosamine	3.5
Mannose	2.3
Fucose	0.6

[a] From Prince *et al.* (1987); integer values calculated for $M_r = 44K$ and 83.4 per cent protein but measured values for Cys and ThrP are given in parentheses.

OSTEONECTIN

General properties

Osteonectin is one member of a group of homologous extracellular matrix proteins secreted by a wide variety of cell types. For example, foetal bovine osteonectin shows 92 per cent sequence identity with the mouse SPARC glycoprotein, secreted by parietal endoderm cells (Engel *et al.*, 1987). Another member of the group is BM-40, secreted by basement membrane-producing cells.

Many, but not all, mineralising tissues have osteonectin as a major component of the extracellular matrix. It accounts for almost a third of the true non-collagenous matrix protein in developing lamellar bone of bovine, porcine and human origin, but is much less abundant in rat bone and is virtually absent from rat incisors (Sodek *et al.*, 1986). Immunohistochemical studies have shown that osteonectin, in mineralising tissues, is closely

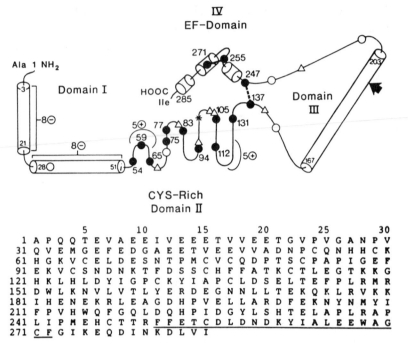

Figure 8.13   Primary and predicted secondary structure of SPARC (Engel *et al.*, 1987): △, sites of phosphorylation; ✱, site of glycosylation; ←, site of endogenous cleavage Leu-197–Leu-198; ○, Met; ●, Cys. The underlined residues in the primary sequence form the predicted EF-hand in domain IV.

associated with the collagen fibrils, and *in vitro* experiments show that osteonectin will bind strongly, but possibly non-specifically, to denatured collagen and to hydroxyapatite (Otsuka *et al.*, 1984; Romberg *et al.*, 1985). Nevertheless, the biological function of osteonectin remains an enigma.

The complete amino acid sequence of the SPARC protein is available, as deduced from cDNA sequences (Mason *et al.*, 1986a, b); it has one site of glycosylation (Asn-98) and 7 Ser residues, all of which are potential sites of phosphorylation, and a total of 285 amino acid residues, giving $M_r = 33\,062$ for the unglycosylated, unphosphorylated protein. The predicted secondary structure (Engel *et al.*, 1987) has a number of interesting features (figure 11.13). These are four regions of different character along the sequence, suggesting four functional domains. Domain I, comprising the first 52 residues, features two sequences of 14–15 residues, each containing 7–8 Glu residues. Although the two sequences are predicted to be α-helical, at physiological pH, the α-helices are not expected to be stable because of the high negative charge density. Domain II comprises about 85 residues with short β-strands alternating with β-turns. Of the eleven Cys residues in this domain, ten are postulated to form disulphide linkages, internal to the domain, which stabilise its structure. Near both ends of domain II are two clusters of positively charged residues that could interact with the acidic clusters in domain I. The sites of phosphorylation are nearly all in domain II, but apart from the sequence -Asp-Ser-Ser-, the Ser residues are not clustered along the primary sequence, though they may well, of course, be closely positioned in the folded protein. Domain III is predominantly α-helical, and domain IV contains a sequence that is expected to form an EF-hand calcium ion binding site. It is unusual to find only one EF-hand in a protein, since they are usually stacked in pairs; the milk protein α-lactalbumin provides a second example of a protein with a single high-affinity binding site resembling the EF-hand structure. Another unusual feature of the EF-hand sequence is the presence of two Cys residues that are predicted to be close enough to form a stabilizing disulphide linkage. A high-affinity ($pK \approx 6.5$) binding site for Ca^{2+} has been demonstrated for osteonectin (Romberg *et al.*, 1985).

The CD spectra of osteonectin and BM-40 have been reported, but differ in several respects, chiefly in the calculated proportion of α-helical structure and in the sensitivity of the protein conformations to Ca^{2+} (Engel *et al.*, 1987; Romberg *et al.*, 1985). In order to explain the observed dependence of the CD spectrum of BM-40 on calcium concentration, Engel *et al.* (1987) suggest that the two predicted α-helices in domain I are stabilised by binding about seven Ca^{2+} in sites with $pK > 5$, each of the sites being each formed from two Glu side chains. In contrast, Romberg *et al.* (1985) found a largely unordered structure for osteonectin, with no dependence of secondary structure on the concentration of calcium.

Interaction of osteonectin with calcium phosphate

The most likely region of the protein for interaction with a calcium phosphate phase is the phosphorylated domain II, though if the speculations of Engel *et al.* (1987) on the high-affinity binding sites of domain IV are correct then this too could contribute to binding. As a site for interaction with a calcium phosphate crystal surface, domain II is unusual compared with the more flexible binding domains of caseins, the phosphophoryns and similar phosphoproteins. The disulphide-stabilised β-strand plus β-turn structure may have the rigid structure that makes binding to a surface slow, but strong, given complementary stereochemistry in the adsorbent and adsorbate.

Romberg *et al.* (1985, 1986) found that osteonectin bound to hydroxyapatite in a specific manner ($K = 8 \times 10^{-8}$ M), with 1 molecule per 40 unit cells on the surface of their preparation. The ability of osteonectin to inhibit the seeded growth of hydroxyapatite from supersaturated solution was monitored by means of the uptake of base required to maintain a constant pH. The concentration of osteonectin that reduced the growth rate by half was only 1.6×10^{-7} M, suggesting that the protein binds preferentially at lattice growth sites. On a molar basis, osteonectin is therefore about five times more potent than bone Gla protein (osteocalcin) in inhibiting hydroxyapaptite growth.

Termine *et al.* (1981) found that little ^{45}Ca-labelled HAP would bind to collagen-coated scintillation vials, but when osteonectin was added, binding of the HAP crystals increased. Treatment of the osteonectin with an anti-osteonectin serum inhibited HAP binding, as did fibronectin, but the mechanism for the latter effect was suggested to be a competition between osteonectin and fibronectin for binding to the collagen (Termine *et al.*, 1981). Collagen and osteonectin also appear to act synergically in the nucleation of calcium phosphate from metastable solution.

SUMMARY, SPECULATIONS AND CONCLUSIONS

In this section, we consider the function of phosphoproteins in mineralising systems in relation to what is known about their structure. Little information is available on the X-ray crystal structure of phosphoproteins. In pepsinogen (James and Sielecki, 1986; Williams *et al.*, 1986) the single site of phosphorylation is in a region of weak and diffuse electron density, suggesting considerable dynamic mobility or conformational disorder. In solution, the narrow linewidth of the ^{31}P resonance revealed by NMR spectroscopy is consistent with high mobility of this SerP side chain. In a small number of proteins containing oligoseryl sequences, it is again found that these regions are likely to be flexible, and on the surface of globular proteins (Bernstein *et al.*, 1977). The numerous studies reviewed here all indicate that, with the exception of statherin, phosphorylated residues in solution are relatively mobile.

More definitive structural information will have to await X-ray crystal structure determination of a multi-phosphorylated phosphoprotein. We know of only one such protein that has been crystallised and is being studied: riboflavin binding protein from hen eggs (Zanette *et al.*, 1984). This protein is of particular interest because it has a C-terminal peptide very similar in primary and predicted secondary structure to the N-terminal phosphopeptide of β-casein (Holt and Sawyer, 1988; Fenselau *et al.*, 1985). Protein flexibility in solution is the outstanding characteristic to emerge from studies on highly phosphorylated phosphoproteins. The SerP (and ThrP) residues may form ion pairs with basic residues such as Lys or Arg in a number of instances, but phosphorylation appears to destabilise secondary and tertiary structure, rather than to promote the higher levels of ordering. In particular, clustered SerP residues in the α_{s1}- and α_{s2}-caseins, phosvitins and (probably) phosphophoryns could act as hinges, allowing the whole proteins to adopt the open structures characteristic of this group in free solution. This is not to say, however, that the flexible proteins are not capable, under certain circumstances, of adopting more defined and stable conformations. One possibility, as yet little investigated, is that the flexible phosphoproteins adopt more regular conformations when bound to calcium phosphate.

Whereas, in general, sites of phosphorylation can be the source of flexibility in the larger scale structure of the phosphoproteins, an intriguing exception is osteonectin (figure 8.13). In this protein, the domain where sites of phosphorylation are concentrated is also highly cross-linked by disulphide bonds. Also in this protein, the longer-range flexibility that could be induced by phosphorylation is likely to be prevented. Another possibility, however, is that the disulphide linkages acting with other sources of conformational stability such as hydrogen-bonding, ion pair formation, etc., serve to hold the phosphorylated domain itself in a fairly fixed conformation, to generate a structure which can bind in a stereospecific way to particular surfaces of crystalline calcium phosphates. Since this protein can bind to collagen as well as to the calcium phosphate, the possibility of inducing oriented crystal growth must be considered.

Hitherto, the stereospecific interaction of proteins with crystals has been considered more in relation to Gla-proteins and proteins rich in Asp and/or Glu residues as exemplified by the notable work of Addadi and co-workers. Phosphorylation increases the binding affinity to calcium phosphates, and the clustering of phosphorylated residues in the amino acid sequence leads to even stronger binding. Neighbouring Asp or Glu residues can further enhance the affinity for binding, as is illustrated by the acidic Pro-rich proteins of saliva, where the effect of the substitution Asp-4 for Asn-4 has been studied. Thus, clustering of phosphorylated residues in acidic regions of the polypeptide chain can be regarded as a means of generating a very strong linkage between the protein and calcium phosphate. Such linkages can be broken at low free-Ca^{2+} concentrations in the surrounding aqueous phase, as has been demonstrated for caseins in the native bovine casein micelle (figure 8.6). But under normal physiological conditions in an extracellular fluid, the binding of a polyphosphorylated peptide to calcium phosphate can be regarded as essentially irreversible. We suggest that proteins able to bind irreversibly to calcium phosphate are unlikely to function actively in the remodelling of mineralised structures.

Phosphoproteins are able to bind Ca^{2+} under physiological conditions. The work of Cookson *et al.* (1980) has shown that the bound Mn^{2+} ions are delocalised along an 'ion shuttle' when binding to a cluster of neighbouring phosphorylated residues occurs. The idea of an 'ion shuttle' seems an excellent one, and, considered in the light of the work of Lee *et al.* (1983), could act to facilitate the nucleation of calcium phosphate from supersaturated solution. An equally valid proposition, however, is that the phosphoproteins bind to the spontaneously forming clusters of calcium and phosphate ions in metastable solutions, preventing their growth to the critical size required for nucleation and hence allowing time for dispersion of the cluster. At our present level of understanding, we can see no fundamental difference between a phosphoprotein acting as a nucleator and promoter of phase separation, on the one hand, and its acting as a stabiliser of metastable supersaturated solutions, on the other: the same molecule could act in both ways, depending on its concentration and the composition and degree of supersaturation of the aqueous phase. Perhaps there are subtle details of protein structure, yet to be discerned, that predispose a phosphoprotein to one role or the other. Holt and Sawyer (1988) have suggested that the Ca^{2+}-sensitive caseins act to control the precipitation of calcium phosphate in the Golgi vesicles of the mammary secretory cell. Either calcium phosphate nucleates on the phosphoproteins or phosphoproteins wrap themselves around nuclei above the critical size for stability. In either case, the result is a highly dispersed, amorphous calcium phosphate with a metastable aqueous phase, which remains supersaturated with respect to the basic crystalline calcium phosphates and even to brushite and monetite. Because of the highly dispersed nature of the micellar calcium phosphate, the surface free energy could significantly reduce the overall free energy of formation of the phase. By isolating the calcium phosphate clusters in the protein matrix of the casein micelle, they cannot act as heterogeneous nucleation catalysts for subsequent precipitation, destroying the co-operative nature of the phase transition. In the terms used by Williams (1975), a potentially catastrophic first-order phase transition is converted to a more easily controlled process of second-order type.

Phosphoproteins may play a general role in biology in maintaining fluids in a state of supersaturation or in controlling stone formation or ectopic calcification. The role may not be limited to calcium phosphate phases, as evidenced by the presence of phosphoproteins or phosphopeptides in pancreatic calcium carbonate and urinary calcium oxalate stones (De Carlo *et al.*, 1984; Montalto *et al.*, 1984). On the other hand, the formation of a calcium phosphate–phosphoprotein complex could be of general use in transporting calcium phosphate in a relatively high-energy, easily re-soluble, form. In milk, the casein micelle allows calcium phosphate to be transported from mother to young. In the extrapallial fluid of moluscs (Marsh, 1986), a calcium phosphate–phosphoprotein complex is again found, even though shell mineralisation is with $CaCO_3$. Unfortunately, the mechanisms of transport of calcium to the mineralisation front in bone are not clear: the involvement of matrix vesicles, which have some similarities to the Golgi vesicles of mammary secretory cells, is recognised, at least in the earliest stages of mineralisation. Speculations on the role of phosphoproteins have concentrated on their possible action at the sites of mineralisation (Veis, 1985; Wuthier, 1986; Glimcher, 1984), rather than on transport to that site or control of the stability of the supersaturated extracellular fluid away from the sites.

The roles of phosphoproteins in maintaining the stability of supersaturated solutions and in transporting high-energy calcium phosphate are not totally disconnected. In a supersaturated liquid, spontaneous solute concentration fluctuations lead to the formation of nuclei. Phosphoproteins can stabilise those nuclei, and the complex can then be removed from the supersaturated fluid to a region where the complex can be dissolved.

We now consider the characteristic features of phosphoprotein structures in relation to the kinetics, stereochemistry and thermodynamics of binding to calcium phosphate. To illustrate the arguments we contrast the behaviour of two extreme hypothetical types of phosphoprotein: one a rigid molecule with a fixed constellation of phosphorylated and other charged residues at its binding site, and the other a highly flexible molecule with the same primary structure.

The rigid phosphoprotein would be expected to bind most strongly and in a stereospecific way to calcium phosphate phases and crystal faces that present a complementary constellation of surface charges. The flexible molecule can adapt its conformation to a wider range of surfaces, including those of amorphous phases, but the loss of conformational entropy on binding may make the overall free energy of binding less than that of the rigid molecule to its complementary surface. However, given a sufficient number of phosphorylated residues, the binding is likely, in both instances, to be strong. The thermodynamic and stereochemical properties of phosphoproteins therefore indicate strong and possibly irreversible binding to all, or selected, crystal faces to be features of any possible biological function. Before considering the kinetics of binding it is appropriate to point out that the Gla-proteins may be superior agents in the modulation of crystal growth, by selective binding to particular phases or crystal faces for two reasons. First, phosphorylation appears to destabilise protein conformation, making it less likely to achieve the rigid geometry required for a stereospecific interaction. Second, the weaker binding of carboxyl groups may allow growth sites on the crystal surface to be blocked or unblocked by small changes of solution composition (e.g., Ca^{2+} or pH) or by the concentration of Gla-protein.

The interaction of the flexible and rigid phosphoproteins are differentiated most clearly by the kinetics of adsorption. Consider the Arrhenius equation:

$$\text{rate of adsorption} = vk \exp(-E_a/RT) \qquad (8.6)$$

where v is an orientation factor, k the rate constant for diffusion to the surface, assumed to be the same for both types of phosphoprotein, and E_a is the activation energy for adsorption. The rigid molecule requires a precise orientation and the desolvation of a large surface area for formation of the transition complex, making the rate of binding slow. The flexible molecule, on the other hand, can react with the surface, residue by residue, in a series of steps of low activation energy. Moreover, in whatever orientation the molecule approaches the surface, it can adapt its conformation in a way appropriate for adsorption. The advantage of a flexible conformation is therefore in allowing a faster reaction with the surface of calcium phosphate crystals. Of particular value, however, may be the ability to react rapidly with the small calcium phosphate ion clusters that are the precursors of nuclei, in order to stabilise metastable supersaturated solutions.

Phosphoproteins can modify the precipitation of calcium phosphate in many different ways. In exploring the relation between structure and function, the need is for discriminating experiments that focus on a particular mechanism or stage of precipitation. Although numerous studies have been performed on the subject of the interaction of phosphoproteins with calcium phosphate, as reviewed here, enough attention has not always been given to defining the solution conditions affecting binding and how these change during precipitation. It is well known, from crystal growth studies, that a critical supersaturation boundary must be exceeded to achieve the formation of nuclei and phase separation within an experimentally practicable period of time. Very small changes in concentration around this boundary drastically alter precipitation kinetics, even if the same phase is formed. For example, ion binding by the phosphoprotein may be the most significant influence on precipitation kinetics at higher protein concentrations, leading to reduced supersaturation and apparently inhibited precipitation. Another disadvantage of experiments involving spontaneous precipitation of calcium phosphate is that changes of phase occur frequently. Well-defined experiments are required in which solution conditions are carefully controlled and binding occurs only to a single phase. It is also clear that a more extensive knowledge of the thermodynamics of binding of phosphoproteins and phosphopeptides to different calcium phosphate phases will enhance our understanding of the biological function of these types of molecules.

REFERENCES

Addadi, L. and Weiner, S. (1985). Interactions between acidic proteins and crystals: Stereochemical requirements in biomineralization. *Proc. Natl Acad. Sci. USA*, **82**, 4110–14

Addadi, L., Berkovitch-Yellin, Z., Weissbuch, I., Mil, J. van, Shimon, L. J. W., Lahav, M. and Leiserowitz, L. (1985). Growth and dissolution of organic crystals with 'tailor-made' inhibitors – Implications in stereochemistry and materials science. *Angew. Chem. Int. Ed. Engl.*, **24**, 466–85

Andrews, A. L., Atkinson, D., Evans, M. T. A., Finer, E. G., Green, J. P., Phillips, M. C. and Robertson, R. N. (1979). The conformation and aggregation of bovine β-casein A. 1. Molecular aspects of thermal aggregation. *Biopolymers*, **18**, 1105–21

Azen, E. A. (1978). Genetic protein polymorphisms in human saliva: an interpretive review. *Biochem. Genet.*, **16**, 79–99

Banks, E., Nakajima, S., Shapiro, L. C., Tilevitz, O., Alonzo, J. R. and Chianelli, R. R. (1977). Fibrous apatite grown on modified collagen. *Science*, **198**, 1164–6

Bennick, A. (1975). Chemical and physical characteristics of a phosphoprotein from human parotid saliva. *Biochem. J.*, **145**, 557–67

Bennick, A., Mclaughlin, A. C., Grey, A. A. and Madapallimattam, G. (1981). The location and nature of calcium-binding stites in salivary acidic proline-rich phosphoproteins. *J. Biol. Chem.*, **256**, 4741–6

Bernstein, F. C., Koetzle, T. F. Williams, G. J. B., Meyer, E. F., Brice, M. D., Rodgers, J. R., Kennard, O., Shimanouchi, T. and Tasumi, M. (1977). The Protein Data Bank: a computer-based archival file for macromolecular structures. *J. Molec. Biol.*, **112**, 535–42

Bhandari, D. G., Levine, B. A., Trayer, I. P. and Yeadon, M. E. (1986). ¹H-NMR study of mobility and conformational constraints within the proline-rich N-terminal of the LC1 alkali light chain of skeletal myosin. *Eur. J. Biochem.*, **160**, 349–56

Boskey, A. L. and Posner, A. S. (1973). Conversation of amorphous calcium phosphate to microcrystalline hydroxyapatite. A pH-dependent, solution-mediated, solid–solid conversion. *J. Phys. Chem.*, **77**, 2313–17

Braunlin, W. H., Vogel, H. J., Drakenberg, T. and Bennick, A. (1986). A calcium-43 NMR study of calcium binding to an acidic proline-rich phosphoprotein from human saliva. *Biochemistry, NY*, **25**, 584–9

Braunlin, W. H., Vogel, H. J. and Forsen, S. (1984). Potassium-39 and sodium-23 NMR studies of cation binding to phosvitin. *Eur. J. Biochem.*, **142**, 139–44

Brignon, G., Ribadeau Dumas, B. and Mercier, J.-C. (1976). First elements of the primary structure of bovine α_{s2}-caseins. *FEBS Lett.*, **71**, 111–16

Brignon, G., Ribadeau Dumas, B., Mercier, J.-C., Pelessier, J. P. and Das, B. C. (1977). Complete amino acid sequence of bovine α_{s2}-casein. *FEBS Lett.*, **76**, 274–9

Byrne, B. M., Schip, A. D. van het, Klundert, J. A. M. van de, Arnberg, A. C., Gruber, M. and AB, G. (1984). Amino acid sequence of phosvitin derived from the nucleotide sequence of part of the chicken vitellogenin gene. *Biochemistry, NY*, **23**, 4275–9

Chaplin, L. C., Clark, D. C. and Smith, L. J. (1988). The secondary structure of peptides derived from caseins: a circular dichroism study. *Biochim. Biophys. Acta*, **956**, 162–72

Chernov, A. A. (1984). In *Modern Crystallography III, Crystal Growth* (ed. A. A. Chernov), Springer, Berlin, chh. 1, 4 and 5

Cocking-Johnson, D., Kampen, C. L. van and Sauk, J. J. (1983). Electron-microscopical studies of conformational changes in dentinal phosphophoryn. *Collagen Rel. Res.*, **3**, 505–10

Cookson, D. J., Levine, B. A., Williams, R. J. P., Jontell, M., Linde, A. and Bernard, B. de. (1980). Cation binding by the rat-incisor-dentine phosphoprotein. *Eur. J. Biochem.*, **110**, 273–8

Creamer, L. K., Richardson, T. and Parry, D. A. D. (1981). Secondary structure of bovine α_{s1}- and β-casein in solution. *Archs Biochem. Biophys.*, **211**, 689–96

Curley-Joseph, J. and Veis, A. (1979). The nature of covalent complexes of phosphoproteins with collagen in the bovine dentin matrix. *J. Dent. Res.*, **58**, 1625–33

Dalgleish, D. G. and Parker, T. G. (1980). Binding of calcium ions to bovine α_{s1}-casein and precipitability of the protein–calcium ion complexes. *J. Dairy Res.*, **47**, 113–22

De Carlo, A., Multigner, L., Lafont, H., Lombardo, D. and Sarles, H. (1984). The molecular characteristics of a human pancreatic acidic phosphoprotein that inhibits calcium carbonate crystal growth. *Biochem. J.*, **222**, 669–77

Deber, C. M., Bovey, F. A., Carver, J. P. and Blout, E. R. (1970). Nuclear magnetic reasonance evidence for cis-peptide bonds in proline oligomers. *J. Am. Chem. Soc.*, **92**, 6191–8

Elgavish, G. A., Hay, D. I. and Schlesinger, D. H. (1984). ¹H and ³¹P nuclear magnetic resonance studies of human salivary statherin. *Int. J. Peptide Protein Res.*, **23**, 230–4

Eliopoulos, E., Geddes, A. J., Brett, M., Pappin, D. J. C. and Findlay, J. B. C. (1982). A structural model for the chromophore-binding domain of ovine rhodopsin. *Int. J. Biol. Macromol.*, **4**, 263–68

Engel, J. Taylor, W. Paulsson, M., Sage, H. and Hogan, B. (1987). Calcium binding domains and calcium-induced conformational transition of SPARC/BM-40/Osteonectin an extracellular glycoprotein expressed in mineralized and nonmineralized tissues. *Biochemistry, NY*, **26**, 6958–65

Fenselau, C., Heller, D. N., Miller, M. S. and White, H. B. iii. (1985). Phosphorylation sites in riboflavin binding protein characterized by fast atom bombardment mass spectrometry. *Anal. Biochem.*, **150**, 309–14

Fujisawa, R., Kuboki, Y. and Sasaki, S. (1986). Changes in interaction of bovine dentin phosphophoryn with calcium and hydroxyapatite by chemical modifications. *Calcif. Tiss. Int.*, **39**, 248–51

Glimcher, M. J. (1984). Recent studies of the mineral phase in bone and its possible linkage to the organic matrix by protein-bound phosphate bonds. *Phil. Trans. R. Soc. Lond. B.*, **304**, 479–508

Graham, E. R. B., Malcolm, G. N. and McKenzie, H. A. (1984). On the isolation and conformation of bovine-casein A. *Int. J. Biol. Macromol.*, **6**, 155–61

Griffin, M. C. A., Price, J. C. and Martin, S. R. (1986). Effect of alcohols on the structure of caseins: circular dichroism studies of kappa-casein A. *Int. J. Biol. Macromol.*, **8**, 367–71

Grizzuti, K. and Perlmann, G. E. (1973). Binding of magnesium and calcium ions to the phosphoglycoprotein phosvitin. *Biochemistry, NY*, **12**, 4399–403

Grøn, P. and Hay, D. I. (1976). Inhibition of calcium phosphate precipitation by human salivary secretions. *Archs Oral Biol.*, **21**, 201–5

Grosclaude, F., Mahé, M.-F. and Ribadeau Dumas, B. (1973). Structure primaire de la caséine α_{s1} et de la caséine β bovine. *Eur. J. Biochem.*, **40**, 323–4

Hartman, P. (1973). In *Crystal Growth: An Introduction* (ed. P. Hartman), North Holland, Amsterdam, Chapter 14

Hartman, P. (1982). Crystal faces: structure and growth. *Geol. Mijnbouw*, **61**, 313–20

Hay, D. I., Moreno, E. C. and Schlesinger, D. H. (1979). Phosphoprotein inhibitors of calcium phosphate precipitation from salivary secretions. *Inorganic Perspectives in Biology and Medicine*, **2**, 271–85

Hay, D. I., Schluckebier, S. K. and Moreno, E. C. (1986). Saturation of human salivary secretions with respect to calcite and inhibition of calcium carbonate precipitation by salivary constituents. *Calcif. Tiss. Int.*, **39**, 151–60

Hay, D. I., Carlson, E. R., Schluckebier, S. K., Moreno, E. C. and Schlesinger, D. H. (1987). Inhibition of calcium phosphate precipitation by human salivary acidic proline-rich proteins: structure–activity relationships. *Calcif. Tiss. Int.*, **40**, 126–32

Holt, C. (1982). Inorganic constituents of milk. III. The colloidal calcium phosphate of cow's milk. *J. Dairy Res.*, **49**, 29–38

Holt, C. (1983). Swelling of Golgi vesicles in mammary secretory cells and its relation to the yield and quantitative composition of milk. *J. Theor. Biol.*, **101**, 247–61

Holt, C. and Sawyer, L. (1988). Primary and predicted secondary structures of the caseins in relation to their biological function. *Protein Engineering*, **2**, 251–9

Holt, C., Davies, D. T. and Law, A. J. R. (1986). Effects of colloidal calcium phosphate content and free calcium ion concentration in the milk serum on the dissociation of bovine casein micelles. *J. Dairy Res.*, **53**, 557–72

Holt, C., van Kemenade, M. J. J. M., Harries, J. E., Nelson, L. S., Jr, Bailey, R. T., Hukins, D. W. L., Hasnain, S. S. and de Bruyn, P. L. (1989a). Preparation of amorphous calcium magnesium phosphates at pH 7 and characterization by X-ray absorption and Fourier transform infrared spectroscopy. *J. Cryst. Growth*, **92**, 239–52

Holt, C., van Kemenade, M. J. J. M., Nelson, L. S., Jr, Hukins, D. W. L., Bailey, R. T., Harries, J. E., Hasnain, S. S. and de Bruyn, P. L. (1989b). Amorphous calcium phosphates prepared at pH 6.5 and 6.0. *Mater. Res. Bull.*, **23**, 55–62

Humphrey, R. S. and Jolley, K. W. (1982). ^{31}P-NMR studies of bovine β-casein. *Biochim. Biophys. Acta*, **708**, 294–9

James, M. N. G. and Sielecki, A. R. (1986). Molecular structure of an aspartic proteinase zymogen, porcine pepsinogen, at 1.8 A resolution. *Nature, Lond.*, **319**, 33–8

Jenness, R. and Holt, C. (1987). Casein and lactose concentrations in milk of 31 species are negatively correlated. *Experientia*, **43**, 1015–18

Jontell, M. and Linde, A. (1983). Non-collagenous proteins of predentine from dentinogenically active bovine teeth. *Biochem. J.*, **214**, 769–76

Van Kemenade, M. J. J. M. (1988). Influence of casein on precipitation of calcium phosphates. Thesis, University of Utrecht, Utrecht, The Netherlands

Van Kemenade, M. J. J. M., and de Bruyn, P. L. (1987). A kinetic study of precipitation from supersaturated calcium phosphate solutions. *J. Colloid Interface Sci.*, **118**, 564–85

Van Kemenade, M. J. J. M., and de Bruyn, P. L. (1989). The influence of casein on the kinetics of hydroxyapatite precipitation. *J. Colloid Interface Sci.* (in press)

Knoop, A.-M., Knoop, E. and Wiechen, A. (1979). Sub-structure of synthetic casein micelles. *J. Dairy Res.*, **46**, 347–50

Kousvelari, E. E., Baratz, R. S., Burke, B. and Oppenheim, F. G. (1980). Immunochemical identification and determination of proline-rich proteins in salivary secretions, enamel pellicle, and glandular tissue specimens. *J. Dent. Res.*, **59**, 1430–38

Kuhn, N. J. and White, A. (1977). The role of nucleoside diphosphatase in a uridine nucleotide cycle associated with lactose synthesis in rat mammary-gland Golgi apparatus. *Biochem. J.*, **168**, 423–33

Landis, W. J., Sanzome, C. F., Brickley-Parsons, D. and Glimcher, M. J. (1984). Radioautographic visualization and biochemical identification of O-phosphoserine- and O-phosphothreonine-containing phosphoproteins in mineralizing embryonic chick bone. *J. Cell Biol.*, **98**, 986–90

Lee, S. L., Glonek, T. and Glimcher, M. J. (1983). ^{31}P nuclear magnetic resonance spectroscopic evidence for ternary complex formation of fetal dentin phosphoprotein with calcium and inorganic orthophosphate ions. *Calcif. Tiss. Int.*, **35**, 815–18

Lee, S. L., Veis, A. and Glonek, T. (1977). Dentin phosphoprotein: an extracellular calcium-binding protein. *Biochemistry, NY*, **16**, 2971–9

Linde, A. (1985). In *The Chemistry and Biology of Mineralized Tissues* (ed. W. T. Butler), EBSCO-media, Birmingham, Alabama, pp. 344–55

Liu, S. T., Hurivitz, A. and Nancollas, G. H. (1982). The influence of polyphosphate ions on the precipitation of calcium oxalate. *J. Urol.*, **127**, 351–5

Lyster, R. L. J., Mann, S., Parker, S. B. and Williams, R. J. P. (1984). Nature of micellar calcium phosphate in cows' milk as studied by high-resolution microscopy. *Biochim. Biophys. Acta*, **801**, 315–17

MacDougal, M., Zeichner-David, M., Bringas, P. and Slavkin, H. (1985). In *The Chemistry and Biology of Mineralized Tissues* (ed. W. T. Butler), EBSCO-media, Birmingham, Alabama, pp. 177–81

Madsen, H.-E. L. and Thorvardarson, G. (1984). Precipitation of calcium phosphate from moderately acid solution *J. Cryst. Growth*, **66**, 369–76

Marsh, M. E. (1986). Biomineralization in the presence of calcium-binding phosphoprotein particles. *J. Exp. Zool.*, **239**, 207–20

Mason, I. J., Murphy, D., Munke, M., Francke, U., Elliott, R. W. and Hogan, B. L. M. (1986a). Developmental and transformation-sensitive expression of the SPARC gene on mouse chromosome 11. *EMBO J.*, **5**, 1831–7

Mason, I. J., Tatlor, A., Williams, J. G., Sage, H. and Hogan, B. L. M. (1986b). Evidence from molecular cloning that SPARC, a major product of mouse embryo parietal endoderm, is related to an endothelial cell 'culture shock' glycoprotein of M_r 43,000. *EMBO J.*, **5**, 1465–72

Mercier, J.-C. and Gaye, P. (1983). In *Biochemistry of Lactation* (ed. T. B. Mepham), Elsevier, Amsterdam, pp. 177–227

Mercier, J.-C., Grosclaude, F. and Ribadeau Dumas, B. (1971). Structure primaire de la caséine α_{s1}-bovine. Séquence complète. *Eur. J. Biochem.*, **23**, 41–51

Mercier, J.-C., Brignon, G. and Ribadeau Dumas, B. (1973). Structure primaire de la caséine κ-bovine. Séquence complète. *Eur. J. Biochem.*, **35**, 222–35

Meyer, J. L. and Eanes, E. D. (1978). A thermodynamic analysis of the secondary transition in the spontaneous precipitation of calcium phosphate. *Calcif. Tiss. Res.*, **25**, 209–16

Montalto, G., Multigner, L., Sarles, H. and De Carlo, A. (1984). Protein inhibitors of crystallization. Characterization and potential role in calcium lithiasis. *Néphrologie*, **5**, 155–7

Moreno, E. C., Kresak, M. and Hay, D. I. (1982). Adsorption thermodynamics of acidic proline-rich human salivary proteins onto calcium apatites. *J. Biol. Chem.*, **257**, 2981–9

Moreno, E. C., Varughese, K. and Hay, D. I. (1979). Effect of human salivary proteins on the precipitation kinetics of calcium phosphate. *Calcif. Tiss. Int.*, **28**, 7–16

Nawrot, C. F., Campbell, D. G., Schroeder, J. K. and Valkenburg, M. van (1976). Dental phosphoprotein-induced formation of hydroxylapatite during *in vitro* synthesis of amorphous calcium phosphate. *Biochemistry, NY*, **15**, 3445–9

Neville, M. C. and Staiert, P. A. (1983). Calcium requirement for lactose synthesis by isolated Golgi vesicles from mouse mammary gland. *J. Cell Biol.*, **97**, 442a

Oppenheim, F. G., Offner, G. D. and Troxler, R. F. (1982). Phosphoproteins in the parotid saliva from the subhuman primate Macaca fascicularis. *J. Biol. Chem.*, **257**, 9271–82

Orci, L. Ravazzola, M. and Anderson, R. G. W. (1987). The condensing vacuole of exocrine cells is more acidic than the mature secretory vesicle. *Nature, Lond.*, **326**, 77–9

Otsuka, K., Yao, K.-L., Wasi, S., Tung, P. S., Aubin, J. E., Sodek, J. and Termine, J. D. (1984). Biosynthesis of osteonectin by fetal porcine calvarial cells *in vitro*. *J. Biol. Chem.*, **259**, 9805–12

Parker, T. G. and Dalgleish, D. G. (1981). Binding of calcium ions to bovine β-casein. *J. Dairy Res.*, **48**, 71–6

Payens, T. A. J. and Vreeman, H. J. (1982). In *Solution Behavior of Surfactants* (eds K. L. Mittal and E. J. Fendler), Plenum Press, New York, 543–71

Perlmann, G. E. (1973). Phosvitin, a phosphoglycoprotein. *Israel J. Chem.*, **11**, 393–405

Perlmann, G. E. and Grizzuti, K. (1971). Conformational transition of the phosphoprotein phosvitin. Random conformation→β structure. *Biochemistry, NY*, **10**, 258–64

Prescott, B., Renugopalakrishnan, V., Glimcher, M. J., Bhushan, A. and Thomas, G. J., Jr (1986). A Raman spectroscopic study of hen egg yolk phosvitin: structures in solution and in the solid state. *Biochemistry, NY*, **25**, 2792–98

Prince, C. W., Oosawa, T., Butler, W. T., Tomana, M., Bhown, A. S., Bhown, M. and Schrohenloher, R. E. (1987). Isolation, characterization, and biosynthesis of a phosphorylated glycoprotein from rat bone. *J. Biol. Chem.*, **262**, 2900–7

Raap, J., Kerling, K. E. T., Vreeman, H. J. and Visser, S. (1983). Peptide substrates for chymosin (rennin): Conformational studies of κ-casein and some κ-casein related oligopeptides by circular dichroism and secondary structure prediction. *Archs Biochem. Biophys.*, **221**, 117–24

Renugopalakrishnan, V., Horowitz, P. M., and Glimcher, M. J. (1985). Structural studies of phosvitin in solution and in the solid state. *J. Biol. Chem.*, **260**, 11406–13

Renugopalakrishnan, V., Uchiyama, A., Horowitz, P. M., Rapaka, R. S., Suzuki, M., Lefteriou, B. and Glimcher, M. J. (1986). Preliminary studies of the secondary structure in solution of two phosphoproteins of chicken bone matrix by circular dichroism and Fourier transform–infrared spectroscopy. *Calcif. Tiss. Int.*, **39**, 166–70

Ribadeau Dumas, B., Brignon, G., Grosclaude, F. and Mercier, J.-C. (1972). Structure primaire de la caséine β bovine. Séquence complète. *Eur. J. Biochem.*, **25**, 505–14

Rollema, H. S., Vreeman, H. J. and Brinkhuis, J. A. (1984). In *22nd Congress Ampère on Magnetic Resonance and Related Phenomena* (eds K. A. Muller, R. Kind and J. Roos), Zurich Ampère Committee, Zurich, 494–5

Romberg, R. W., Werness, P. G., Lollar, P., Riggs, B. L. and Mann, K. G. (1985). Isolation and characterization of native adult osteonectin. *J. Biol. Chem.*, **260**, 2728–36

Romberg, R. W., Werness, P. G., Riggs, B. L. and Mann, K. G. (1986). Inhibition of hydroxyapatite crystal growth by bone-specific and other calcium-binding proteins. *Biochemistry, NY*, **25**, 1176–80

Rosenstein, R. W. and Taborsky, G. (1970). Nonphosphorylated serine residues in phosvitin. *Biochemistry, NY*, **9**, 658–9

Saitoh, E., Isemura, S. and Sanada, K. (1985). Inhibition of calcium-carbonate precipitation by human salivary proline-rich phosphoproteins. *Archs Oral Biol.*, **30**, 641–3

Sawyer, L., Fothergill-Gilmore, L. A. and Russell, G. A. (1986). The predicted secondary structure of enolase. *Biochem. J.*, **236**, 127–30

Schlesinger, D. H. and Hay, D. I. (1977). Complete covalent structure of statherin, a tyrosine-rich acidic peptide which inhibits calcium phosphate precipitation from human parotid saliva. *J. Biol. Chem.*, **252**, 1689–95

Schlesinger, D. H. and Hay, D. I. (1986). Complete covalent structure of a proline-rich phosphoprotein, PRP-2, an inhibitor of calcium phosphate crystal growth from human parotid saliva. *Int. J. Peptide Protein Res.*, **27**, 373–79

Schmidt, D. G. (1982). In *Developments in Dairy Chemistry, Vol. 1* (ed. P. F. Fox), Applied Science Publishers Ltd, Barking, UK, 61–86

Slattery, C. W. and Evard, R. (1973). A model for the formation and structure of casein micelles from subunits of variable composition. *Biochim. Biophys. Acta*, **317**, 529–38

Sleigh, R. W., Mackinlay, A. G. and Pope, J. M. (1983). NMR studies of the phosphoserine regions of bovine α_{s1}- and β-casein. *Biochim. Biophys. Acta*, **742**, 175–83

Sodek, J., Domenicucci, C., Zung, P., Kuwata, F. and Wasi, S. (1986). In *Cell Mediated Calcification and Matrix Vesicles* (ed. S. Yousuf Ali), Elsevier, Amsterdam, 135–41

Stetler-Stevenson, W. G. and Veis, A. (1983). Bovine dentin phosphophoryn: Composition and molecular weight. *Biochemistry, NY*, **22**, 4326–35

Stetler-Stevenson, W. G. and Veis, A. (1987). Bovine dentin phosphophoryn: Calcium ion binding properties of a high molecular weight preparation. *Calcif. Tiss. Int.*, **40**, 97–102

Taborsky, G. (1970). Effect of freezing and thawing on the conformation of phosvitin. *J. Biol. Chem.*, **245**, 1054–62

Termine, J. D. and Posner, A. S. (1970). Calcium phosphate formation *in vitro*. I. Factors affecting initial phase separation. *Archs Biochem. Biophys.*, **140**, 307–17

Termine, J. D. and Conn, K. M. (1976). Inhibition of apatite formation by phosphorylated metabolites and macromolecules. *Calcif. Tiss. Res.*, **22**, 149–57

Termine, J. D., Eanes, E. D. and Conn, K. M. (1980). Phosphoprotein modulation of apatite crystallization. *Calcif. Tiss. Int.*, **31**, 247–51

Termine, J. D., Kleinman, H. K., Whitson, S. W., Conn, K. M., McGarvey, M. L. and Martin, G. R. (1981). Osteonectin, a bone-specific protein linking mineral to collagen. *Cell*, **26**, 99–105

Traub, W. and Perimann, G. E. (1972). X-ray study of phosvitin, the phosphoglycoprotein in hens' egg yolk. *Israel J. Chem.*, **10**, 655–58

Uchiyama, A., Lefteriou, B. and Glimcher, M. J. (1985). In *The Chemistry and Biology of Mineralized Tissues* (ed. W. T. Butler), EBSCO-media, Birmingham, Alabama, 182–4

Udich, H.-J., Hoft, H. D. and Bornig, H. (1986). Effect of phosphoprotein on precipitation and crystallization of calcium phosphate salts. An *in vitro* study using an agar gel matrix model. *Biomed. Biochim. Acta*, **45**, 703–11

Veis, A. (1985). In *The Chemistry and Biology of Mineralized Tissues* (ed. W. T. Butler), EBSCO-media, Birmingham, Albama, 170–6

Vogel, H. J. (1983). Structure of hen phosvitin: A ^{31}P NMR, ^{1}H NMR, and laser photochemically induced dynamic nuclear polarization ^{1}H NMR study. *Biochemistry, NY*, **22**, 668–74

West, D. W. and Clegg, R. A. (1981). Golgi vesicles isolated from rat mammary tissue contain endogenous caseins and 0.1 mM free calcium. *Biochem. Soc. Trans.*, **9**, 468

Williams, R. J. P. (1975). Phases and phase structure in biological systems. *Biochim. Biophys. Acta*, **416**, 237–86

Williams, S. P., Bridger, W. A. and James, M. N. G. (1986). Characterization of the phosphoserine of pepsinogen using ^{31}P nuclear magnetic resonance: Corroboration of X-ray crystallographic results. *Biochemistry, NY*, **25**, 6655–59

Wong, R. S. C. and Bennick, A. (1980). The primary structure of a salivary calcium-binding proline-rich phosphoprotein (protein C), a possible precursor of a related salivary protein A. *J. Biol. Chem.*, **255**, 5943–8

Wuthier, R. E. (1986). In *Cell Mediated Calcification and Matrix Vesicles* (ed. S. Yousuf Ali), Elsevier, Amsterdam, 47–55

Zanette, D., Monaco, H. L., Zanotti, G. and Spadon, P. (1984). Crystallization of hen eggwhite riboflavin binding protein. *J. molec. Biol.*, **180**, 1185–7

9
Phospholipids and calcification

Adele L. Boskey

INTRODUCTION

Phospholipids are predominantly found within the membranes of cells and subcellular organelles. On average, the phospholipids account for 50 per cent of the membrane lipid, the other half being cholesterol. Together, the lipids and the proteins within membranes control cell function (Seelig and MacDonald, 1987). The phospholipids are known to play a role determining cell shape, controlling the flux of ions into and out of the cell, mediating the fusion of cells, and regulating cell metabolism. Phospholipids are also involved in the activation of certain enzymes, and provide a reservoir for the storage of compounds, or precursors of these compounds, which control cell function (e.g., prostaglandins, leukotrienes, diacylglycerides, acetylcholine, etc.).

Certain membrane phospholipids serve as promoters of hydroxyapatite formation. This chapter reviews recent evidence linking each of these functions – structure, fluidity, fusion, metabolism and nucleation – to events in the calcification process.

DEFINITIONS AND PROPERTIES

Phospholipids are phosphorylated derivatives of polyalcohols; 1,2-diacylglycerols (phosphatides), 1-alkenyl-acyl glycerols (plasmologens), or sphingosine (sphingomyelin). The phosphate group in the diacylglycerol derivatives is frequently linked (figure 9.1) to a nitrogenous base such as choline (phosphatidylcholine PC), ethanolamine (phosphatidylethanolamine PE), or serine (phosphatidylserine PS). Similarly, in phosphatidylinositol (PI), it is the sugar myo-inositol that is linked to the phosphate. The phospholipids containing bases are zwitterionic. PE and PC, which have no

A

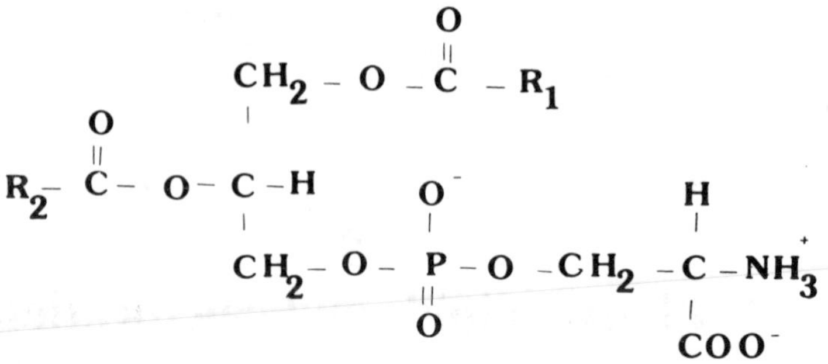

B

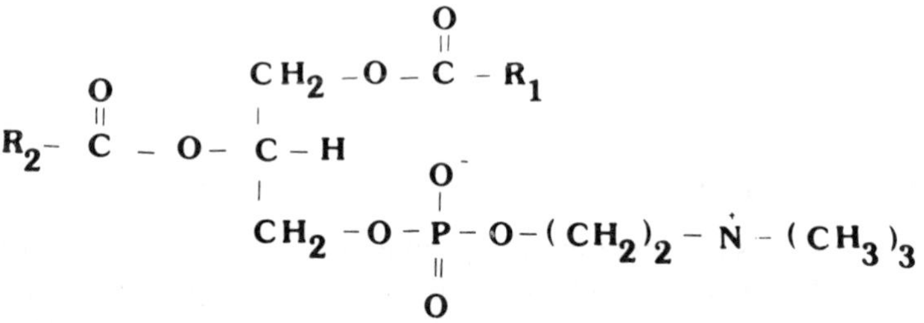

Figure 9.1 The structure of (A) phosphatidylserine, PS, and (B), phosphatidylcholine, PC, at physiologic pH. Note that PS has a net charge of -1 and PC has a net charge of 0 at this pH. R_1 and R_2 are the acyl or alkyl chains of the fatty acid attached to the glycerol (OH) backbone. In membrane phospholipids R_2 is frequently arachidonic acid, the precursor of prostalandins, leukotrienes, and thromboxanes. In the lyso-phosphatides the fatty acid is absent from the 2-position, leaving a free –OH.

net charge at physiologic pH, are neutral phospholipids, whereas PS has a negative charge and is acidic. PI and phosphatidic acid, PA, which has no moiety linked to the phosphate, are also acidic. Cardiolipin, the most acidic of the phosphatides, consists of two molecules of PA covalently linked together through a molecule of glycerol. It is the acidic phospholipids, phosphatidylserine and phosphatidylinositol, which are most intimately related to the calcification process.

The phospholipids are amphipathic, consisting of hydrophobic fatty acid side chains and polar hydrophilic head groups (phosphate). In membranes (figure 9.2), the phospholipids assemble so that their charged, polar head groups are exposed to the aqueous phases inside or outside the 5–15 nm thick membrane, while the non-polar fatty acids in the alkyl and acyl side chains are buried in the membrane bi-layer (Singer and Nicholson, 1972). Membrane-associated proteins, as illustrated in the figure, may be partially or fully inserted into the bilayer. Details of membrane structure and function are reviewed elsewhere (Cullis *et al.*, 1985; Kohler and Klein, 1977; Singer and Nicholson, 1972).

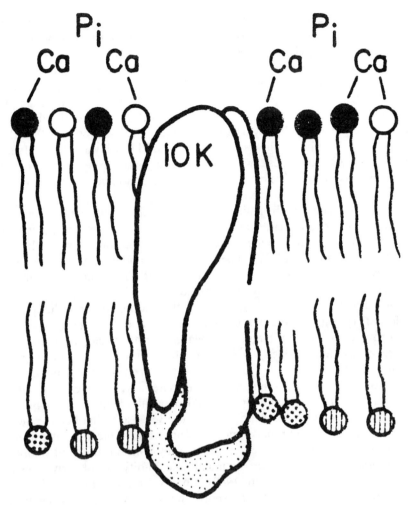

Figure 9.2 Two-dimensional model of a portion of a plasma membrane, showing the polar (balls) head groups on the surfaces, and the hydrophobic acyl and alkyl chains forming the bilayer. Proteins buried in the membrane (shaded) may protrude into either the cytoplasmic or the extracellular surfaces, or may be totally buried in the membrane. This model represents a portion of the membrane containing the calcifiable proteolipid with its 10*K* apo-protein. The presence of the apo-protein orients the phospholipids, facilitating binding of calcium and inorganic phosphate to acidic phospholipids, leading to mineralisation, as described in the text. (Figure kindly supplied by Dr Boyan.)

Within membranes, phospholipids interact both non-covalently and covalently with proteins. The covalently linked proteolipids (Folch-Pi and Stoffyn, 1972; Schlesinger, 1981) contain hydrophobic proteins and thus are usually buried within the membrane. Because of their hydrophobic properties, they are generally extractable with lipid solvents or detergent.

Proteolipids are distinct from lipoproteins, containing more lipid than protein, being exclusively intrinsic membrane proteins, and being very hydrophilic. A specific proteolipid isolated from calcified tissues that can act as a promoter of hydroxyapatite formation, will be discussed later.

The non-covalent interactions with membrane phospholipids can alter the conformation and modify the function of proteins. For example, alkaline phosphatase plays an essential role in calcification, binds to the membrane via phosphatidylinositol (Low and Zilversmit, 1980) and is inhibited by the phospholipids PE, PS, PC and PI (Farley and Jorch, 1983). In contrast, Na–K ATPase, which may play a parallel role in regulation of phosphate concentration, is activated by phospholipids (Warren *et al.*, 1974).

The membranes are dynamic structures. Phospholipids undergo internal motion of their fatty-acid side chains, glycerol backbone and polar head groups. Such motion is believed to allow the transport of water through membranes (Traube, 1973). Phospholipids also undergo lateral movement and translation (flip-flop) across the bilayer. This motion facilitates changes in shape and fluidity of the membrane.

Membrane fluidity is determined by the motion of phospholipids of different types in discrete regions of the membrane. Phospholipids are not uniformly distributed in membrane bilayers – rather, they have an asymmetric distribution, which varies with cell and membrane type (Op den Kamp, 1979). In most plasma membranes, phosphatidylcholine and sphingomyelin are predominantly in the outer layer, while phosphatidylserine, phosphatidylethanolamine, and phosphatidylinositol are principally in the inner surface of the membrane. Because of the heterogeneous structure of the membrane, some areas are more subject to alteration in shape or permeability. In general, increasing concentrations of lysophosphatides and cholesterol increase membrane fluidity; sterol derivatives can have the same effect (Nelson, 1980). Changes in membrane fluidity alter membrane permeability, ion transport, and receptor responses. However, there is not always a direct relationship between fluidity and ion permeability (Rossignol *et al.*, 1985). Extreme alterations in fluidity can be toxic to cells (Holmes *et al.*, 1983). In calcifying tissues, alterations in membrane fluidity are important for calcium and proton transport into and out of the cell. For example, the fluidity of the basal membrane of the ameloblast is thought to allow calcium transport towards developing enamel (Reith, 1983). Changes in membrane fluidity and interaction of phospholipids with calcium facilitate exocytosis (Nayar *et al.*, 1982) and the formation of vesicles. The significance of extracellular matrix vesicles in calcification will be apparent later.

In addition to the abilities of phospholipids to interact with cholesterol and proteins forming enclosed, bilayer structures, the phospholipids also interact with cations and cationic molecules (Hauser *et al.*, 1976; Joos and

Carr, 1967; Hauser and Phillips, 1979; Hendrickson and Fullington, 1965; Holwerds *et al.*, 1981). Calcium binding to phospholipids markedly alters membrane and lipid properties. In some cases, the presence of inorganic phosphate amplifies the effect. Membrane fusion, essential to cell division, exocytosis, and other processes, requires calcium binding and is facilitated by the presence of inorganic phosphate (Fraley *et al.*, 1980). Calcium transport, through a model PS membrane, is similarly accelerated by the binding of calcium and phosphate to the phosphatidylserine in the membrane (Yaari *et al.*, 1982).

The phospholipids most directly involved in the calcification process are the acidic phospholipids, which function as hydroxyapatite nucleators and facilitate calcium transport. Those phospholipids that determine cell properties, control exocytosis and vesicle formation, and serve as precursors of metabolic intermediates play an indirect but equally important role.

DISTRIBUTION OF PHOSPHOLIPIDS IN CALCIFIED AND CALCIFYING TISSUES

Lipids are relatively minor components in the calcified tissues, accounting, on average, for less than 1 per cent of the dry weight of the tissue. Phospholipids account for 20–30 per cent of the total lipid extractable from these tissues. Despite their low concentration, a role for phospholipids in the calcification process is suggested by the histological association of lipids with early mineral deposition, and by the increase in the content of certain phospholipids in actively mineralising tissues.

Extraction of phospholipids from calcified tissues is impeded by the interaction of the lipids with the mineral. The acidic phospholipids, because of their negative charge, bind to hydroxyapatite (Primes *et al.*, 1982), making it difficult to extract the lipids with typical lipid solvents. Two distinct methods have been applied in the analyses of calcified tissue phospholipids. In the first method, extraction by stirring in lipid solvents is followed by extraction in acidified solvents, the acid being used to decalcify the tissue. In the second, sonication in lipid solvents and buffer is used to disrupt the lipids from the mineral surface. The use of these techniques, coupled with analytical methods for the determination of phospholipid composition, has revealed the presence of unique phospholipid-containing macromolecules in the calcifying tissues.

Anatomic localisation of the macromolecules in these calcifying tissues has similarly been hampered by the lack of reagents specific for phospholipids and by the loss of lipids caused by most fixation techniques (Weibull *et al.*, 1983). The classic studies of Irving (1958; 1959; 1963), showing a concentration of sudanophilic (lipid-containing) material at the mineralisation fronts in dentine, cartilage, and bone, can be challenged by observations that the lipid stains cross-react with non-collageneous proteins such as

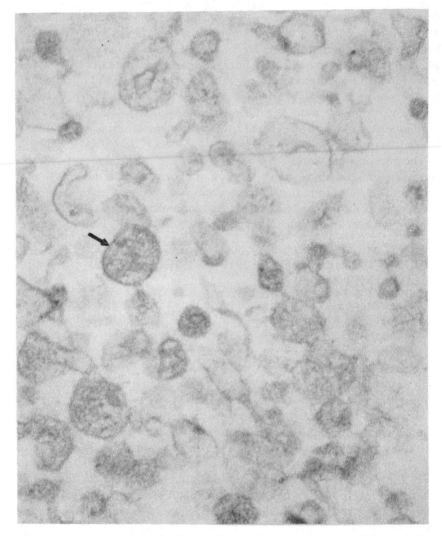

Figure 9.3 Matrix vesicle fraction from confluent, third-passage costochondral growth plate cartilage cells. Arrow shows trilaminar membrane which is characteristic of matrix vesicles. This preparation was also shown to have enriched alkaline phosphatase activity. (Figure courtesy of Drs Boyan and Swain.)

the phosphoproteins, or may be subject to other interpretations. In all calcified tissues studied to date, however, the phospholipids appear distributed between membranes of cells and cellular organelles, cell debris, and, in some tissues but not all, matrix vesicles.

Matrix vesicles (Anderson, 1969; 1980) are extracellular, membrane-bound bodies (figure 9.3) reported to be the site of initial mineral deposition in cartilage (Anderson, 1969; Ali, 1976), mantle dentine

(Katchburian, 1973), and woven bone (Bernard, 1969). *In vitro*, hydroxy-apatite mineral deposits in isolated matrix vesicles (Ali, 1976; Hsu and Anderson, 1977; Vaananen, 1980), in part because of the sequestration of calcium by the acidic phospholipids in their membranes, and in part because of the enzymatic activities associated with the vesicles. The mechanism through which matrix vesicles facilitate hydroxyapatite deposition is discussed later.

Two related phospholipid-containing species, both matrix vesicle components, concentrated in the calcified/calcifying tissues, are the complexed acidic phospholipids and the calcifiable proteolipids. Anghileri (1972) was the first to identify acidic phospholipid–calcium phosphate complexes, also called complexed acidic phospholipids, in calcifying tumours. Studies by Boskey and co-workers (for review, see Boskey, 1981) demonstrated that these complexes were found only in calcifiable and calcified tissues. Wuthier and Gore (1977) showed that the complexed acidic phospholipids were components of cell and matrix vesicle membranes. The complexes, whose chemistry was reviewed by Wuthier (1982), consist predominantly of acidic phospholipids, with lesser amounts of calcium and inorganic phosphate. Studies by Boyan and Boskey (Boyan-Salyers and Boskey, 1981; Boyan and Boskey, 1984) proved that within calcified tissues, the complexed acidic phospholipids were found associated with calcifiable proteolipids, with the proteolipids accounting for as much as 80 per cent of the complexed acidic phospholipids in a calcifying tissue.

Calcifiable proteolipids were first characterised in oral bacteria (Takazoe *et al.*, 1970). As illustrated in figure 9.2, they consist of a hydrophobic apo-protein which associates with acidic phospholipids. As would be anticipated, there are high proportions of calcifiable proteolipids in matrix vesicle membranes (Boyan-Salyers *et al.*, 1978). Proteolipid-mediated calcification in bacteria has been extensively studied as a model of membrane-mediated calcification (Boyan *et al.*, 1984). Results of these studies, as well as investigations of other proteolipids, provide insight into the functions of the lipid and protein components of these hydrophobic macromolecules. From these studies, it has been suggested that the protein portion of the proteolipid is responsible for the organisation of the lipid structure (Boggs *et al.*, 1977). This organisation, in turn, facilitates complexed acidic phospholipid formation on the membrane surface (Boyan *et al.*, 1986). The proteolipids may enhance mineralisation, both in this way and by serving as ionophores, increasing proton transport (Boyan *et al.*, 1986; Swain and Boyan, 1988). The apo-protein associated with the complexed acidic phospholipids in several species appears on SDS-gels to be a 10 000 MW protein (Boyan *et al.*, 1982). Antibodies (Boyan *et al.*, 1982) against the bacterial 10 000 MW apo-protein cross-react with several higher-MW protein isolates from *Bacterionema matruchotii*-complexed acidic phospholipid and proteolipid fractions (Boyan, personal

Table 9.1 Complexed acidic phospholipid content of some calcified and calcifiable tissues

	Content[a]	Acid phospholipids[b]
Fetal calf[c]		
Articular cartilage	0.43	PS, PI
Growth plate		
Reserve zone	3.3	PS, PI
Proliferating zone	13.2	PS, PI
Hypertrophic zone	30.2	PS, PI
Primary spongiosa	1.5	PS, PI
Normal (6–8 weeks old) rat[d]		
Epiphysis	16	PS, PI
Cancellous bone	6.6	PS, PI
Cortical bone	6.1	PS, PI
Intramembranous bone	5	PS, PI
Dystrophic HA deposits		
Tumoral calcinosis[e]	2.8	PS, PI, PC
Parotid stones[f]	7	PS, PI, CDL
Submandibular stones[g]	6.8	PS, PI, SPH, PE
Atherosclerotic placque[h]	8	PS, PI, CDL

[a] μg per mg demineralised dry weight.
[b] Principal phospholipid constituents of the isolated complexed acidic phospholipids.
[c] From Boskey *et al.* (1980).
[d] From Boskey and Marks (1985); Boskey *et al.* (1984); Boskey (1985); Boskey and Wientroub (1986); Boskey and Timchak (1983).
[e] From Boskey *et al.* (1983b).
[f] From Boskey *et al.* (1983a).
[g] From Boskey *et al.* (1981).
[h] From Dmitrovsky and Boskey (1985).

communication). This confirms the relationship between proteolipid and complexed acidic phospholipids, since the antibodies do not react with acidic phospholipids.

Table 9.1 lists the complexed acidic phospholipid contents and compositions of a variety of normal and pathologically calcified tissues. Neither non-calcifying tissues, nor tissues which contain pathologic calcium phosphate deposits other than hydroxyapatite, contain significant levels of these lipids. The composition of these complexes is remarkably comparable to that of the phospholipids which are released from the calcified tissues after demineralisation (Wuthier, 1982). Changes in the distribution and concentration of these complexes during mineralisation suggest they are involved in the mineralisation process.

Calcification of cartilage during the process of endochondral ossification provides a dynamic model for characterising factors involved in physiologic mineral deposition. The relationship between lipids and calcification of cartilage was first suggested on the basis of the accumulation of the lipid staining dye, Sudan black B, at the mineralisation front of the growth plate (Irving, 1963). Shapiro (1970a, b) and Wuthier (1968) later characterised the phospholipids associated with calcifying cartilage and bone, demonstrating the need for acid decalcification to extract the majority of the acidic phospholipids. Boskey *et al.* (1980) showed a progressive increase in the content of the complexed acidic phospholipids, going from the resting zone to the hypertrophic zone (where mineralisation commences) in bovine growth plates. This pattern was comparable to that reported by Wuthier (1968) for mineral-bound lipids.

A role for lipids in bone mineralisation was first suggested by Enlow and Conklin (1964). As in calcified cartilage, the acidic phospholipids phosphatidylserine, phosphatidylinositol, and phosphatidic acid, but not cardiolipin (a mitochondrial lipid), were extracted from bone in greater amounts after decalcification (Wuthier, 1968; Shapiro, 1970a, b). The complexed acidic phospholipids of mineralised mammalian tissues were first identified in compact bone (Boskey and Posner, 1976a). Younger, developing endochondral and endosteal bone contained higher proportions of the complexed acidic phospholipids than more mature tissues. Bones formed by intramembranous ossification contained lower amounts of these lipids than the endosteal and endochodral bones of the same animals (Boskey and Wientroub, 1986). Calcifiable proteolipids were similarly found in compact bones; an age dependence was not reported (Ennever *et al.*, 1978).

On the basis of the distribution of the complexed acidic phospholipids in the growth plate (Boskey *et al.*, 1980), and in an implant model of endochondral bone formation where maximal complexed acidic phospholipid contents occurred prior to detectable cartilage calcification (Boskey and Reddi, 1983) it was hypothesised that formation of the complexed acidic phospholipids occurred as a prelude to mineral deposition. More recently, using labelled inorganic phosphate to study phospholipid metabolism during cartilage calcification in a chick limb bud mesenchymal cell system (Mont *et al.*, 1987), this hypothesis has been confirmed.

The presence of a lipid-staining material at the dentine–predentine interface was the first suggestion that lipids were also involved in dentine calcification (Irving, 1959). This intense staining was associated with the presence of acidic phospholipids by biochemical analyses (Shapiro and Wuthier, 1966). As seen in table 9.2, the phospholipid composition of dentine and predentine are distinct, with the dentine phospholipids, similar to those in the other mineralised tissues, containing elevated amounts of acidic phospholipids (Shapiro and Wuthier, 1966; Dirksen and Marinetti, 1970; Prout *et al.*, 1973; Odutuga and Prout, 1974; Wuthier, 1984). Again, like bone and cartilage, complexed acidic phospholipids, proteolipids, and extracellular matrix vesicles are components of the newly forming dentine matrix (Haynes *et al.*, 1982).

The recent development of a malachite green aldehyde osmium tetroxide stain, specific for the visualisation of phospholipids at the EM level, revealed an abundance of phospholipids, not part of matrix vesicles, in dentine and predentine. These phospholipids appeared in close association

Table 9.2   Phospholipid composition[a] of mineralised and mineralising tissues

	PC	PE	SPH	PS	PI	CDL
Growth plate[b]	38*	25*	4	11	5	5
Cancellous bone[c]	36*	27*	6	10	6	3
Cortical bone[d]	49*	24*	5	9	8	6
Intramembranous bone[e]	49*	24*	4	6	8	8
Enamel pre[f]	43	11	7	6	11	6
Enamel cell[f]	32	18	9	11	9	9
Predentine[g]	55	21	5	9	3	4
Dentine[g]	55	23	11	6	5	1

[a] Major phospholipid components as a percentage of total lipid phosphorus.
* lyso-phosphatides have been combined with indicated values. PC = phosphatidylcholine. PE = phosphatidylethanolamine. SPH = sphingomyelin. PS = phosphatidylserine. PI = phosphatidylinositol. CDL = cardiolipin.
[b] Immature rat; average calculated from Boskey and Timchak (1983), Boskey (1985), Boskey and Wientroub (1986).
[c] Immature rat; from Boskey and Timchak (1983) and Boskey (1985).
[d] Immature rat; from Boskey and Timchak (1983), Boskey and Wientroub (1986).
[e] Immature rat; from Boskey and Wientroub (1986).
[f] Immature rat; from Goldberg et al., (1983).
[g] Fetal calf; from Manzoli and Gelli (1968).

with collagen fibrils, suggesting that the matrix phospholipids might be involved in mineralisation (Goldberg and Septier, 1985). Similar association of lipid and type I collagen has been noted in other mineralising tissues (Lelous et al., 1982; Ennever et al., 1984); although specific phospholipid stains have not yet been applied to tissues other than dentine and enamel. In the future, combination of these stains with an anti-calcifiable proteolipid antibody could provide additional insight into the role of these lipids in the control of mineralisation.

Enamel formation and mineralisation involves distinct cell types and bears little resemblance to the formation of dentine or bone. The functions of the cells in enamel formation are discussed elsewhere (Warshawsky and Smith, 1974). Complexed acidic phospholipids, calcifiable proteolipids, and matrix vesicles are not thought to have a role in enamel formation. However, there are phospholipids found in developing enamel (Dirkson and Marinetti, 1970; Fincham et al., 1972; Prout et al., 1973; Prout and Odutuga, 1974a, b, c; Odutuga and Prout, 1974; Goldberg et al., 1983). Using p-phenyldiamine to enhance lipid staining of freeze-substituted sections at the EM level, Goldberg et al. (1983) demonstrated the presence of abundant cellular debris in the enamel surface zones, and suggested that the enamel lipids were derived from cellular components. Autoradiographic studies demonstrated that these lipids were membrane-associated components, rather than true 'matrix' components. Although these cell fragments have not been shown to play a direct role in mineralisation of enamel, the authors suggested that they may supply enzyme activity needed for matrix maturation (Goldberg et al., 1984).

The presence of complexed acidic phospholipids and proteolipids in all the calcified tissues (except enamel) did not a priori indicate they played a role in mineralisation. This role was demonstrated by *in vitro* studies, discussed below, which showed these lipids acted as promoters of hydroxyapatite formation, and was confirmed by *in vivo* studies (Raggio *et al.*, 1986).

PHOSPHOLIPIDS IN DISEASE STATES WHERE CALCIFICATION IS ALTERED

Insight into the importance of phospholipids in calcification has also been provided by studies of abnormal tissues. The alteration of lipid composition in diseased tissues provides insight into both the function of the lipids and the pathogenesis of the disease. For example, the buildup of cholesterol, leading to a decrease in membrane fluidity, in osteonecrotic bone (Boskey *et al.*, 1983a) and other necrotic tissues (Papahadjopoulos, 1974) demonstrated the importance of proper membrane fluidity for cell function. Analysis of the complexed acidic phospholipid content of parotid and submandibular stones revealed the presence of complexes containing large amounts of cardiolipin, predominantly a bacterial and mitochondrial phospholipid only in the parotid stones (Boskey *et al.*, 1981; Boskey *et al.*, 1983a), verifying the concept that bacteria could serve as nidii for these stones. In non-calcified atherosclerotic placques, the detection of complexed acidic phospholipids (Dmitrovsky and Boskey, 1985) suggested a mechanism by which the well-documented accumulation of phospholipids facilitated calcification.

The most extensively studied calcified tissue abnormality, in which alterations in phospholipids have been associated with the disease, is vitamin-D-dependent rickets. Impaired calcification of cartilage (rickets) and bone (osteomalacia) is the hall-mark of vitamin-D deficiency. It was in rachitic chicks and pigs that Wuthier first noted the accumulation of mineral-associated acidic phospholipids (Wuthier, 1971). The extended growth plates of vitamin-D- and phosphate-deficient animals are the sites of abundant non-mineralised matrix vesicles (Simon *et al.*, 1973; Anderson *et al.*, 1975) and cells containing abnormal lipid droplets (Matthews *et al.*, 1970). The lesions in the bones of these animals (Atkin *et al.*, 1985) are more extensive than those in animals that are only vitamin-D deficient (Boskey and Wientroub, 1986).

Lipid extracts of the vitamin-D- and phosphate-deficient animals' cartilage and bones differ from extracts from normal animals, having elevated cholesterol, decreased lyso-phosphatide, and slightly decreased complexed acidic phospholipid and proteolipid contents (Boskey and Timchak, 1983; Ritter and Boyan-Salyers, 1980). Treatment with vitamin D_3 and phosphate produces a rapid (24–48 h) increase in complexed acidic phospholipid content, and a correction of the other lipid abnormalities (Boskey, 1985). The altered lipid compositions in the untreated animals are characteristic of membranes with decreased fluidity (Stubbs and Smith, 1984). The resultant altered membrane permeability could, in part, account for the defective osteoid which exists in these animals (Sampath *et al.*, 1984). Vitamin D stimulates phospholipase A_2 activity in matrix vesicles and chondrocytes (Boyan and Schwartz, personal communication), and in intestinal cells (O'Doherty, 1979), providing an explanation for the increase in lyso-phosphatides in treated animals.

The increase in complexed acidic phospholipid content when vitamin-D-deficient animals are given vitamin D is accompanied by gradual elimination of the defects in matrix mineralisation (Boskey, 1985); this further supports the hypothesis that increases in complexed acidic phospholipid content precede, and then facilitate, initial mineralisation. A single treatment of normo-phosphatemic vitamin-D-deficient rats with 1,25-dihydroxyvitamin D, and to a lesser extent with metabolites that can be converted to 1,25-dihydroxyvitamin D, similarly produces a significant increase in complexed acidic phospholipids in calcifying cartilage and bone. In these vitamin-D-treated animals, the complexed acidic phospholipid content is directly related to serum levels of 1,25-dihydroxyvitamin D (Boskey *et al.*, 1988). Thus, 1,25-dihydroxyvitamin D appears to be the metabolite responsible for altering bone and cartilage phospholipid metabolism. This suggestion is supported by studies that demonstrate that this metabolite, and not 24,25-dihydroxyvitamin D, stimulates phosphatidylserine synthesis in osteoblast-like cells (Matsumoto *et al.*, 1985). This vitamin D metabolite similarly alters phospholipid composition in renal brush border membranes (Elgavish *et al.*, 1983).

Vitamin D may act directly as a steroid hormone, promoting synthesis of proteins involved in phospholipid metabolism. It may also act indirectly, increasing intracellular calcium levels, which in turn may also effect these enzymes. Vitamin D may also directly alter membrane properties by inserting itself into the membranes (Holmes *et al.*, 1983); however, to produce a detectable effect, concentrations greater than those used in animal experiments would be required. Recent data indicate that vitamin D is not acting solely by correcting hypocalcemia, since vitamin-D-depleted chicks given a diet enriched in calcium, and having a serum Ca content equivalent to normal, have bone-complexed acidic phospholipid contents comparable to those in rachitic animals (Boskey and Dickson, 1988).

Bones of vitamin-D-repleted chicks with low serum phosphate also have reduced contents of complexed acidic phospholipids. Although the content of the complexed acidic phospholipids in these animals is not as low as in the rachitic chick, the importance of phosphate as well as vitamin D for the metabolism of phospholipids associated with mineralisation is apparent. To separate the effects of vitamin D and phosphate, studies are currently being done on the lipid composition in an animal model of vitamin-D-resistant rickets, the hypophosphatemic mouse. These studies, coupled with studies at the cellular level, should provide greater insight into the regulation of phospholipid metabolism by vitamin D, and the relevance of this regulation to the calcification process.

PHOSPHOLIPID METABOLISM

Until recently, there have been few studies of phospholipid metabolism in connective tissue cells. The discovery of the phospho-inositide pathway, which is involved in the regulation of multiple cellular events, created a flow of activity designed to understand how cell membranes regulate cell function (Berridge, 1984). This, and the evidence that changes in membrane phospholipid composition altered cell function, led to more extensive investigations into the metabolism of phospholipids in osteoblasts, chondroblasts, and other connective tissue cells (Cornell and Horwitz, 1980). Most of the current knowledge of the metabolism of phospholipids comes from studies in other tissues.

Phospholipid synthesis in the connective tissues cells appears to be identical to that in other tissues (Schuster *et al.*, 1975; Wuthier and Cummins, 1974). Specific reactions, however, which are dependent on calcium levels, might be altered in vitamin-D-deficient animals. Reacylation of phosphatides, in which acyl-groups are replaced on lyso-phosphatides, or exchanged for other fatty acids is a calcium-dependent reaction modulated by the calcium-binding protein calmodulin (Ansell and Spanner, 1982). Inhibition of calmodulin activity in growing rats resulted in growth plate abnormalities accompanied by altered proportions of cartilage membrane lyso-phosphatides (Boskey *et al.*, 1984). The base exchange enzyme (Hubscher, 1962) also has a calcium requirement. Phosphatidyl-serine and phosphatidylethanolamine exchange bases with free serine or ethanolamine using this enzyme. This enzyme, considering the importance of phosphatidylserine in formation of complexed acidic phospholipids and in regulation of calcium transport, may be a key enzyme in controlling phospholipid metabolism in calcifying tissues. Studies of the action of this enzyme in isolated osteoblast, chondroblast, or ondotoblast populations have not yet been reported. In fact, the only detailed studies of phospholipid metabolism in calcifying tissues are the initial study demonstrating the selectivity of phospholipid synthesis in chick cartilage (Eisenberg *et al.*, 1970), and an investigation of phospholipid synthesis by isolated chondrocytes and matrix vesicles showing that vesicles are not capable of synthesising phospholipids *de novo* (Wuthier *et al.*, 1978).

Turnover of phospholipids is dependent on the activities of phospholipase A_2, phospholipase C and phospholipase D (figure 9.4). Each of these enzymes is dependent on calcium (Elsbach *et al.*, 1985; Rakhimov *et al.*, 1980; Billah *et al.*, 1981), and, as noted above, phospholipase A_2 activity in

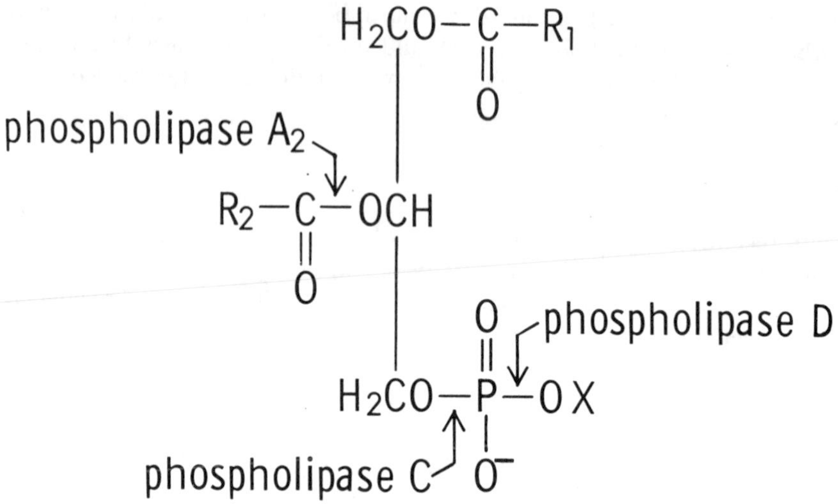

$$H_2CO-\underset{\underset{O}{\|}}{C}-R_1$$

phospholipase A_2

$$R_2-\underset{\underset{O}{\|}}{C}-OCH$$

phospholipase D

$$H_2CO-\underset{\underset{O^-}{|}}{\overset{\overset{O}{\|}}{P}}-OX$$

phospholipase C

Figure 9.4   Phospholipase activities are summarised using this schematic diagram of a typical phosphatide. All of the enzymes shown, phospholipase A_2, phospholipase C and phospholipase D require calcium.

chondrocytes has been shown to be stimulated by vitamin D. Elevated levels of phospholipase A_2 are found in the hypertrophic cells of the growth plate (Wuthier, 1973), suggesting that altered phospholipid turnover may occur parallel to the onset of calcification. In this respect, it is interesting to note that the complexed acidic phospholipids are not as good a substrate for phospholipase A_2 as phosphatidylserine itself.

Intracellular phospholipid metabolism is controlled, in part, by hormones. Receptor binding by certain agonists causes the hydrolysis of membrane phosphatidylinositol 4,5-diphosphate by a specific phospholipase C (Berridge, 1984). This releases two second messengers, inositol 1,4,5-triphosphate and diacylglycerol. Inositol triphosphate causes the release of calcium from intracellular stores (mitochondria, endoplasmic reticulum). Calcium release from mitochondria is a key event in endochondral ossification (Brighton and Hunt, 1978; Shapiro and Greenspan, 1969). Thus this pathway that facilitates calcium release is apt to be important in connective-tissue cells. Diacylglyceride activates a tyrosine kinase (protein kinase C), triggering a cascade of other events in the cell. Like other second messengers, inositoltriphosphate and diacylglycerol can be rapidly removed and resynthesised by specific enzymes. The phospholipase C that starts this pathway is specific for phosphatides containing arachidonic acid in the 2 position; the turnover of diacylglycerol can therefore include the production of another set of second messengers, prostaglandins, leukotrienes, and thromboxanes. Prostaglandins have been shown to stimulate

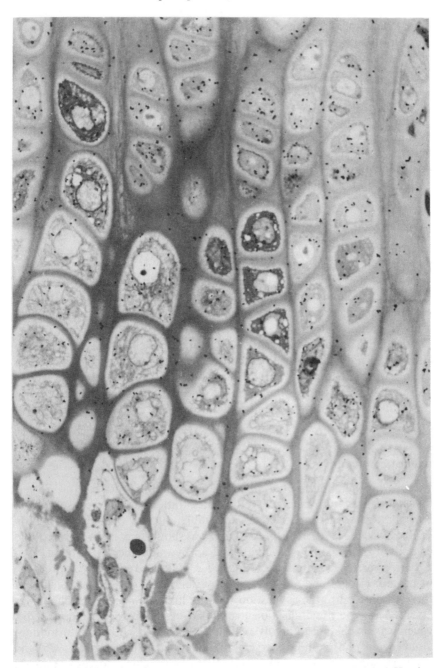

Figure 9.5   Autoradiograph of a mouse growth plate labelled with tritiated inositol. Heaviest label (24 h after i.p. injection) is seen in cells in the hypertrophic and degenerating zones, suggesting the importance of phosphatidylinositol at sites of initial calcification. (Courtesy of Drs Neufeld and Tonna.)

bone formation and resorption (Kumegawa *et al.*, 1984).

Agonists relevant to mineral homeostasis that activate phospholipase C include parathyroid hormone (Meltzer *et al.*, 1982); however, at the time of writing, there are no published studies of the role of inositide phospholipid metabolism in the regulation of mineralisation. Neufeld and Tonna (1987) have demonstrated that hypertrophic cells pick up more tritiated inositol than other growth plate cells (figure 9.5). Since it is the hypertrophic cells whose mitochondria lose calcium prior to matrix calcification, one might speculate that future studies will demonstrate the importance of this pathway in the release of calcium from connective tissue cells as a prelude to initial mineralisation.

IN VITRO STUDIES

The role of phospholipids in promoting biological calcification has principally been studied in three related *in vitro* systems. Phospholipid suspensions in calcium phosphate solutions were used initially to demonstrate that acidic phospholipids could promote mineral deposition and to investigate the mechanism by which they did so. Matrix vesicle calcification was similarly studied in cell-free solutions, as well as in cell and organ culture. These studies provided insight into the *in vivo* action of matrix vesicles, but left unresolved many questions concerning the mechanism of action of these extracellular membrane-bound bodies. Most recently, the use of phospholipid liposomes, which can be considered models of matrix vesicles, have begun to provide more detailed insight into the mechanism of vesicle action.

Acidic phospholipids

A crude phospholipid preparation isolated from the oral bacteria, *Bacterionema Matruchotti*, was the first lipid preparation shown to cause calcium phosphate precipitation from a metastable calcium phosphate solution (Takazoe *et al.*, 1970). This preparation was shown to contain a proteolipid composed of acidic phospholipids and an hydrophobic apo-protein. Calcification in a carbonate-buffered, pH 7.2, solution required the presence of protein (Vogel and Ennever, 1971; Ennever *et al.*, 1974). Results of these studies led to the suggestion that the hydrophobic environment was essential for the mineralisation event (Vogel and Boyan-Salyers, 1976), which was postulated to involve calcium-phosphate salt bridge formation. Crude acidic phospholipid extracts from dentine (Odutuga *et al.*, 1975) and compact bones (Ngoma and Davis, 1976) were shown to cause mineral deposition in the absence of protein. The nature of the calcium phosphate mineral phase was not determined in any of these experiments.

Following separation of the complexed acidic phospholipids from the total lipid extract of compact bone, the complexed acidic phospholipids, but not the non-complexed fraction, were shown to cause the formation of a poorly crystalline hydroxyapatite (Boskey and Posner, 1976b). Phosphatidylserine, phosphatidylinositol, and cardiolipin, but not phosphatidic acid, phosphatidylethanolamine, phosphatidylcholine, nor the lysophosphatides, caused mineral deposition when 0.25–5 mg/ml lipid were dispersed in metastable calcium phosphate solutions (Boskey and Posner, 1976b). Phosphatidylserine and phosphatidylinositol, dispersed in these metastable calcium phosphate solutions, formed Ca-phospholipid phosphate complexes, which behaved identically to bone-derived complexed acidic phospholipids. In contrast, the calcium salts of these acidic phospholipids, or acidic phospholipids initially suspended in solutions of high calcium content, were unable to cause hydroxyapatite formation when returned to the metastable calcium phosphate solution (Boskey and Posner, 1982).

Phospholipases, which hydrolyse phospholipids removing specific moieties, provided further insight into the phospholipid structure required for the formation of complexed acidic phospholipids and the formation of hydroxyapatite. Phospholipase D, which removes serine or inositol from phosphatidylserine or phosphatidylinositol, prevented hydroxyapatite formation by PS and PI, but had no effect on hydroxyapatite formation by complexed acidic phospholipids (Boskey and Posner, 1977). This suggested that O–P–O serine and O–P–O inositol linkages were protected in the complexed acidic phospholipids. Phospholipase C, which removes phosphoserine and phosphoinositol, preventing hydroxyapatite formation by the acidic phospholipids, comparably had no effect on hydroxyapatite formation by the complexed acidic phospholipids.

Phospholipase A_2, which hydrolyses the fatty acid in the 2-position of the glycerol backbone, had a time-dependent effect. PS was rapidly hydrolysed by phospholipase A_2, while Ca–PS–P had a much slower rate of hydrolysis. Although unpublished Laser–Raman studies did not reveal any interaction between inorganic phosphate and fatty acid groups, the phospholipase A_2 data again suggest a protective effect, which may explain why the complexed acidic phospholipids can persist in tissues with high phospholipase A_2 activity (Wuthier, 1973), while the acidic phospholipids themselves cannot.

Hydroxyapatite formation, induced by complexed acidic phospholipids, has been used as a model of initial mineralisation in studies showing the inhibitory effects of diphosphonates (Boskey et al., 1979), magnesium (Boskey and Posner, 1980), and the lack of effects of the bone-gla protein (Boskey, et al., 1985).

Synthetic proteolipids, consisting of the basic protein lysozyme, and phosphatidylinositol (Vogel et al., 1973) were also shown to cause calcium phosphate mineral formation in calcium phosphate solutions. The lysozyme–phosphatidylinositol suspensions formed structures similar to those of extracellular matrix vesicles. They, and the lipid dispersions used in the *in vitro* studies discussed above, while providing clues into how matrix vesicle lipids might facilitate mineralisation, did not explain all of the observed features of matrix vesicle calcification.

Matrix vesicles

Tissue slices of cartilage bind ^{45}Ca (Anderson and Reynolds, 1973) and show the accumulation of mineral crystals on the surface of extracellular matrix vesicle membranes (Ali, 1976). Details of matrix-vesicle-mediated calcification were reviewed by Wuthier (1982). In addition to the histo-chemical observation that matrix vesicles serve as the site of initial calcification of both physiologic and dystrophic hydroxyapatite deposits (Anderson, 1980) *in vitro*, in tissue and organ culture matrix vesicles also appear to be the site of initial mineral deposition (Chin *et al.*, 1986; Murphree *et al.*, 1982; Escarot-Charrier *et al.*, 1983).

The *in vitro* study of matrix-vesicle-mediated calcification is advantageous, since culture conditions can be modulated to control the rate and extent of calcification. However, most investigators have used these systems to better characterise the role of specific enzymes in calcification, or to demonstrate that specific cell types produce matrix vesicles. Several laboratories have demonstrated that both hypertrophic (Glaser and Conrad, 1981; Golub *et al.*, 1983; Wuthier *et al.*, 1985) and resting (Boyan *et al.*, 1989) or other non-cartilage, connective tissue cells (Rifas *et al.*, 1982; Vaananen *et al.*, 1983) produce matrix vesicles in culture. However, the composition of vesicles from different sites, although similar to those in their respective tissues (table 9.3) are different. Whether they have different functions *in situ* remains to be determined.

One of the uncertainties concerning *in situ* and *in vitro* calcification concerns the nature and site of formation of the first mineral. Since phosphatidylserine is concentrated on the internal membrane of the vesicle (Majeska *et al.*, 1979), one would anticipate that the complexed acidic phospholipids are also inside the vesicle wall. The complexed acidic phospholipids promote direct hydroxyapatite formation, yet both amorphous calcium phosphate and hydroxyapatite have been reported to be the initial calcium phosphate mineral phase with isolated vesicles (Wuthier, 1982).

In addition to the uncertainty of the nature of the first mineral to deposit associated with the vesicles, several other questions arise. Although many investigators believe the function of matrix vesicles is to provide a protected environment for initial mineral deposition, other functions in the calcification process have been suggested. One suggestion, supported by the studies of Hirschman *et al.* (1983), Katsura *et al.* (1980), Fujiwara *et al.*

(1981) and Katsura and Yamada (1986) was that the vesicles contain (and transport) enzymes that modify the extracellular matrix, facilitating extravesicular calcification. Whether vesicles are formed specifically, rather than as a co-event during matrix maturation, is also not known. The manner in which calcium and phosphate accumulate in the vesicle is also uncertain. If vesicles are released pre-loaded with phosphate, as Wuthier's data suggest (Wuthier, 1977), and if initial mineralisation occurs within the vesicle, then how does calcium get inside? Once mineral deposits in the vesicle, how does the mineral get from inside the vesicle to an oriented position in the extracellular matrix? Answers to several of these questions are being suggested by studies using liposomes as vesicle models.

Liposomes

Liposomes are uni- or multilamellar structures prepared synthetically from lipid mixtures. Generally, they are made by dispersing lipid films of known composition in aqueous solutions. These solutions can contain material to be encapsulated; hence their applicability as drug delivery systems (Hauser, 1982). Liposomes can be prepared with uniform sizes (Enoch and Strittmatter, 1979; Gains and Hauser, 1982; Aurora *et al.*, 1985) or as polydisperse mixes. Thus they are highly applicable as models of extracellular matrix vesicles. In fact, not only has calcium phosphate deposition been studied in liposomes; liposomes have also been used to study iron oxide deposition (Mann *et al.*, 1986).

Eanes and colleagues (1984, 1985, 1987), using liposomes prepared from phosphatidylcholine, dicetylphosphate and cholesterol, caused mineral formation inside vesicles (figure 9.6) containing 25 or 50 mM phosphate; a phosphate concentration comparable to that reported to exist in matrix vesicles by Wuthier (1977). Calcium was transported into the vesicles from the external solution (1.33 mM Ca) in which the vesicles were suspended by a calcium ionophore (x-537A). When the liposomes contained Mg (0.8 mM) as well as phosphate, the presence of amorphous calcium phosphate was detected by X-ray diffraction within the ionophore treated vesicles (Eanes *et al.*, 1984). This is not surprising, since this non-crystalline phase is the initial phase precipitated in highly supersaturated solutions (Boskey and Posner, 1973), and since Mg stabilises this phase, retarding, or even preventing, its conversion to poorly crystalline hydroxyapatite (Boskey and Posner, 1974). In the absence of magnesium, hydroxyapatite was found both within and outside the liposomes (Eanes *et al.*, 1984), indicating, since the liposomes were not leaky prior to internal mineral deposition, that the formation of crystalline mineral within the liposomes caused their membranes to rupture, exposing the crystals to the external solution. When this external solution was metastable with respect to hydroxyapatite, crystal proliferation continued in the external solution

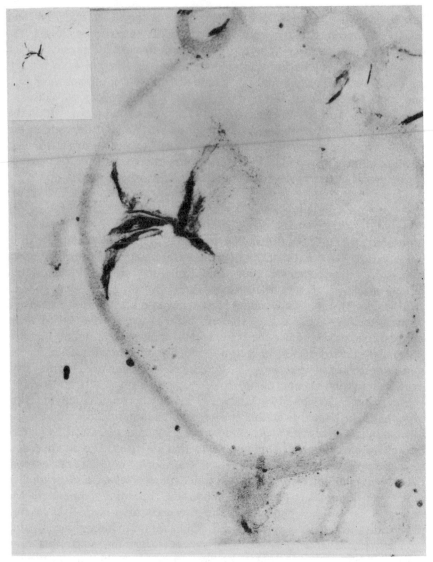

Figure 9.6   Electron micrographs of an osmium-fixed thin section showing hydroxyapatite crystals inside a liposome prepared from 7:2:1 (mole/mole) phosphatidylcholine:dicetyl phosphate, and cholesterol. Insert is a higher-power view of a similar preparation. (Courtesy of Drs Heywood and Eanes.)

following liposome rupture (Eanes and Hailer, 1985).

With phosphatidylserine included in the liposomes (Eanes and Hailer, 1987), less calcium phosphate was formed within the liposomes, in part because PS adsorbed to the crystal surfaces, inhibiting crystal proliferation. Mineral proliferation, promoted by PS in metastable calcium phosphate solutions was not noted, perhaps because transport of Ca into the membrane resulted in the formation of Ca–PS salts, which, as discussed previously, do not cause mineral deposition. In addition, the presence of Mg in the inside of the liposome may have competed for Ca binding sites on the PS, preventing the formation of calcium–PS complexes (Boskey and Posner, 1980; Newton *et al.*, 1978). Preliminary studies in our laboratory suggest that much more mineral formation occurs in situations in which the liposomes contain preformed complexed acidic phospholipids (Ca–PS–Pi) than those in which the membranes contain only PS.

The above models answer some questions about matrix-vesicle-mediated calcification, but leave others unanswered. These model vesicles differ from matrix vesicles in their composition (see table 9.3) and structure. *In situ*, calcium transport into the vesicles would be facilitated either by Ca-transport proteins in the vesicle membrane or by lyso-phosphatides, which are naturally occurring ionophores (Tyson *et al.*, 1976). Calcium, along with phosphate, might be present in the vesicles when they are released from the cell membrane. Certainly, the presence of complexed acidic phospholipids in vesicle membranes (Wuthier and Gore, 1977) suggests they may have been formed prior to vesicle release.

In vitro studies with liposomes of composition closer to that of matrix vesicles, albeit without proteins, may shed further light on these questions. However, the observed data do explain why some investigators find amorphous calcium phosphate and others hydroxyapatite within isolated

Table 9.3 Phospholipid composition of matrix vesicles isolated from tissues and cell culture

| | | % of total lipid P | | |
| | Bovine growth plate[a] | Chick growth plate[b] | | Cultured chick growth plate[c] |
		NCL	CPLX	
SPH	14.9	23.9	4.6	31.1
PC	33.8	32.3	10.3	28.8
LPC	—	10.6	9.6	3.0
PE	20.9	9.2	1.0	21.3
LPE	—	7.0	3.5	0.8
PS	13.2	6.3	30.0	12.8
LPS	—	1.3	13.3	—
PI	8.3	1.6	12.5	3.2
PA	2.6	—	—	0.9
CDL	2.9	5.6	8.4	1.0
PG				0.5

[a] Peress *et al.* (1977).
[b] Wuthier and Gore (1977).
NCL = non-complexed lipid fraction. CPLX = complexed acidic phospholipid fraction.
[c] Wuthier *et al.* (1985).

Phospholipids: SPH = sphingomyelin. PC = phosphatidylcholine.
PE = phosphatidylethanolamine. PS = phosphatidylserine. PI = phosphatidylinositol.
PA = phosphatidic acid. CDL = cardiolipin. LX = lysophosphatides.

vesicles and tissue slices. They do demonstrate how mineral proliferations can occur outside the vesicle.

DISCUSSION

Phospholipids convey to the membranes they are found in many abilities. The ability to transport water and ions, the ability to move, alter their shapes, and form vesicles, and the ability to activate enzymes are all dependent on phospholipids. Deposition of hydroxyapatite on a calcifiable matrix requires the presence of cells. The cells secret and modify the matrix, transport ions and enzymes needed for the formation of mineral, and are the origin of matrix vesicles that create a site for initial calcification. All these cell-mediated events are dependent on phospholipids. Alterations in phospholipid metabolism can markedly alter the function of cells, and the mineralisation process.

In calcifying tissues, phospholipids associated with proteolipids form complexes that can cause hydroxyapatite formation. Studying isolated cells, membranes, or model membranes *in vitro* has provided insight into how these phospholipids directly affect calcification. Thus, calcification is dependent on phospholipids because of their functions in regulating cellular activity, and because of their action as hydroxyapatite nucleators. For the unconvinced, it should be noted that the fluid aspirated from the growth plate of rachitic rats contains a lipid-soluble factor that causes *de novo* hydroxyapatite deposition in cartilage-like fluids (Howell *et al.*, 1978); the phospholipid composition of the 'nucleational factor' is identical to that of the calcifiable proteolipid found in the growth plates of these animals (Boyan *et al.*, 1988).

ACKNOWLEDGEMENTS

Dr Boskey's research described in this review was supported by NIH grant DE-04141.

REFERENCES

Ali, S. Y. (1976). Analysis of matrix vesicles and their role in the calcification of epiphyseal cartilage. *Fed. Proc.*, **35**, 142

Ali, S. Y., Sajdera, S. W. and Anderson, H. C. (1970). Isolation and characterization of calcifying matrix vesicles from epiphyseal cartilage. *Proc. Nat. Acad. Sci., U.S.*, **67**, 1513–20

Anderson, H. C. (1969). Vesicles associated with calcification in the matrix of epiphyseal cartilage. *J. Cell Biol.*, **41**, 59–72

Anderson, H. C. (1980). Calcification Processes. *Path. Ann.*, **15**, 45–75

Anderson, H. C. and Reynolds, J. J. (1973). Pyrophosphate stimulation of calcium uptake into cultured embryonic bones. Fine structure of matrix vesicles and their role in calcification. *Devel. Biol.*, **34**, 211–37

Anderson, H. C., Cecil, R. and Sajdera, S. W. (1975). Calcification of rachitic rat cartilage in vitro by extracellular matrix vesicles. *Am. J. Path.*, **79**, 237–54

Anghileri, L. J. (1972). Phospholipid–calcium complexes in experimental tumors. *Experientia*, **28**, 1086–9

Ansell, G. B. and Spanner, S. (1982). In *Phospholipids* (eds A. Neuberger and L. L. M. van Deenen), Elsevier, Amsterdam, pp. 1–43

Atkin, I., Pita, J. C., Ornoy, A., Agundez, A., Castiglione, G. and Howell, D. S. (1985). Effects of vitamin D metabolites on healing of low phosphate vitamin D-deficient induced rickets in rats. *Bone*, **6**, 113–23

Aurora, T. S., Li, M., Cummins, H. Z. and Haines, T. H. (1985). Preparation and characterization of monodisperse unilamellar phospholipid-vesicles with selected diameters of from 300 to 600 nm. *Biochim. Biophys. Acta*, **820**, 250–8

Bernard, G. W. (1969). The ultrastructural interface of bone crystals and organic matrix in woven and lamellar endochondral bone. *J. Dent. Res.*, **48**, 781–8

Berridge, M. J. (1984). Inositol triphosphate and diacylglycerol as second messengers. *Biochem. J.*, **220**, 345–60

Billah, M. M., Lapetina, E. G. and Cuatrecasas, P. (1981). Phosphatidic acid – a possible mechanism for the production of arachidonate acid. *J. Biol. Chem.*, **256**, 5399–403

Boggs, J., Wood, D., Moscarello, M. and Papahadjapolous, D. (1977). Lipid phase separation induced by hydrophobic protein in phosphatidylserine-phosphatidylcholine vesicles. *Biochem.*, **16**, 2325–33

Boskey, A. L. (1981). In *The Chemistry and Biology of Mineralized Connective Tissues* (ed. A. Veis), Elsevier, North Holland, pp. 531–7

Boskey, A. L. (1985). Lipid changes in the bones of the healing vitamin D deficient, phosphate deficient rat. *Bone*, **6**, 173–8

Boskey, A. L. and Dickson, I. (1988). Influence of Vitamin D status on the content of complexed Acidic phospholipids in Chick Diaphyseal Bone. *J. Bone Min. Res.*, **4**, 365–71

Boskey, A. L. and Marks, S. C. Jr (1985). Mineral and matrix alterations in the bones of incisors-absent (ia/ia) osteopetrotic rat. *Calcif. Tiss. Intl.*, **37**, 287–92

Boskey, A. L. and Posner, A. S. (1973). Conversion of amorphous calcium phosphate to microcrystalline hydroxyapatite. *J. Phys. Chem.*, **77**, 2313–7

Boskey, A. L. and Posner, A. S. (1974). Magnesium stabilisation of amorphous calcium phosphate. *Mat. Res. Bull.*, **9**, 907–16

Boskey, A. L. and Posner, A. S. (1976a). Extraction of a calcium-phospholipid phosphate complex from bone. *Calcif. Tiss. Res.*, **19**, 273–83

Boskey, A. L. and Posner, A. S. (1976b). In vitro nucleation of hydroxyapatite by a bone Ca–PL–PO$_4$ complex. *Calcif. Tiss. Res.*, **22S**, 197–201

Boskey, A. L. and Posner, A. S. (1977). The role of synthetic and bone extracted Ca-phospholipid-PO$_4$ complexes in hydroxyapatite formation. *Calcif. Tiss. Res.*, **23**, 251–8

Boskey, A. L. and Posner, A. S. (1980). Effect of magnesium on lipid-induced calcification: an in vitro model for bone mineralization. *Calcif. Tiss. Intl.*, **32**, 139–43

Boskey, A. L. and Posner, A. S. (1982). Optimal conditions for Ca-acidic phospholipid phosphate complex formation. *Calcif. Tiss. Intl.*, **34**, s1–s7

Boskey, A. L. and Reddi, A. H (1983). Changes in lipids during matrix induced endochondral bone formation. *Calcif. Tiss. Intl.*, **35**, 549–54

Boskey, A. L. and Timchak, D. M. (1983). Phospholipid changes in the bones of the vitamin D deficient, phosphate deficient, immature rat. *Metab. Bone Dis. Rel. Res.*, **5**, 81–5

Boskey, A. L. and Wientroub, S. (1986). The effect of vitamin D deficiency on rat bone lipid composition. *Bone*, **7**, 277–81

Boskey, A. L., Goldberg, M. R. and Posner, A. S. (1977). Calcium–phospholipid–phosphate complexes in mineralizing tissues. *Proc. Soc. Exp. Biol. Med.*, **157**, 588–91

Boskey, A. L. Goldberg, M. R. and Posner, A. S. (1979). Effect of diphosphonates on hydroxyapatite formation induced by calcium–phospholipid–phosphate complexes. *Calcif. Tiss. Intl.*, **27**, 83–8

Boskey, A. L. Posner, A. S., Lane, J. M., Goldberg, M. R. and Cordella, D. M. (1980). Distribution of lipids associated with mineralization in the bovine epiphyseal growth plate. *Arch. Biochem. Biophys.*, **199**, 305–11

Boskey, A. L., Boyan-Salyers, B. D., Burstein, L. S. and Mandel, I. D. (1981). Lipids associated with salivary stone mineralization. *Arch. Oral. Biol.*, **26**, 779–85

Boskey, A. L., Burstein, L. S. and Mandel, I. (1983a). Phospholipids associated with parotid sialoliths. *Arch. Oral. Biol.*, **28**, 655–67

Boskey, A. L., Vigorita, V., Stuchin, S., Sencer, O. S. and Lane, J. M. (1983b). Chemical characterization of the mineral deposits in tumoral calcinosis. *Clin. Orthop.*, **178**, 258–69

Boskey, A. L., Lewinson, D. and Bullough, P. G. (1984). The effects of trifluoperazine on calcifying tissue in the immature rat. *Proc. Soc. Exp. Biol. Med.*, **176**, 154–63

Boskey, A. L., Wians, F. H. and Hauschka, P. V. (1985). The effect of osteocalcin on in vitro lipid-induced hydroxyapatite formation and seeded hydroxyapatite growth. *Calcif. Tiss. Intl.*, **37**, 57–62

Boskey, A. L., DiCarlo, E. D., Gilder, H., Donnelly, R. and Wientroub, S. (1988). The effect of short-term treatment with vitamin D metabolites on bone lipid and mineral composition in healing vitamin D-deficient rats. *Bone*, 185–94

Boyan, B. and Boskey, A. L. (1984). Co-isolation of proteolipids and calcium–phospholipid–phosphate complex. *Calcif. Tiss. Intl.*, **36**, 214–18

Boyan, B., Dereszewski, G., Hinman, B., Florence, M. and Griffith, G. (1982). In *Fifth International Workshop on Calcified Tissues, Kiryat Anavim, Israel*, Excerpta Medica, Amsterdam, 12–17

Boyan, B. D., Howell, D. S., Pita, J. C., Blanco, L. and Cieslak, S. (1988). Characterization of a calcification induced in epiphyseal cartilage extracellular fluid. *J. Biol. Chem.*, *Bone*, **9**, 185–94

Boyan, B. D., Landis, W. J., Knight, J., Dereszewski, G. and Zeagler, J. (1984). Microbial hydroxyapatite formation as a model of *Scanning Electron Microsc.*, **4**, 1793–1800

Boyan, B. D., Schwartz, Z., Swain, L. D., Carnes, D. L., Jr and Zislis, T. (1989). Differential expression of phenotype by reserve zone and growth region chondrocytes *in vitro*. *Bone*, in press

Boyan, B. D., Swain, L. and Renthal, R. (1986). Proton transport by calcifiable proteolipids. In *Cell Mediated Calcification and Matrix Vesicles* (ed. S. Y. Ali), Elsevier Bioscience BV, 199–204

Boyan-Salyers, B. D. (1981). In *The Chemistry and Biology of Mineralized Connective Tissues* (ed. A. Veis), Elsevier–North Holland, 539–42

Boyan-Salyers, B. D. and Boskey, A. L. (1981). Relationship between proteolipids and calcium–phospholipid–phosphate complexes in Bacterionema matruchotii calcification. *Calcif. Tissue Intl.*, **30**, 167–74

Boyan-Salyers, B. D., Vogel, J., Riggan, L., Summers, F. and Howell, R. (1978). Application of a microbial model to biologic calcification. *Metab. Bone Dis. Rel. Res.*, **1**, 143–7

Brighton, C. T. and Hunt, R. M. (1978). Electron microscopic pyroantimonate studies of matrix vesicles and mitochondria in the rachitic growth plate. *Metab. Bone Dis. Rel. Res.*, **1**, 199–204

Chin, J. E., Schalk, E. M., Kemick, M. L. S. and Wuthier, R. E. (1986). Effect of synthetic human parathyroid hormone on the levels of alkaline phosphatase activity and formation of alkaline phosphatase-rich matrix vesicles by primary cultures of chicken epiphyseal growth plate chondrocytes. *Bone Mineral*, **1**, 427–36

Cornell, R. B. and Horwitz, R. F. (1980). Apparent coordination of the biosyntheses of lipids in cultured cells: its relationship to the regulation of membrane sterol phospholipid ration and cell cycling. *J. Cell. Biol.*, **86**, 810–19

Cullis, P. R., Hope, M. J., de Kruijff, B., Verkleij, A. J. and Tilcock, C. P. S. (1985). In *Phospholipids and Cellular Regulation* (ed. J. F. Kuo), vol. I, CRC Press, Boca Raton, pp. 1–37

Dirkson, T. R. and Marinetti, G. V. (1970). Lipids of bovine enamel and dentine and human bone. *Calcif. Tiss. Res.*, **6**, 1–10

Dmitrovsky, E. and Boskey, A. L. (1985). Calcium–acidic phospholipid–phosphate complexes in human atherosclerotic aortas. *Calcif. Tiss. Intl.*, **37**, 121–5

Eanes, E. D. and Hailer, A. W. (1985). Liposome-mediated calcium phosphate formation in metastable solutions. *Calcif. Tiss. Intl.*, **37**, 390–4

Eanes, E. D. and Hailer, A. W. (1987). Calcium phosphate precipitation in aqueous suspensions of phosphatidylserine-containing anionic liposomes. *Calcif. Tiss. Intl.*, **40**, 43–8

Eanes, E. D., Hailer, A. W. and Costa, J. L. (1984). Calcium phosphate formation in aqueous suspensions of multilamellar liposomes. *Calcif. Tiss. Intl.*, **36**, 421–30

Eisenberg, E., Wuthier, R. E., Frank, R. B. and Irving, J. T. (1970) Time study of *in vivo* incorporation of ^{32}P orthophosphate into phospholipids of chicken epiphyseal tissues. *Calcif. Tiss. Res.*, **6**, 32–48

Elgavish, A., Rifkind, J. and Saktor, B. (1983). In vitro effects of vitamin D_3 on the phospholipids of isolated renal brush border membranes. *J. Membr. Biol.*, **72**, 85–91

Elsbach, P., Weiss, J., and Kao, L. (1985). The role of intramembrane Ca^{2+} in the hydrolysis of the phospholipids of Escherichia coli by Ca^{2+} dependent phospholipase. *J. Biol. Chem.*, **260**, 1618–22

Enlow, D. H. and Conklin, J. L. (1964). A study of lipid distribution in compact bone. *Anat. Rec.*, **148**, 279

Ennever, J., Riggan, L. J. and Vogel, J. J. (1984). Proteolipid and collagen calcification *in vitro*. *Cytobiol*, **39**, 155–6

Ennever, J., Vogel, J. J. and Levy, B. M. (1974). Lipid and bone matrix calcification *in vitro*. *Proc. Soc. Exp. Biol. Med.*, **145**, 1386–8

Ennever, J., Vogel, J. J., Rider, L. J. and Boyan-Salyers, B. D. (1976). Microbiologic calcification by proteolipid. *Proc. Soc. Exp. Biol. Med.*, **152**, 147–50

Ennever, J., Vogel, J. J. and Riggan, L. J. (1978). Phospholipids of a bone matrix calcification nucleator. *J. Dent. Res.*, **57**, 731–4

Enoch, H. G. and Strittmatter, P. (1979). Formation and properties of 1000 A diameter, single-bilayer phospholipid vesicles. *Proc. Natl Acad. Sci. U.S.*, **76**, 145–9

Escarot-Charrier, B., Glorieux, F. H., van der Rest, M. and Pereira, G. (1983). Osteoblasts isolated from mouse calvariae initiate matrix mineralisation in culture. *J. Cell. Biol.*, **96**, 639–43

Farley, J. R. and Jorch, U. M. (1983). Differential effects of phospholipids on skeletal alkaline phosphatase (EC3.1.3.1) activity in extracts, in situ and in circulation. *Arch. Biochem. Biophys.*, **22**, 477–88

Fincham, A. G., Burkland, G. A. and Shapiro, I. M. (1972). Lipophilia of enamel matrix. A chemical investigation of the neutral lipids and lipophilic proteins of enamel. *Calcif. Tiss. Res.*, **9**, 247–59

Folch-Pi, J. and Stoffyn, P. J. (1972). Proteolipids from membrane systems. *Anals. N.Y. Acad. Sci.*, **195**, 86–107

Fraley, R., Wilschut, J., Duzgunes, N., Smith, C. and Papahadjopoulos, R. (1980). Studies on the mechanism of membrane fusion, role of phosphate in promoting calcium induced fusion of phospholipid vesicles. *Biochem.*, **19**, 6021–9

Fujiwara, T., Katsura, N. and Kawanura, M. (1981). Study of protease associated with matrix vesicles. *J. Dent. Res.*, **60B**, 1232 (abstract)

Gains, N. and Hauser, H. (1982). Characterisation of small unilamellar vesicles produced in unsonicated phosphatidic acid and phosphatidylcholine–phosphatidic acid dispersions by pH adjustments. *Biochim. Biophys. Acta.*, **731**, 31–6

Glaser, J. H. and Conrad, H. E. (1981). Formation of matrix vesicles by cultured chick embryo chondrocytes. *J. Biol. Chem.*, **256**, 12607–11

Goldberg, M. and Escaig, F. (1984). An autoradiographic study of the *in vivo* incorporation of [^{3}H]-palmitic acid into the dentine and enamel lipids of rat incisors, with a comparison of rapid-freezing freeze-substitution fixation and aldehyde fixation. *Arch. Oral. Biol.*, **29**, 691–5

Goldberg, M. and Escaig, F. (1987). Rapid freezing and malachite green–acrolein–osmium tetroxide freeze-substitution fixation improve visualization of extracellular lipids in rat incisor pre-dentin and dentin. *J. Histochem. Cytochem.*, **35**, 427–33

Goldberg, M. and Septier, D. (1985). Improved lipid preservation by malachite green-glutaraldehyde fixation in rat incisor predentine and dentine. *Arch. Oral Biol.*, **10**, 717–726

Goldberg, M., Lelous, M., Escaig, F. and Boudin, M. (1983). Lipids in the developing enamel of the rat incisor, parallel histochemical and biochemical investigation. *Histochem.*, **78**, 145–56

Goldberg, M., Escaig, F. and Septier, D. (1984). In *Tooth Enamel IV* (eds. R. W. Fearnhead and S. Suga), Elsevier Science, Amsterdam 125–30

Golub, E. E., Schattschneider, S. C., Berthold, P., Burke, A. and Shapiro, I. (1983).

Induction of chondrocyte vesiculation in vitro. *J. Biol. Chem.*, **258**, 616–21

Hauser, H. (1982). Methods of preparation of lipid vesicles: assessment of their suitability for drug encapsulation. *Trends Pharmacol. Sci.*, **3**, 274–7

Hauser, H. and Phillips, M. C. (1979). Interactions of the polar groups of phospholipid bilayer membranes. *Progr. Surface Membr. Sci.*, **13**, 297–413

Hauser, H., Darke, A. and Phillips, M. C. (1976). Ion-binding to phospholipids. Interaction of calcium with phosphatidyl serine. *Eur. J. Biochem.*, **62**, 335–44

Haynes, H., Boyan, B., Hinman, B. and Leal, D. (1982). Proteolipid isolated from rat incisor dentine and predentine matrix vesicles. *J. Dent. Res.*, **61**, 193–5

Hendrickson, H. S. and Fullington, J. G. (1965). Stabilities of metal complexes of phospholipids: Ca(II), Mg(II), and Ni(II) complexes of phosphatidyl serine and triphosphoinositide. *Biochem.*, **4**, 1599–605

Hirschman, A., Deutsch, D., Hirschman, M., Bab, I. A., Sela, J. and Muhlrad, A. (1983). Neutral protease activities in matrix vesicles from bovine fetal alveolar bone and dog osteosarcoma. *Calcif. Tiss. Intl.*, **35**, 791–7

Holmes, R. P., Mahfouz, M., Travis, B. D., Yoss, N. L. and Keenan, M. J. (1983). The effect of membrane lipid composition on the permeability of membranes to Ca^{2+}. *Ann. N.Y. Acad. Sci.*, **414**, 44–56

Holwerda, D. L., Ellis, P. D. and Wuthier, R. E. (1981). Carbon-13 and phosphorus-31 nuclear magnetic resonance studies on the interaction of calcium with phosphatidylserine. *Biochem.*, **20**, 814–23

Howell, D. S., Blanco, L., Pita, J. C. and Muniz, O. (1978). Further characterization of a nucleational agent in hypertrophic cell extracellular cartilage fluid. *Metab. Bone Dis. Rel. Res.*, **1**, 155–61

Hubscher, G. (1962). VI. The effect of metal ions on the incorporation of L-serine into phosphatidylserine. *Biochim. Biophys. Acta*, **57**, 551–61

Hsu, H. T. and Anderson, H. C. (1977). A simple and defined method of studying calcification by isolated matrix vesicles. Effect of ATP and vesicle phosphatase. *Biochim. Biophys. Acta*, **500**, 162–72

Irving, J. T. (1958). A histologic stain for newly calcified tissue. *Nature*, **181**, 704–5

Irving, J. T. (1959). A histologic staining method for sites of calcification in teeth and bone. *Arch. Oral Biol.*, **1**, 89–96

Irving, J. T. (1963). The sudanophil material at sites of calcification. *Arch. Oral Biol.*, **8**, 735–45

Joos, R. W. and Carr, C. W. (1967). The binding of calcium to mixtures of phospholipids. *Proc. Soc. Exp. Biol. Med.*, **124**, 126–8

Katchburian, E. (1973). Membrane-bound bodies as initiators of mineralization of dentine. *J. Anat.*, **116**, 285–302

Katsura, N. and Yamada, K. (1986). Isolation and characterization of a metalloprotease associated with chicken epiphyseal cartilage matrix vesicles. *Bone.*, **7**, 137–43

Katsura, N., Sakata, M., Fujiwara, T., Kawamura, M. and Tomita, K. (1980). Degradation of cartilage proteoglycan by matrix vesicles. *J. Dent. Res.*, **59B**, 920

Kohler, S. J. and Klein, M. (1977). Orientation and dynamics of phospholipid head groups in bilayers and membranes determined from ^{31}P nuclear magnetic resonance chemical shielding tensors. *Biochemistry*, **16**, 519–27

Kumegawa, M., Ikeda, E., Tanaka, S., Haneji, T. J., Yora, T., Sakagishi, Y., Minami, N. and Hiramatsu, M. J. (1984). The effects of Prostaglandin E_2, parathyroid hormone, 1,25 dihydroxycholecalciferol, and cyclic nucleotide analogs on alkaline phosphatase activity in osteoblastic cells. *Calcif. Tiss. Intl.*, **36**, 72–6

Lelous, M., Boudin, D., Salomon, S. and Polonvski, J. (1982). The affinity of type I collagen for lipid *in vivo*. *Biochim. Biophys. Acta*, **708**, 26–32

Low, M. G., and Zilvermat, D. B. (1980). Role of phosphatidylinositol in attachment of alkaline phosphatase to membranes. *Biochem.*, **19**, 390–5

Majeska, R. J., Holwerda, D. L., and Wuthier, R. E. (1979). Localization of phosphatidylserine in isolated chick epiphyseal cartilege matrix vesicles with Trinitrobenzenesulfonate. *Calcif. Tiss. Intl.*, **27**, 41–5

Mann, S., Hannington, J. P. and Williams, R. J. P. (1986). Phospholipid vesicles as a model system for biomineralization. *Nature*, **324**, 565–7

Manzoli, F. A. and Gelli, M. (1968). Quantitative determination of lipids in dental pulp (bos taurus) during development. *Arch. Oral. Biol.*, **13**, 705–12

Matthews, J. L., Martin, J. H., Sampson, H. W., Kunin, A. S. and Roan, J. H. (1970). Mitochondrial granules in the normal and rachitic rat epiphyses. *Calcif. Tiss. Res.*, **5**, 91–9

Matsumoto, T., Kawanobe, Y., Morita, K. and Ogata, E. (1985). Effect of 1,25-Dihydroxyvitamin D$_3$ on phospholipid metabolism in a clonal osteoblast-like rat osteogenic sarcoma cell line. *J. Biol. Chem.*, **260**, 13704–9

Meltzer, E., Weinreb, S., Bellorin-Font, E. and Hruska, K. A. (1982). Parathyroid hormone stimulation of renal phosphoinositide metabolism is a cyclic nucleotide-independent effect. *Biochim. Biophys. Acta*, **712**, 258–304

Mont, M. A., Boskey, A. L., Ryaby, J. T., Mularchuk, P., Bendo, J., diCarlo, E. and Binderman, I. (1987). Application of a culture system for analysis of differentiation and mineralization of mesenchymally-derived cells. *Orthopaed. Trans.*, 33rd ORS, 440 (abstract)

Murphree, S., Hsu, H. T. and Anderson, H. C. (1982). In vitro formation of crystalline apatite by matrix vesicles isolated from rachitic rat epiphyseal cartilage. *Calcif. Tiss. Intl.*, **34**, S62–S68

Nayar, R., Hope, M. J. and Cullis, P. R. (1982). Phospholipids as adjuncts for calcium-ion stimulated release of chromaffin granule contents-implications for mechanisms of exocytosis. *Biochem.*, **21**, 4583–9

Nelson, D. H. (1980). Corticosteroid-induced changes in phospholipid membranes as mediators of their action. *Endocrin. Rev.*, **1**, 180–99

Neufeld, E. B. and Tonna, E. A. (1987). Tritiated inositol autoradiographic studies of Phosphatidylinositol syntheses and distribution in mouse skeletal/dental tissues. *Anat. Rec.*, **218**, 98 (abstract)

Newton, C., Pangborn, W., Nir, S. and Papahadjopoulos, D. (1978). Specificity of Ca. *Biochim. Biophys. Acta*, **506**, 281–5

Ngoma, Z. and Davis. R. (1976). Mineralization et induction crystalline in vitro par les lipides extraits des l'os compact boivin. *Path. Biol.*, **24**, 307–11

O'Doherty, P. J. A. (1979). 1,25 Dihydroxyvitamin D$_3$ increases the activity of the intestinal phosphatidylcholine deacylation–reacylation cycle. *Lipids*, **14**, 75–7

Odutuga, A. A. and Prout, R. E. S. (1974). Lipid analysis of human enamel and dentine. *Arch. Oral Biol.*, **19**, 729–31

Odutuga, A. A., Prout, R. E. S. and Hoare, R. J. (1975). Hydroxyapatite precipitation in vitro by lipids extracted from mammalian. *Arch. Oral Biol.*, **20**, 311–15

Op den Kamp, J. A. F. (1979). Lipid asymmetry in membranes. *Ann. Rev. Biochem.*, **48**, 47–91

Papahadjopoulos, D. (1974). Cholesterol and cell membrane function: A hypothesis concerning the etiology of atherosclerosis. *J. Theor. Biol.*, **43**, 329–37

Peress, N. S., Anderson, H. C. and Sajdera, S. W. (1974). The lipids of matrix vesicles from bovine fetal epiphyseal cartilage. *Calcif. Tiss. Res.*, **14**, 275–81

Primes, K. J., Sanchez, R. A., Metzner, E. K. and Pazel, K. M. (1982). Large scale purification of phosphatidylcholine from egg yolk phospholipids by column chromatography on hydroxyapatite prepared by the Tiselius method. *J. Chromat.*, **236**, 519–22

Prout, R. E. S. and Odutuga, A. A. (1974a). Lipid composition of dentine and enamel of rats maintained on a diet deficient in essential fatty acids. *Arch. Oral Biol.*, **19**, 725–8

Prout, R. E. S. and Odutuga, A. A. (1974b). The effects on the lipid composition of enamel and dentine of feeding a corn oil supplement to rats deficient in essential fatty acids. *Arch. Oral Biol.*, **19**, 955–8

Prout, R. E. S. and Odutuga, A. A. (1974c). In vitro incorporation of [1-^{14}C-] linoleic acid into the lipids of enamel and dentine of normal and essential fatty acid deficient rats. *Arch. Oral Biol.*, **19**, 1167–70

Prout, R. E. S., Odutuga, A. A. and Tringe, F. C. (1973). Lipid analysis of rat enamel and dentine. *Arch. Oral Biol.*, **18**, 373–80

Raggio, C. L., Boyan, B. D. and Boskey, A. L. (1986). In vivo hydroxyapatite formation induced by lipids. *J. Bone Mineral Res.*, **1**, 409–15

Rakhimov, M. M., Mad'yarow, Sh. R., Kholodkova, T. P., Babaev, M. U., Rashidova, S. Sh., Kalendareva, T. I., Almatov, K. T., Mirasalikhova, N. M. and Mirkhodzhaev,

U. Z. (1978). Influence of calcium ions on the enzymatic hydrolysis of phospholipids as a function of the physical state of the substrate. *Biokhimiya*, **43**, 433–45

Reith, E. J. (1983). A model for transcellular transport of calcium based on membrane fluidity and movement of calcium carriers within the more fluid microdomains of the plasma membrane. *Calcif. Tiss. Intl.*, **35**, 129–34

Rifas, L., Shen, V. and Mitchell, V. (1982). Selective emergence of differentiated chondrocytes during serum-free culture of cells derived from fetal rat calvaria. *J. Cell Biol.*, **92**, 493–504

Ritter, N. M. and Boyan-Salyers, B. D. (1980). A comparison of proteolipid concentration and calcification in normal and rachitic chick epiphyseal cartilage. *Fed. Proc.*, **39**, 661 (abstract)

Rossignol., M., Uso, T. and Thomas, P. (1985). Relationship between fluidity and ionic permeability of bilayers from natural mixtures of phospholipids. *J. Membr. Biol.*, **87**, 269–75

Sampath, T. K., Wientroub, S. and Reddi, A. H. (1984). Extracellular matrix proteins involved in bone induction are vitamin D dependent. *Biochem. Biophys. Res. Commun.*, **124**, 829–35

Schlesinger, M. (1981). Proteolipids. *Ann. Rev. Biochem.*, **50**, 193–206

Schuster, G. S., Dirksen, T. R. and Harms, W. S. (1975). Effect of exogenous lipid on lipid syntheses by bone and bone cell culture. *J. Dent. Res.*, **54**, 131–9

Seelig, J. and Macdonald, P. M. (1987). Phospholipids and proteins in Biological Membranes. ^{2}H NMR as a method to study structure, dynamics and interactions. *Acc. Chem. Res.*, **20**, 221–8

Shapiro, I. M. (1970a). The association of phospholipids with inorganic bone. *Calcif. Tiss. Res.*, **5**, 13–20

Shapiro, I. M. (1970b). The phospholipids of mineralized tissues. I. Mammalian compact bone. *Calcif. Tiss. Res.*, **5**, 21–9

Shapiro, I. M. and Greenspan, J. S. (1969). Are mitochondria directly involved in Biological Mineralization? *Calcif. Tiss. Res.*, **3**, 100–2

Shapiro, I. M. and Wuthier, R. E. (1966). A study of the phospholipids of bovine dental tissues II. Developing bovine dental pulp. *Arch. Oral Biol.*, **11**, 501–12

Simon, D. R., Berman, I. and Howell, D. S. (1973). Relationship of extracellular matrix vesicles to calcification in normal and healing rachitic epiphyseal cartilage. *Anat. Rec.*, **176**, 167–80

Singer, S. J. and Nicholson, G. L. (1972). The fluid mosaic model of the structure of cell membranes. *Science*, **175**, 720–31

Stubbs, C. D. and Smith, A. D. (1984). The modification of mammalian membrane polyunsaturated fatty acid composition in relation to membrane fluidity and function. *Biochim. Biophys. Acta*, **779**, 89–137

Swain, L. D. and Boyan, B. D. (1988). Ion translocating properties of calcifiable proteolipids. *J. Dent. Res.*, **67**, 526–30

Takazoe, I., Vogel, J. J. and Ennever, J. (1970). Calcium hydroxyapatite nucleation by lipid extract of Bacterionema Matruchotti. *J. Dent. Res.*, **49**, 395–8

Trauble, H. (1973). Phase transitions in lipids. *Biomembranes*, **3**, 197–227

Tyson, C. A., Zande, H. V. and Green, D. E. (1976). Phospholipids as ionophores *J. Biol. Chem.*, **251**, 1326–32

Vaananen, H. K. (1980). Calcium incorporation in matrix vesicles isolated from chicken epiphyseal cartilage. *Calcif. Tiss. Intl.*, **30**, 227–32

Vannanen, H. K., Morris, D. C. and Anderson, H. C. (1983). Calcification of cartilage matrix in chondrocyte cultures derived from rachitic rat growth plate cartilage. *Metab. Bone Dis. Rel. Res.*, **5**, 87–92

Vogel, J. J. and Boyan-Salyers, B. D. (1976). Acidic lipids associated with the local mechanism of calcification. *Clin. Orthop.*, **118**, 230–41

Vogel, J. J. and Ennever, J. (1971). The role of lipoprotein in the intracellular hydroxyapatite formation in Bacterionema Matruchotti. *Clin. Orthoped. Rel. Res.*, **78**, 218–22

Vogel, J. J., Campbell, M. M. and Ennever, J. (1973). Calcification of a lysozyeinositol phosphatide. *Proc. Soc. Exp. Biol. Med.*, **143**, 677–81

Warren, G. B., Toon, P. A., Birdsail, N. J. M., Lee, A. G. and Metcalfe, J. C. (1974).

Titrations of the activity of pure adenosine triphosphate-lipid complexes. *Biochem.*, **13**, 5501–8

Warschawsky, H. and Smith, C. E. (1974). Morphological classification of rat incisor ameloblasts. *Anat. Rec.*, **179**, 423–46

Weibull, C., Christiansson, A. and Carlemalm, E. (1983). Extraction of membrane lipids during fixation dehydration and embedding of Acholeplasma Laidlawn-cells for electron microscopy. *J. Microsc.*, **129**, 201–7

Wuthier, R. E. (1968). Lipids of mineralizing epiphyseal tissues in the bovine fetus. *J. Lipid Res.*, **9**, 68–78

Wuthier, R. E. (1971). Zonal analysis of phospholipids in the epiphyseal cartilage and bone of normal and rachitic chickens and pigs. *Calcif. Tiss. Res.*, **8**, 36–53

Wuthier, R. E. (1973). The role of phospholipids in biologic calcification. *Clin. Orthoped.*, **90**, 191–200

Wuthier, R. E. (1977). Electrolytes of isolated epiphyseal chondrocytes, matrix vesicles, and extracellular fluid. *Calcif. Tiss. Res.*, **23**, 125–33

Wuthier, R. E. (1982). The role of phospholipid–calcium–phosphate complexes in biological mineralization. In Anghileri, L. J. and A. M. Tuffet-Anghileri (eds), *The Role of Calcium in Biological Systems*, vol. I, CRC Press, Boca Raton, 41–70

Wuthier, R. E. (1984). In Linde, A. (ed.) *Dentin and Dentingenesis*, vol. II, CRC Press, Boca Raton, 93–106

Wuthier, R. E., Chin, J. E., Hale, J. E., Register, T. C., Hale, L. V. and Ishikawa, Y. (1985). Isolation and characterization of calcium accumulating matrix vesicles from chondrocytes of chicken epiphyseal growth plate cartilage in primary culture. *J. Biol. Chem.*, **260**, 15972–9

Wuthier, R. E. and Cummins, J. W. (1974). In vitro incorporation of ^{3}H serine into phospholipid of proliferating and calcifying epiphyseal cartilage and liver. *Biochim. Biophys. Acta*, **337**, 50–9

Wuthier, R. E. and Gore, S. (1977). Participation of inorganic ions and phospholipids in isolated cell, membrane and matrix vesicle fractions. Evidence for Ca: Pi: acidic phospholipid complexes. *Calcif. Tiss. Res.*, **24**, 163–71

Wuthier, R. E., Majeska, R. J. and Collins, G. M. (1977). Biosynthesis of matrix vesicles in epiphyseal cartilage. I. In vivo incorporation of ^{32}P orthophosphate into phospholipids of chondrocyte, membrane and matrix vesicle fractions. *Calcif. Tiss. Res.*, **23**, 135–9

Wuthier, R. E., Wians, F. H., Giancola, S. and Dragic, S. S. (1978). In vitro biosynthesis of phospholipids by chondrocytes and matrix vesicles of epiphsyseal cartilage. *Biochem.*, **17**, 1431–6

Yaari, A. M., Shapiro, I. M. and Brown, C. E. K. (1982). Evidence that phosphatidylserine and inorganic phosphate may mediate transport during calcification. *Biochem. Biophys. Res. Commun.*, **105**, 778–84

Index